THE
OTHER
SIDE
OF
VACCINES

Kate William

ISBN: 978 107 214 4717
Self-published by Kate William

ACKNOWLEDGEMENT

First and foremost, thanks be to God, for His amazing grace, and mercies, new each morning. He deserves all the glory.

To my husband, for your support, and encouragement, and love. Thanks for sharing this amazing adventure called 'life' with me!

To my children, whose innocence, and enthusiasm, and endless curiosity, fill me with joy, and help me see life with new eyes.

To my parents and family, for your love and assistance – and listening patiently to my long rants!

To my friends and followers, for your generous sharing of stories and information, and for your endless support and encouragement.

To all those who stand for truth, no matter the cost.

Thankyou.

"And have no fellowship with the unfruitful works of darkness, but rather reprove them"
(Ephesians 5:11)

TABLE OF CONTENTS

INTRODUCTION

I never dreamed that, one day, I'd write a book about vaccines (of all things!)

When my first son was born in 2005, I knew very little about vaccines. I didn't know what was in them. I didn't know how they were produced. I didn't even really know how they worked.

All I knew was that 'everybody' got them, and it never crossed my mind to question, or investigate further.

As the months passed, my baby boy seemed to be sick every other week. If it wasn't fevers, it was coughing, and if it wasn't coughing, it was vomiting and if it wasn't all that, it was hand-foot-and-mouth disease.

Everybody told me it was normal. It's the family day care, they said! It's all those germs, they said!

I worked in a medical centre at the time, and my son was a regular patient.

Then, in 2009, my second son was born, and life would never be the same.

While I was pregnant (still working in the medical centre), the great 'Swine Flu Panic' was underway. Our medical centre was in utter chaos, as people lined up outside the door, panicked over every little sniffle, or twinge of a sore throat. Nurses rushed about in full protective gear, and a temporary triage station was set up outside. It was in this environment of fear and panic, that I was convinced to have a flu vaccine, because – somehow – it would protect me from 'swine flu'. I was between 7 and 8 months pregnant.

It still didn't cross my mind to question or opt out.

Not long after being vaccinated, I began to suffer from a terrible double ear infection, and was prescribed antibiotics. It took weeks to get the pain and infection under control.

My son was born soon after.

He was vaccinated at birth, with the standard Hepatitis B vaccine, along with Vitamin K. It still hadn't crossed my mind to question or investigate...but that day was coming.

Soon after birth, it became obvious that he was a very irritable, colicky baby. At eight weeks, I took him to the neighbourhood health clinic to have his vaccines. Within 48 hours, my irritable, colicky baby was even more so - as a red, itchy rash broke out on his arm. The doctor diagnosed ringworm, but soon it spread all over his torso and legs, despite the use of anti-fungal creams.

A second doctor diagnosed eczema, and prescribed corticosteroid creams. I began sleeping beside him, and we would doze on and off through the night, between my rocking him, and rubbing his back, as he squirmed and yowled in discomfort.

Two months later, in a sleep deprived haze, I took him back to the neighbourhood clinic to have his next round of vaccines. Within days, the eczema flared up worse than ever, and my baby boy was utterly miserable - unable to sleep for more than 10 – 15 minutes at a time.

Although I noticed that his symptoms had progressively worsened after each vaccine, his doctors never mentioned that vaccines might be involved, and I simply put it out of my mind.

I took him to several doctors, hoping to get answers, but nothing seemed to work. We trialled medication for silent reflux, thinking that might help his digestive issues, but to no avail. Finally, one nurse said in exasperation "Some babies are just difficult! You'll have to wait for him to grow out of it".

I couldn't accept that my baby was 'just difficult' and so I began to search for answers outside of the conventional medical system. I took him to a naturopath who, within minutes, declared that he was suffering from internal thrush (candida overgrowth).

He administered a homeopathic remedy, and gave me detailed instructions of what I had to change in our diets and lifestyle. He explained how the body attempts to detoxify through the skin, if the liver and bowels are not working sufficiently. He asked if my son had been vaccinated...Well, yes actually. A lightbulb was starting to come on now.

He encouraged me to investigate vaccines, before I consented to any more.

Within a month, my baby boy was sleeping through the night (for the first time), his skin was clear, and he turned into a happy, delightful little boy.

My son was due for his six-month vaccines at the time. I simply never made that appointment. I began researching, instead.

That was almost a decade ago, and I still haven't stopped researching.

Our family completely changed our diet and personal care habits, and the results were astounding. We simply stopped getting sick – no more coughs, no more headaches, no more allergies, no more aching legs, no more hyperactivity. It was incredible. I couldn't understand why doctors had never told me that changing our diet could change our life.

The more I learnt, the more I had to know. And the more I knew, the more I had to tell people! I began to read the medical journals and studies for myself. I got up early to research, before my children woke up. I stayed up late at night when everyone else was in bed.

In 2016, I had the idea to write up all the reasons why I choose not to vaccinate. I originally pictured it as a blog, or social media, post. I began writing, and after several days, I had listed 101 reasons why I choose not to vaccinate. I decided I should add some detail to each point, so I began to put together some references.

By this point, I was living in the Pacific Islands, with a small baby...and no electricity. Once per week, I would organize someone to look after the baby, and I would get a lift into town, to the internet café. There, I would pay $2 per hour, to perch into a little booth, in front of an old computer, and start researching, jotting down notes and references in a notebook. After a month or two, I realised this was going to be a lot bigger than a blog post, and started to envision an e-book.

As it continued to grow, I decided to make a full book. At one point, about 6 months in, my USB stick was somehow corrupted, and many of my files lost. I spent a week pondering if I really wanted to continue...and then realized that I *couldn't not*. So, I started again.

It's taken almost three years, in which time I've had another baby, moved countries, lost my laptop during a severe cyclone which ripped part of the roof off our home, and flooded all our possessions. I had to wait six months before I was able to get another computer and take up where I'd left off.

It's been a journey, you could say!

Over the past decade, I have met the most amazing individuals, heard the most heartbreaking stories, and learnt the most mind-blowing things!

I hope you find the information herein useful. There are two sides to every story – and the vaccine issue is no different. The media has ensured we've heard one side of the story.

This is the *other* side.

1.

VACCINE THEORY

The vaccination program is a world-wide, multi-billion-dollar industry that supplies billions of vaccines every year. The general consensus is that vaccines are safe and effective and, furthermore, are the sole reason that epidemics of dreaded diseases like smallpox and polio have been eradicated.

That's what I once thought, too. But a closer inspection of the facts reveals a rather different picture.

In order to clearly see this picture, we must go back to the basics, the foundation on which this massive industry was built apon. Now bear with me, because this is really, really, *really* important. Once you understand these concepts, you will look at the field of vaccinology with new eyes!

Vaccines are built upon a foundation made up of three theories. They are:

- a.) Infectious diseases cause illness, and can spread to others (referred to as the 'Germ Theory')
- b.) Antibodies can protect us from being infected with those diseases.
- c.) If enough people have immunity, the group is protected from outbreaks ('herd immunity')

The ordinary person just assumes, like I once did, that the experts got it right - they checked and re-checked and it was proven beyond any shadow of a doubt, and we no longer have to even consider them theories, but they are established facts.

As it turns out, there may be another side to these theories...

a) The Germ Theory

The Germ Theory is the current paradigm that dominates modern medicine today. According to the theory, each disease is caused by a specific microbe or pathogen. Although not the first proponent of the 'Germ Theory', it was the experiments of Louis Pasteur (1822-1895) that convinced much of Europe that diseases were caused by 'germs'.

Pasteur was not a doctor, but a chemist. Although he is hailed as a hero today, it was discovered after his death that he committed fraud and scientific misconduct in some of his most famous works [1].

Among other things, he developed the first rabies vaccine in 1885. He administered it to an 11-year-old boy (unlawfully, since he had no medical license) who was mauled by a dog. The boy survived with no signs of rabies. Funnily enough, the dog also survived...with no signs of rabies.

Although the chances of the boy contracting rabies were estimated to be only 10% anyway [2], the boy's good health was chalked up to the 'success' of Pasteur's vaccine, and this laid the foundation for what would become a global, multi-billion-dollar industry.

The first Pasteur Institute was established on the basis of this success, for "*the study of virulent and contagious diseases*" [3], and still remains a highly influential organization today, with a global network of institutes around the world.

The 'germ theory' was furthered by the work of German doctor Robert Koch (1843-1910), who believed each specific disease must be caused by a specific agent ('germ'), and to this end, he developed a set of postulates, which are still regarded as the 'gold standard in medical microbiology' [4].

Koch's Postulates are:

1. The organism must always be present, in every case of the disease.
2. The organism must be isolated from a host containing the disease and grown in pure culture.
3. Samples of the organism taken from pure culture must cause the same disease when inoculated into a healthy, susceptible animal in the laboratory.
4. The organism must be isolated from the inoculated animal and must be identified as the same original organism first isolated from the originally diseased host.

Unfortunately, even Koch was unable to fulfil his own postulates, much less those coming along behind him, yet the 'germ theory' continued unabated and eventually became entrenched as a foundational 'truth' of modern medicine.

There were some eminent voices of dissent, though – one was Rudolf Virchow (1821-1902), founder of the 'cell theory', who believed that diseases were the result of abnormal cellular activity, and not from outside pathogens [5-6].

Another was Antoine Bechamp (1816-1908), an eminent French scientist - he believed that pathogens were the result of disease, and not the cause of it.

It was later shown that Pasteur had plagiarized Antoine Bechamp's work, and taken credit for some of his discoveries and ideas [7].

Nevertheless, the 'Germ Theory' had so captivated the imagination of the scientific world, that by the time of his death, Bechamp's illustrious career and discoveries were reduced to a short, dismissive obituary, published in the British Medical Journal which stated that he was *'associated with bygone controversies as to priority which it would be unprofitable to recall"* [8].

The discovery in 1914, that certain types of bacteria can mutate into other forms depending on the environment they are placed in [9], should have been pause for thought (and a re-visit to Bechamp's earlier work, suggesting that 'germs' were the result of disease, and not the cause of it), however the 'germ theory' of disease has not only continued unabated, but has only grown in power and influence, to the point where voices of dissent are ridiculed as 'science deniers'.

More recent work shows that bacteria also changes form over it's life-cycle, which has huge implications for how diseases are recognized and tested [10].

When it comes to viruses, a number of new scientific discoveries, when looked at through the 'germ theory' lens, only raise more questions than they answer. One example is the discovery that viruses make up about 8% of the human genome [11] – one such viral gene was found to be essential for establishing the human placenta after conception takes place [12]. Researchers have also discovered that three-day-old human embryos – which consist of just 8 cells – produce retroviruses that are vital to the genetic activity of the developing embryo [13].

In light of all this, we must ask – why do viruses seem to co-exist within our very DNA, without causing disease? Why do healthy people carry viruses and bacteria in their gut, or on their skin, with no symptoms of illness? If viruses can only re-produce in living cells, where did the first virus come from, and why did that cell begin to manufacture that virus? Are there 'good' viruses, and 'bad' viruses, like they now believe there are 'good' and 'bad' bacteria? Why do cell-cultures in laboratory settings first need to have toxins added to them, before they will produce viruses?

A full analysis of the germ theory is beyond the scope of this book, but these are a few points to encourage the reader to think critically about how disease is portrayed to us.

Other theories exist in the realm of what is now known as 'alternative' medicine, namely that all disease results from an acute exposure to poisons, or a gradual build-up of toxicity and/or nutritional deficiency, and is the result of the body's self-regulating and self-healing mechanisms.

The role of bacteria and viruses in this scenario is not as a pre-curser or 'villain', but to scavenge and 'clean up' in the wake of this cleansing/healing process.

b)Antibody Theory

The second part of the theory that forms the foundation of vaccines is the belief that specific antibodies protect us from disease.

We're told by official health bodies that vaccines prompt our bodies to produce antibodies, which then protect us when we encounter that disease in the environment. When Edward Jenner first started vaccinating people, nobody had ever heard of 'antibodies' – they were not discovered until a century later, and were originally referred to as 'anti-toxins'.

Knowledge and science, however, have continued to evolve, and we now know that the immune system is so incredibly complex that even immunologists can barely grasp it. What has become obvious over the years, is that antibodies have very little, if any, role in the state we refer to as 'immunity'. Here's why:

1. Numerous cases where antibodies had no influence on disease susceptibility.

It was demonstrated over 60 years ago, that people with high levels of antibodies still got the disease for which they were supposedly immune to, while others with low to no detectable antibodies came through disease outbreaks with no sign of the disease to which they should have been susceptible [14].

Here are a number of examples in the scientific literature, where antibodies (or lack thereof) bore little or no relation to immunity:

- Before the introduction of mass polio vaccination, it was discovered that some 85% of children under the age of 5 years had little or no antibodies to poliovirus, yet only 1 in 170 of those with 'no immunity' became ill during polio epidemics [15].

- In 1968, around the same time that measles vaccination was being introduced, it was discovered that children with congenital aggama-globulinemia (an inability to produce antibodies) contracted measles and subsequently displayed the usual symptoms, followed by immunity, yet they only had insignificant traces of antibodies in circulation [16].

- Animal experiments published in 2013 revealed that mice with high levels of antibodies could still succumb to fatal infection with vesicular stomatitis virus (VSV). They found that even though B-cells were essential, survival after infection "*did not require antibodies or other aspects of traditional adaptive immunity*" [17].

- Even though 95% of children had measles antibodies after vaccination, vaccine efficacy was not more than 68%. In other words, 27% of people who got measles were supposedly 'immune' [18].

- In 1992, three patients with *severe* tetanus were described in the Journal of Neurology. All three patients had levels of tetanus antibodies at least 100 times greater than the 0.01 IU/ml considered to provide immunity. One of those patients died [19].

- Seven infants with clinical symptoms of tetanus, were found to have tetanus antibody levels 4 - 13 times higher than 0.01

IU/ml. A further two infants, also with clinical symptoms of tetanus, whose mothers were given multiple tetanus boosters during pregnancy, had levels 100-400 times higher than the level supposed to give protection [20].

- During the 1990's, large scale clinical trials of a HIV vaccine were conducted in Thailand, among intravenous drug users. The vaccines were deemed to be 'effective' in that they induced an antibody response, however, a decade later, the randomized, double-blind, placebo-controlled results showed that vaccine recipients had the same rate of HIV infection and disease progression, as those who had received a placebo [21].

Even the CDC noted they had found no proof that pertussis antibody levels correlated with protection from the disease:

"The findings of efficacy studies have not demonstrated a direct correlation between antibody responses and protection against pertussis disease" [22].

Modern medicine is viewed by many as being on the cutting edge of science, and yet, the discovery that antibodies are not responsible for immunity was made almost 80 years ago. The discovery, by immunologist Dr Merrill W Chase, seemed to attract little fanfare at the time, and has been largely forgotten over the years, despite his illustrious career at Rockefeller University, and publishing at least 150 scientific papers [23].

Dr Chase, working in his laboratory, tried to induce immunity into a guinea pig, by vaccinating it with blood serum (which includes antibodies) from another guinea pig. The experiment failed to produce immunity. However, when he used white blood cells, the immunity from the second guinea pig was transferred to the first [23].

It became common knowledge that B-cells (a type of white blood cell) produces antibodies, which, despite Dr. Chase's discovery, were assumed to provide immunity. Animal experiments, mentioned earlier, showed that it was not the antibodies produced by B-cells that cause immunity, but a different chemical produced by B-cells – one that maintains macrophages (another type of white blood cell) [24].

2. Vitamin D is necessary for a robust immune system – yet Vitamin D *limits* antibody production.

According to vaccine logic, the more antibodies you have, the more protected you are, but in a *normally* functioning immune system, antibody production is tightly restricted (for good reason – more on that later).

It's now common knowledge that Vitamin D is necessary for a healthy immune system, yet Vitamin D *limits* antibody production [25-26].

It begs the question, why, if antibodies really are as vital as we have been led to believe...

3. Presence of antibodies *enhances* some diseases.

In 1977, researchers revealed that the presence of antibodies to dengue fever enhanced infection with other strains of dengue fever [27].

They found that "*dengue replicates readily in cultures of peripheral blood leukocytes (PBL) prepared from immune simian or human donors, but poorly or not at all in leukocytes from non-immune hosts.*"

Note that their definition of 'immune simian or human donors' refers to those with evidence of *antibodies*.

This finding was later replicated, and expanded upon, by other researchers [28], and the perplexing phenomena came to be called 'antibody-dependent enhancement of viral infection' [29].

Scientists say that antibody-dependent enhancement "*is exploited by a variety of viruses and has been associated with disease exacerbation*" [29].

It was recently discovered that Zika virus infection is also enhanced by the presence of antibodies for dengue fever [28], due to cross-reactivity - both viruses apparently belong to the family known as 'flaviviruses'.

Antibody-enhancement of infection has also been found with coxsackievirus strains [30]. The presence of antibodies to one strain of coxsackievirus was shown to increase percentage of infected cells by 10 to 50-fold in subsequent infections with other strains [31].

Respiratory Syncytial Virus (RSV) infection has also been shown to be enhanced by the presence of prior antibodies [32], as has Ebola [33], HIV [34], Severe Acute Respiratory Syndrome (SARS) [35], and malaria [36].

4. Antibodies are too late to prevent infection.

The immune system is comprised of two parts – cellular immunity (also known as non-specific, innate, or Th1, immunity) and humoral immunity (also known as specific, adaptive, or Th2, immunity).

Cellular immunity, which involves phagocytes and cytotoxic T-cells, is the first line of defence. Humoral immunity, which involves B-cells, is the last line of defence.

The following graph, although simplistic, gives the basic idea...

Th1 immune system	Th2 immune system
A.k.a. 'Cellular' or 'non-specific' immunity	A.k.a. 'specific' or 'adaptive' immunity
First line of defence	Last line of defence
Features lymphocytes	Features antibodies
Stimulated by natural infection	Stimulated by vaccination

Cellular immunity, which utilises T-cells, is the first line of defence against foreign invaders and pathogens.

We don't know exactly how many potential pathogens or poisons the cellular immune system effectively deals with every day, because they are dealt with early, and seldom produce symptoms [37], however it is estimated to be in the millions [38].

If we are constantly being bombarded with millions of 'germs' every day of our life, but we are healthy for the most part, then

a) those germs are either not harmful, or infectious, and/or b) aspects of our Th1 immune system deal with them, without even activating the immune response that creates symptoms.

The humoral immune system, which involves antibody production, is highly specific, and the *last line of defence*. This part of the immune system, which is located in the bone marrow, is what vaccines are specifically designed to target.

Upon first exposure, it takes the body up to 14 days to reach peak antibody production [39], unless we are talking about HIV, which can purportedly take up to 30 months following infection to develop specific antibodies [40].

Yet, they tell us that infectious organisms are replicating at a tremendous rate. Take the H5N1 avian influenza, for example - it is said to be highly virulent, and have a staggering mortality rate above 60% in humans. This virus replicates so rapidly, that it reaches peak virus titers in the lungs, within 48hrs after infection, about ~10^7 PFU/gram, which means about 10,000,000 plaque forming units per gram [41].

Upon second exposure though, the antibody response is rather quicker, because the naïve B-cells have now become 'memory' B-cells. The aim is that the vaccine 'primes' the immune system through training the B-cells, so that it recognizes the invader when we are next exposed to it, and gets those antibodies into action much faster.

But there is one small problem. Even a 'primed' immune system produces antibodies rather too late to prevent infection by a virulent marauder. Upon secondary (or later) exposures, it still takes the body between 3 - 5 days to reach peak antibody levels [42-43].

At best, antibodies may attempt to play 'catch-up' to the invading pathogen.

The definition of immunity, according to the Oxford Dictionary, is *"The ability of an organism to resist a particular infection or toxin by the action of specific antibodies or sensitized white blood cells"* [44].

Given the rather tardy response by antibodies, it might be more accurate to define immunity as the ability of an organism to resist a particular infection or toxin, by the action of the innate immune system. If the innate immune system fails, you have an infection on your hands.

5. Antibodies are highly inflammatory.

When you discover that significant amounts of antibodies are produced too late to be effective in preventing infection, perhaps you may question why this would be so?

Is it some defect in the immune system? Some fatal flaw of nature?

Probably not.

Nature, it would seem, has a good reason for this state of affairs.

When antibodies are produced, and then bind with the antigen, together they form 'antigen-antibody complexes', also known as 'immune complexes' - intermediate sized molecules which then act as an antigen in their own right, and must be removed by the innate immune system [45].

Basically, the innate immune system has to 'mop up' the after-effects of the humoral immune system activation.

One of the ways the innate immune system tries to clear the immune complex, is via the complement system, which works through promoting inflammation, such as heat (fever), swelling, redness and, consequently, pain [46].

In other words, the symptoms we generally associate with *illness,* may be the side-effects of our body trying to rid itself of antibodies.

Because the complement system can be highly damaging to host tissue, not to mention highly uncomfortable, its use is tightly regulated in a normally-functioning immune system.

When there is an *over-production of antibodies*-turned-immune-complexes, the body cannot effectively clear them, leading to inflammation and damage in specific tissues, such as kidneys, lungs and often, these immune complexes end up lodged in the small blood vessels and joints.

This process has been labelled 'Type III Hypersensitivity', and these reactions can occur hours, days or even *years* after exposure to the original antigen [47].

Some examples of Type III hypersensitivity reactions are systemic lupus erythematosus (SLE), vasculitis, skin rashes, fever, arthralgia (pain in the joints), and malaise - the latter four are sometimes grouped under the name 'serum sickness' [48].

Serum sickness was first noted in the late 19th and early 20th centuries, following administration of diptheria antitoxin. It was found to be caused by the body's immune response to a foreign protein (horse serum) contained in the antitoxin [49].

More recently, researchers induced symptoms of serum sickness in dogs, by injecting them with human albumin. All of the dogs showed delayed reactions, 5 - 13 days later, including lethargy, edema, vasculitis, vomiting and lack of appetite. Despite treatment, 2 of the 6 dogs died [50].

Note that vaccines intended for injection into humans may also contain proteins from other species. Therefore, it is hardly surprising that some of the adverse reactions reported, following vaccination, include autoimmune diseases and hypersensitivity reactions [51], vasculitis, skin rashes, fever, arthralgia, malaise...and serum sickness [52-53].

These delayed reactions could be vastly under-reported, given they can occur weeks (or possibly months, or even years) following receipt of vaccines.

6. High antibody production comes with a cost.

As previously discussed, there are two 'arms' of the immune system. In a properly functioning immune system, the two arms of the immune system work in harmony, and there is balance, known as immunostasis.

However, when one arm of the immune system becomes dominant, the other becomes suppressed, leading to immune malfunction, and increased susceptibility to disease [54-56].

The issue with vaccination, is that it primarily stimulates antibody production, causing the adaptive immune system to become dominant. Its more complicated than that, but this is the basic explanation. Another mechanism, by which vaccines could potentially induce Th2 dominance, is via oxidative stress, caused by additives, such as mercury or aluminium [57-58].

This inevitably leads to suppression of innate immunity – and there are numerous studies showing that vaccines can do just that [59-61].

Such an imbalance has far-reaching consequences for health and disease, since immune system imbalance - specifically Th2 dominance - has been implicated in a number of disease states.

- In 2002, an in-depth, controlled study of tuberculosis-infected patients, and their household contacts and community controls, in Gambia and Senegal, found that those who were infected had significantly lower Th1 markers, and raised Th2 markers, compared with healthy controls. After months of treatment, levels of Th1 markers had nearly quadrupled, signaling a shift toward higher Th1 activity, and lower Th2 activity. Researchers noted that this shift was not observed in those who had poor clinical outcomes [62].

- Asthma is generally regarded as an inflammatory condition, and there is evidence that it is characterized by a Th2-dominant state, with Th2 cytokines being over-expressed, whilst their Th1 counterparts are under-expressed [63].

- It is thought that Th2 cells are responsible for triggering hypersensitivity disorders, such as allergy, eczema, hayfever and urticaria [64].

 - Th1 cytokine levels are typically lower in patients with advanced cancer, while Th2 markers are either unchanged, or higher [65]. Samples taken from non-small cell lung cancer and basal cell carcinoma expressed a noticeable imbalance towards Th2 functioning [66]. Prostate cancer patients were also found to have low Th1 markers, and heightened Th2 markers [67].

 - A study of 20 autistic children found consistently elevated levels of Th2 cytokines, and consistently lowered levels of Th1 cytokines [68].

There is a very famous disease that is characterised by this exact immune system malfunction – that is, impaired cellular response (macrophages) with an enhanced antibody response...

It's called AIDS.

AIDS patients preferentially make antibodies, at the expense of cellular immunity [69]. This is the classic immune system imbalance, leading to Th2 dominance, that we have just explored.

If antibodies were actually responsible for immunity, this would spell good news indeed for those diagnosed with AIDS. They would be *less likely* to suffer infections, than the average person. Unfortunately, this is quite obviously not the case. Research shows the higher the levels of antibodies, the quicker the disease progresses [70].

What if a person has the hallmarks of AIDS - such as low CD4+ count and symptoms of immunodeficiency...but test negative to HIV? Obviously, they cannot be diagnosed with AIDS, because that does not fit into the currently accepted paradigm. Instead, they are diagnosed with 'idiopathic lymphocytopenia', also dubbed by some as 'HIV-negative AIDS' [71].

The million-dollar question, of course, is what would cause the immune system to be so skewed to cause AIDS/idiopathic lymphocytopenia?

Maybe vaccines [72]?

It makes sense, when we consider the net effect of vaccination on the immune system.

Schuil, et al (1998), described the case of a 4-year-old girl with a history of encephalitis following MMR vaccination, who was later diagnosed with idiopathic CD4+ T lymphocytopenia. They deduced that the vaccine caused problems because the girl was immuno-deficient, but perhaps the vaccine caused the immunodeficiency, too, given it was only diagnosed afterwards [73].

Is it possible that everything we thought we knew about HIV/AIDS is wrong? From the beginning, there have been high-profile, outspoken critics of the HIV/AIDS theory, the most well-known being Peter Duesberg, a Professor of Molecular and Cell Biology at the University of California, Berkeley [74].

Duesberg maintains that HIV is simply a 'passenger' virus, but the true cause of the immune changes seen in AIDS, is recreational drug use, malnutrition, and chemotherapy drugs – all of which skew the immune system towards Th2 dominance, (much like repeated vaccination does) [75].

Another is Kary Mullis, who won the 1993 Nobel prize in Chemistry, for his invention of polymerase chain reaction (PCR) technique which, ironically, is used to search for HIV fragments in AIDS patients. Mullis believed that a type of 'immune overload' was responsible for the disease known as AIDS [76].

It seems highly plausible that repeated vaccination could at least contribute to such a state of 'immune overload'.

Unfortunately, efforts to medically rectify Th1/Th2 imbalance have been ineffective at best, and downright dangerous at worst. In 2006, TeGenero Immuno Therapeutics went bankrupt after a Phase 1 clinical trial of the immunomodulatory drug TGN1412 resulted in all six (100%) volunteers being rushed to hospital, four of them with massive organ failure.

The drug was supposed to stimulate the innate immune system. Treating doctors later confirmed that all six volunteers had suffered from a 'cytokine storm and, ironically, their white blood cell counts had virtually vanished within hours of injection [77].

Studies on animals suggest that vaccination during infancy not only skews the immune system towards a Th2 bias - as we have already discussed - but that effect may be permanent, affecting immune system status into adulthood [78].

This discovery has led to efforts to develop vaccines that would induce a Th1 response – like the response you get from *natural infection*. Experiments towards this end have involved novel DNA vaccines [79], selected adjuvants [80] and oral administration of bacterial extract [81].

If a Th1 type response is desirable, and natural infection elicits such a response, it really begs the question: Might we be better off diverting the billions of dollars currently spent on vaccine programs, into novel strategies to support normal immune function?

What might national health-care systems look like, if widespread nutritional supplementation was promoted, to support a vigorous first-line Th1 response in the event of pathogenic/toxin exposure?

Studies show that there are numerous approaches that can promote Th1 response, and down-regulate Th2 response. One of these is selenium, which is often deficient in HIV-positive individuals with disease progression [82]. Others include zinc [83], probiotic bacteria [84] and plant sterols [85].

7. The (other) problem with antibodies.

Understanding the full implications of Th1/Th2 skewing caused by vaccination is critical to understanding the vaccine debate.

We've already explored the fact that antibodies are not called into play until after infection has already taken place. According to one immunology textbook, "The induction of an adaptive immune response begins when a pathogen is ingested by an immature dendritic cell in the *infected* tissue" [86].

What this means is that, whether the immune system is 'primed' via vaccines or not, antibodies are still utilized *only after* cells have already become infected.

Now, herein we encounter another problem – the 'elephant in the room', if you will.

Antibodies are rather large, and they don't typically enter cells, although scientists have been trying for at least a decade to genetically-engineer antibodies that can target proteins inside the cell [87-88].

So, while antibodies may bind to antigens *outside* the cell, what happens to cells that have already been infected?

Then you must rely on T-cells to orchestrate the killing of diseased cells, in order to stop the spread of disease - this is known as cell-mediated immunity. This is the natural sequence of events when a Th1-type response is generated, *such as seen in natural infection* [89].

The natural Th-1 type response is to eliminate infection via externalising it - this is the classic disease symptoms we know so well, such as rash, fever, cough, mucus, swelling, etc [90].

Th2 dominance inhibits this natural response, which inevitably must lead to either:

    a) altered disease manifestation, so for example, the vaccinated person who has whooping cough, may have a cough, but without the tell-tale 'whoop' sound [91], or

b) chronic underlying infection, inflammation or auto-immune disease [92-93].

Let's go over this one more time, because it's extremely important.

First: Vaccines are designed to stimulate antibody production.

Second: Antibodies cannot stop infection, nor can they enter cells that are infected.

Third: Due to immune imbalance caused by vaccination, infected cells harbour infection chronically, causing inflammation and auto-immune conditions.

Fourth: Person shows only mild or no signs of acute illness, but becomes progressively burdened down by chronic health issues.

So, what actually happens is that the vaccine has not prevented infection, it has simply prevented the body from *expelling the infection.*

This has massive implications for statistics purporting to prove vaccine efficacy, because the vaccinated may not show the tell-tale symptoms that would result in diagnosis.

This also relates to another problem with the current vaccine paradigm.

It was once believed that vaccination provides lifelong immunity [94].

 One old poster, from the Iowa Department of Health, features a smiling badger, holding up a needle, and the slogan says "Parents, it hurts for a moment, but it protects for a lifetime".

Despite that early optimism, we have since discovered that, not only do some people fail to develop the required levels of antibodies, but those antibodies wane over time. Remember, in the current paradigm, antibodies are the main indicator of 'immunity'.

Enter repeated booster shots.

According to the World Health Organization, 15% of children do not develop the required level of antibodies following measles vaccination, which is why the schedule now includes two doses of the measles-mumps-rubella vaccine [95].

In order to get that 15% of children over the threshold of 'immunity', all children are required to have an extra shot.

Once claimed to offer 'lifelong protection', health authorities now inform us that 'Virtually everyone (more than 99%) will be protected against measles and rubella, for more than 20 years after two doses of MMR' [96].

Herein we encounter another problem - not only do different vaccines wane at different rates, but the same vaccine wanes at different rates in different people. In order to have a high percentage of people with sufficient antibodies at any given time, vaccine programs must cater to the lowest common denominator.

So, for example, if antibodies to polio persisted in twenty percent of people for 30 years, but only persisted for 15 years in the rest of the population, then everyone would be encouraged - and possibly even mandated, in future - to have the vaccine every 15 years, regardless of your own personal antibody status.

The same issue comes up with trivalent or hexavalent vaccines - that is, vaccines with more than one antigen. Take the diptheria-tetanus-pertussis vaccine - the tetanus component is thought to protect most people for at least 25 years, while the diptheria lasts 10 years, and pertussis antibodies wane after only 4-5 years [97].

Over the past few years, the tone has begun to turn towards promoting adolescents and adult booster shots, as the favoured solution to preventing future outbreaks. The first formal adult vaccination schedule was published in 2002 [98].

Once upon a time, a child received one dose of diptheria-tetanus-pertussis vaccine before the age of two years, now a child receives five doses before 5 years of age, then another booster at around age 11years. In adulthood, the tetanus-diptheria booster is recommended every ten years, plus a tetanus-diptheria-pertussis booster during every pregnancy for women, plus a booster if the adult is going to be around an infant, plus a booster if you suffer any kind of open wound or injury [98].

The United States does not have a central database that registers adult vaccinations, but in 2016, the Australian Childhood

Immunization Register was expanded to include adult vaccines, too [99]. Although adult vaccines are not (yet) mandated, a number of employment sectors, and situations, are requiring adults be 'up-to-date' with booster shots.

In the United States, "*CDC does not issue any requirements or mandates for state agencies, health systems, or health care workers regarding infection control practices, including influenza vaccination or the use of masks.*"

"However, some employers require certain immunizations. Hospitals, for example, may require some staff to get the flu vaccine or hepatitis B vaccine or take other precautions such as the use of masks" [100].

Although vaccines may not be mandatory for hospital visitors, they may be pressured into vaccines, just the same. In 2012, Ben Hammond, then a mine-site supervisor, was told by hospital staff that he 'needed' to have a pertussis booster shot, before visiting his newborn son in hospital, who was born eight weeks premature.

Two days later, he began to feel ill, and 12 days later, he was paralysed. He was later diagnosed with Acute Disseminated Encephalomyelitis [101].

c) Herd Immunity Theory

The concept of 'herd immunity' was introduced in the 1920's, before most of today's vaccines were invented. It was coined as a result of mice experiments, and some mathematical equations [102].

Researchers noted that inoculation of a certain percentage of mice in a group, seemed to confer some level of protection to all mice in the group.

Although there were a few inexplicable anomalies, which could not be explained by the theory, the seeds of the idea were sown, and would grow to become accepted dogma.

'Herd immunity' appeared again in the 1930's, when it was noted that measles epidemics in Baltimore, Maryland, seemed to appear, when the proportion of children with immunity fell below 55% [103].

This was before a measles vaccine was in use, so the 'immunity' they referred to was via natural infection.

It was also in the 1930's when E.S Godfrey theorized that 'herd immunity' against diptheria could be achieved via vaccination of 30% of children under 5 years of age [104].

Fast forward to 1992, outbreaks occurred across the developing world - despite overall vaccination coverage of 79% of infants [105].

E.S Godfrey's optimistic prediction turned out to be just one of many to fall short, in the chequered history of herd immunity...

It was boldly proclaimed in 1967, that "*with the isolation of the measles virus and the development and extensive field testing of several potent vaccines, the tools are at hand to eradicate the infection. With the general application of these tools during the coming months, eradication can be achieved in this country in 1967"* [106].

That prediction turned out to be overly optimistic.

Again in 1984, it was forecast that *"as a result of efforts to immunize at least 95% of the population, the US is nearing elimination of measles virus"* [107]. Oops...not quite!

Finally, in 2000, measles was declared 'eliminated' from the US [108]. By 'elimination', they mean *"the absence of continuous disease transmission for 12 months or more in a specific geographic area"* [109].

With the growing number of immunocompromised people who cannot be vaccinated, waning immunity, lack of immunity passed from mother to baby, and pathogenic shift due to selective pressure...it has become patently obvious that 'herd immunity' via a vaccine is an impossible dream.

The obvious failures of 'herd immunity' have been many and varied, over the past several decades. Here's just a couple of examples:

> **1985**: Measles outbreak among adolescents in Corpus Christi, Texas, despite more than 99% vaccination rate [110].

> **2011:** Large measles outbreak in highly vaccinated population, in Quebec, Canada. Those who'd received two doses of vaccine were more susceptible than those who'd only had one dose [111].

2015: Small outbreak of pertussis at Monterey Park School in Salinas, California. The school had a vaccination rate of 99.5%. All four students who were diagnosed with pertussis were vaccinated [112].

In a 2014 analysis published in the Oregon Law Review, scholars concluded that 60 years of widespread vaccination policies *"have not attained herd immunity for any childhood disease"*, and that *"herd immunity is unattainable for most diseases and is therefore an irrational goal"* [113].

Still, the desire to feel like we are helping protect the vulnerable is very compelling – researchers say that about 30% of parents cite 'herd immunity' as motivation for vaccination [114].

Despite tampering with the human immune system for more than a century now, via attempts to artificially induce immunity, even experts understand very little about the immune system.

This is astutely summed up in a quote from Garry Fathman MD, Professor of Immunology and Rheumatology, and Associate Director of the Institute for Immunology, Transplantation and Infection [115]:

"The immune system remains a black box...It's staggeringly complex, comprising at least 15 different interacting cell types that spew dozens of different molecules into the blood to communicate with one another and to do battle. Within each of those cells sit tens of thousands of genes whose activity can be altered by age, exercise, infection, vaccination status, diet, stress, you name it...That's an awful lot of moving parts. And

we don't really know what the vast majority of them do, or should be doing..."

And this from a 2013 study on the mechanisms of vaccine adjuvants [116]:

"Surprisingly, despite the wide use of vaccine adjuvants in billions of doses of human and animal vaccines, the mechanisms of action by which they potentiate immune responses are not well characterized. This is well captured in a famous quote by Janeway (1989) who observed that adjuvants are "the immunologists' dirty little secret".

Many decades after universal childhood vaccination programs were implemented, with great optimism that one shot was going to protect our children for the rest of their lives, it has become abundantly clear that:

a) the promise of 'immunity' via vaccines was not as clearcut as once thought, and
b) we don't know as much about the immune system as we thought we did, and
c) tampering with this system, of which we know little, has profound consequences, which are being ignored by today's vaccination programs.

2.
VACCINE HISTORY

Now that we have established that vaccines don't work quite like we've been told, you may be wondering how diseases that once terrorized Western civilization, are now virtually eradicated. Surely, vaccines must help somehow?

Maybe there's another side to history, too?

Let's go back in time, for a few moments, to the 19th century. During this time, a massive population shift took place, from rural areas to cities, in search of the riches and 'better life' promised by the Industrial Revolution. The misery and chaos that ensued were a perfect breeding ground for poverty, disease, and death…

1. OVERCROWDING

During the 19th century, the population of London swelled by more than six-fold, from 1 million to more than 6 million inhabitants, to become the largest city in the world [1].

All across the western world, as the Industrial Revolution took hold, vast numbers of rural folk moved into towns and cities. For example, in 1750, only 15% of the population lived in towns, but by 1880, a massive 80% of the population were urban dwellers [2].

The Industrial revolution, and city living, promised a better life that, for many, turned into an unimaginable nightmare.

With housing in short supply, unscrupulous landlords turned buildings into tenements, and leased every spare inch to desperate families – dingy, damp cellars, fire-trap attics and under-stair storage rooms, many without any ventilation or light. Just imagine the damp, mouldy air these people were constantly breathing – it's hardly a wonder that tuberculosis and pneumonia were the biggest killers, accounting for one-fifth of all deaths [3].

"Hideous slums, some of them acres wide, some no more than crannies of obscure misery, make up a substantial part of the metropolis ... In big, once handsome houses, thirty or more people of all ages may inhabit a single room" [4].

Disease and death were uncomfortably close in these crowded quarters: *"...the report of a health officer for Darlington in the 1850's found six children, aged between 2 and 17, suffering from smallpox in a one-roomed dwelling shared with their parents, and elder brother and an uncle. They all slept together on rags on the floor, with no bed. Millions of similar cases could be cited, with conditions getting even worse as disease victims died and their corpses remained rotting among families in single-roomed accommodations for days, as the family scraped together pennies to bury them"* [5].

2. LACK OF PLUMBING

Entire streets had to share one outdoor toilet, which was usually in foul condition – cleaning supplies were expensive, and flies hung around in droves (and then made their way through open windows to nearby kitchens etc), and of course, diarrhoea was ever-present.

Sewerage drained into waterways via open channels in the streets and lanes, or simply lay stagnant in stinking cesspools of filth.

Henry Mayhew was an investigative journalist who, in 1849, described a London street with a ditch running down the middle, that contained the only drinking water available to residents. He said it was '*the colour of strong green tea*', and '*more like watery mud than muddy water*'.

'*As we gazed in horror at it, we saw drains and sewers emptying their filthy contents into it; we saw a whole tier of doorless privies (toilets) in the open road, common to men and women built over it; we heard bucket after bucket of filth splash into it*' [6].

3. CONTAMINATED DRINKING WATER

With no environmental laws in place, raw sewage poured into drinking water supplies, as did run-off and toxic waste from factories and animal slaughterhouses.

"*The spill-off from the slaughter-houses and the glue factories, the chemicals of the commercial manufacturers, and all of Chicago's raw sewage had begun to contaminate the drinking water*" [7].

In London, the River Thames, which was the source of drinking water for many Londoners, became a stinking flow of excrement and filth, as human, animal and industrial waste was dumped into it. *"In the heatwave of 1858, the stagnating open sewer outside Westminster's windows fermented and boiled under the scorching sun"* [8].

During a cholera epidemic in London, in 1854, Dr John Snow realized that the only people who seemed to be completely unaffected, were the workers at a local brewery – they were drinking beer instead of water [9]! The discovery that disease could be spread via water was revolutionary at the time, and paved the way for massive sanitary reforms

4. CONTAMINATED FOOD SUPPLY

With slow, unreliable transport, and no refrigeration, food was often past its use-by date. Diseased and rotting meat was made into sausages and ham. *"Pigs are largely fed upon diseased meat which is too far gone, even for the sausage maker, and this is saying a great deal; and as a universal rule, diseased pigs are pickled and cured for ham, bacon etc"* [10].

Milking cows were often fed on 'whisky slops' and other rotting, cheap food, and therefore became diseased. *"New York's milk supply was also largely a by-product of the local distilleries, and the milk dealers were charged with the serious offense of murdering annually eight thousand children"* [11].

Before pasteurization, milk was treated with formaldehyde to prevent souring [12].

'Fresh' produce, when it was available, was not so fresh after all - often slimy, and unfit for human consumption.

"Piles of pickled herrings are exposed to the air 'til the mass approaches a condition of putridity: and this slimy food, with wilted and decayed vegetables, sausages not above suspicion, and horrible pies, composed of stale and unripe fruits, whose digestion no human stomach can accomplish, find ready purchasers. These decaying animals and vegetable remains are daily entombed in the protuberant stomachs of thousands of children, whose pallid expressionless faces and shrunken limbs are the familiar attributes of childhood in these localities" [13].

5. ABSENT MOTHERS

During the 19th century, countless mothers died during, or soon after, childbirth. There were a number of reasons for this: a) Malnutrition was rife, b) Doctors took offense at the idea they had dirty hands, and refused to wash them [14], c) chloroform and forceps were used unnecessarily in uncomplicated labours [15], and d) many girls grew up with deformed hips due to rickets, which later resulted in problems during childbirth, which increased maternal mortality.

If the baby survived past infancy, they could generally look forward to a life of malnutrition, hard labor and improper care, often performed by older siblings.

During the Industrial Revolution, many mothers worked long hours in factories, leaving their young children in the care of hired 'nurse-girls', who were little more than children themselves, between 8-12yrs of age [16].

Many children ended up living on the streets, driven to stealing and pilfering, in order to survive.

"In 1848 Lord Ashley referred to more than thirty thousand 'naked, filthy, roaming lawless and deserted children, in and around the metropolis" [17].

6. CHILD LABOUR & HARD LABOUR

With the Industrial Revolution in full swing, and labour in short supply, children *as young as three and four* were put to work in sweatshops and factories. Many of the jobs involved long hours, working in dangerous conditions, such as around heavy machinery, or working near furnaces.

"Children of all ages, down to three and four, were found in the hardest and most painful labor, while babes of six were commonly found in large numbers in many factories. Labor from twelve to thirteen, often sixteen hours per day was the rule" [18].

"Very often the children are woken at four in the morning. The children are carried on the backs of the older children asleep to the mill, and they see no more of their parents till they go home at night and are sent to bed" (Richard Oastler, interviewed in 1832) [19].

"The smallest child in the factories were scavengers......they go under the machine, while it is going...it is very dangerous when they first come, but they become used to it" (Charles Aberdeen worked in a Manchester cotton factory, written in 1832) [19].

"*Sarah Golding was poorly and so she stopped her machine. James Birch, the overlooker, knocked her to the floor. She got up as well as she could. He knocked her down again. Then she was carried to her house...she was found dead in her bed. There was another girl called Mary......she knocked her food can to the floor. The master, Mr. Newton, kicked her and caused her to wear away till she died. There was another, Caroline Thompson, who was beaten till she went out of her mind. The overlookers used to cut off the hair of any girl caught talking to a lad. This head shaving was a dreadful punishment. We were more afraid of it than any other punishment for girls are proud of their hair*" (An interview in 1849 with an unknown woman who worked in a cotton factory as a child) [19].

Children were forced to do back-breaking work in the most appalling conditions: "*Children began their life in the coal-mines at five, six or seven years of age. Girls and women worked like boys; they were less than half-clothed, and worked alongside men who were stark naked. There were from twelve to fourteen working hours in the twenty-four, and these were often at night...A common form of labour consisted of drawing on hands and knees over the inequalities of a passageway not more than two feet, or twenty-eight inches high a car or tub filled with three or four hundred weight of coal, attached by a chain, and hooked to a leather band around the waist*' [20].

Children were sometimes crushed to death, or had limbs severed, in some of the more dangerous industries, such as underground mining: "*...we occasionally hear of a little boy in the mine run over by a coal car, or kicked to death by a mule, or fatally injured by a piece of falling slate. And in the coal* *breakers little boys are sometimes ground in large crushers that break the coal, caught in the wheels or other machinery, or buried in a stream of coal…"* [21].

One coal-mine reported 349 deaths in a year, 58 of them were children under 13 years of age [22].

The job of cleaning chimneys was often performed by children. It was a dangerous job, and many children died from breathing in soot every day [22].

Basically, millions of children had no childhood, but a monotonous, depressing existence.

"Children had not a moment free, save to snatch a hasty meal, or sleep as best they could. From earliest youth they worked to a point of extreme exhaustion, without open air exercise, or any enjoyment whatever, but grew up, if they survived at all, weak, bloodless, miserable, and in many cases deformed cripples, and victims of almost every disease" [23].

And to make matters worse, many children were constantly exposed to poisons, such as arsenic, lead and mercury, which were being widely used in industries, such as silk and cotton spinning [24].

Adulthood didn't bring much change – hard labour, often for 12-16 hours per day. The terrible conditions and over-work, along with poor diet, aged people quickly: *"Among the labouring classes, life expectation everywhere remained low – little more than 30 years – and from the 1830's photographs show working people looking old by their thirties and forties, as poor nutrition, illness, bad living conditions and gross over-work took their toll'* [25].

7. POLLUTED AIR

Factories spewed soot and waste into the air, unchecked and unregulated. Cities were covered in a layer of grease and grime.

"In manufacturing towns, factory chimneys spewed soot, and everything was covered in grease and grime. Smoke was a major ingredient of the famous London fog, which not only reduced visibility, but posed serious health risks" [26].

It's no surprise that lung and chest complaints were rife. And then there was the ever-present stench of open sewage, rubbish, animal dung etc.

"Refuse, including the rotting corpses of dogs and horses, littered city streets. In 1858, the stench from sewage and other rot was so putrid that the British House of Commons was forced to suspend its sessions" [26].

That episode became known as 'The Great Stink', and (much later) in 1952, atmospheric conditions coupled with coal-fire burning, led to the event now known as 'The Great Smog" – and the premature death of some four thousand people [27].

Even today, an estimated 9000 people die prematurely each year in London alone, due to air pollution [28]. Yet the levels of pollution in Victorian times were up to 50x worse than they are today [29] – how many lives were cut short because of the foul air polluting their lungs?

8. LACK OF BREASTFEEDING

Infant formula was first patented and marketed in 1865, consisting of cow's milk, wheat and malt flour, and potassium bicarbonate – and regarded as 'perfect infant food' [30].

Over the next 100 years, breastfeeding rates dropped to just 25% [31], as social attitudes disdained the practice as being only for the uneducated, and those who could not afford infant formula [32].

Not only did millions of babies miss out on the nurturing of their mother's breast, but their formula was poor quality, and often made with contaminated water in unsterile bottles, and milk quickly spoiled during warm weather without refrigeration.

It's hardly a wonder that so many babies succumbed to diarrheal infections, such as typhoid fever.

9. IMPROPER GARBAGE DISPOSAL

Without a proper disposal system in place, alleys, courtyards, and streets became littered with rubbish and waste – sometimes knee-high, which was not only offensive-smelling, but a great attraction for all kinds of scavengers - rats, pigs, dogs, cockroaches and swarms of flies [33].

10. ANIMALS

Because horses and donkeys were used to transport goods, they also had to be housed in overcrowded cities, often in close quarters to humans, since space was at a premium. Rotting carcases were left to decompose where they lay.

Animal poo was a constant feature of the city streets – by 1890, 300,000 horses were being used in London, creating 1000 tonnes of dung per day [34].

Pigs roamed freely in the streets, ferreting amongst the rubbish – some towns recorded more resident pigs than people.

Animal slaughterhouses were located amongst high-density tenement housing – animals were constantly slaughtered in full view of the surrounding residents, and the sounds and smell of death were constantly in the air.

"The suffering caused to animals by the present system of slaughtering is a source of pain and annoyance to all persons living near to these establishments. The animals are seldom fed from the time they arrive, until they are killed, and constantly give expression to their suffering. Many slaughterhouses are located in the centre of blocks of high-tenement houses, and business of slaughtering, as viewed from the adjacent windows, is in the highest degree demoralising in its effects upon the young" [35].

11. LACK OF SUNLIGHT

Due to the burning of coal, and wood fires, cities were blanketed in a thick, black smog that covered everything in grime.

Even if you weren't working 12-16hr days in factories, you could barely hope to get a little sunshine in your time off, either. The murk was so dense that countless accidents occurred, including horses and carts running into shop-fronts, or over pedestrians, or into each other [36].

Vitamin D deficiency was widespread, and in the late 1800's, studies concluded that up to 90% of children were suffering from rickets [37]. In young girls, this often led to deformed hips, and consequently, later problems in childbirth.

12. MALNUTRITION

Millions of families subsisted on the cheapest food possible. Malnutrition was rife, and up to 500 people per year died of starvation. Even those who could afford to eat regular meals lacked fresh fruit and vegetables [38].

Scurvy (Vitamin C deficiency) claimed many lives – an estimated 10,000 men during the California Gold Rush in the mid-1800's [39]. Even in those who did not have overt signs of scurvy, a state of mild deficiency must have been prevalent, leading to weakened immunity to disease and infection.

13. BAD MEDICINE

If you thought blood-letting and leeches were dubious enough, how about an injection of arsenic [40], or a gargle with mercury [41]?

Smallpox sores were dabbed with corrosives, in order to disinfect them [42].

Treatment for syphilis included mercury rubs, bismuth injections, and arsenic injections – some patients endured more than 100 such injections [40].

It's highly possible that the medical 'treatments' killed more people than the diseases they were intended to treat.

Hospitals were known to be breeding-grounds of disease, and in many cases, over-run by rats. *"This day, the inquest held on the body of the infant that was eaten by rats in Bellevue Hospital, New York, was concluded. The evidence of Mary O'Connor, the mother of the child, and that of numerous other witnesses was taken...and recommended that proper means be taken to rid the hospital of the rats that now infest the institution"* [43].

14. LACK OF BASIC CLEANLINESS

Given that less than 2% of the urban population had running water to their homes [44], and soap/detergents viewed as luxuries, washing of hands, clothes, plates and utensils had to be done with dirty, contaminated water – or not at all.

Note that items such as nappies and sanitary 'rags' also had to be washed – no 'disposables' in those days!

15. MENTAL AND EMOTIONAL STRESS

We now know that stress and fear take a huge toll on the body, resulting in immune system malfunction [45]. Can you imagine the mental anguish of being surrounded by abject poverty, and seeing no way of escape for yourself or your children? Or the panic of watching everybody you love succumb to a dreaded disease, and not having the knowledge, or means, to protect yourself?

Fear and hysteria ran high during disease outbreaks – during a cholera epidemic in the US in 1849 *"thousands fled panic-stricken before the scourge...The streets were empty, except for the doctors rushing from victim to victim, and the coffin makers and undertakers following closely on their heels"* [46].

Not to mention the stress of toiling for long hours in monotonous or dangerous work, with hardly a piece of dry bread to fill your hungry stomach. Given the poor living conditions that millions suffered, it was hardly a wonder that average life expectancy was, tragically, just 15 or 16 years among the working class [47].

Against this backdrop of filth, misery, and disease...came vaccines.

Edward Jenner

Although Edward Jenner is often hailed as the 'father of modern vaccines', the practice began hundreds of years before Jenner was even born.

As early as 1000BC in India, people were injecting dried and ground smallpox scabs, or pus, to try and protect from smallpox [48].

In 1721, a Lady Mary Wortley Montage, wife of the British Ambassador to Constantinople introduced what the Turks called 'ingrafting' to England - where the pus from the sore of a small-pox patient was introduced into the blood of a healthy person via a cut. This, Lady Mary claimed, rendered smallpox entirely harmless [49].

The practice was originally taken up enthusiastically by many in the medical profession, and in 1754, the Royal College of Physicians in London issued a declaration that all opposition to smallpox inoculation had been refuted by experience, and they declared the practice to be *"highly salutary to the human race"* [50].

Over time, however, it became obvious that this 'highly salutary' practice spread smallpox (among other things), and turned healthy vaccinees into reservoirs of infection. This method of inoculation was made illegal by an Act of Parliament in 1840 [51].

By 1840, they had found a 'highly scientific' alternative to inoculation, which was, of course, Edward Jenner's methods.

Twenty years before Jenner's vaccination attempts, a cattle farmer by the name of Benjamin Jesty heard the same folk stories that Jenner must have later heard - that milkmaids infected with cowpox seemed to have immunity to smallpox. Using his wife's knitting needle, and the pus from an infected cow, Jesty 'inoculated' his pregnant wife, and two young sons just near the elbow [52].

Mrs Jesty became quite ill, and Benjamin feared for the life of his wife and unborn child. The two boys however, seemed to be unaffected. His wife survived, but news of Jesty's experiment spread, and villagers were not too impressed [52].

Upon his death in 1816, his tombstone read:

"He was born at Yetminster in this County, and was an upright honest Man; particularly noted for having been the first person known that introduced the Cow pox by Inoculation, and who from his great strength of mind, made the Experiment from the Cow on his Wife and two Sons in the Year 1774" [52].

Edward Jenner, it would seem, had more of a knack for marketing himself, and Jesty was all but lost to history.

In 1796 Edward Jenner 'vaccinated' James Phipps, a boy about eight years old, with the matter taken from the hand of a dairy-maid infected with casual cow-pox.

After waiting six weeks Jenner injected this boy on both arms with smallpox matter, (taken from the arm of a boy with smallpox). Several months later, when Phipps was again injected with smallpox pus, he had, according to Jenner, been 'artificially exposed to the disease a second time and no effect was produced' [53].

Jenner, fully convinced that his method worked, also experimented on his young son, injecting him with both swine pox and later with cowpox. Tragically, he grew up to be developmentally disabled, and died of tuberculosis at age 21 [53].

The boy James Phipps, who was declared immune to smallpox, was unfortunately not immune to tuberculosis, and also passed away from the disease at age 20. Jenner's wife Catherine, and two sisters, also passed away from tuberculosis [54].

Did Jenner's experiments cause, or contribute to, the untimely death of his loved ones?

We cannot say for sure, but smallpox vaccination was later linked to an increase in tuberculosis, then known as consumption [55-56].

What else do we know about the man Edward Jenner, and how did he manage to do what Benjamin Jesty couldn't? It seems Edward Jenner was more gifted in self-promotion and, some would argue, not immune from using slight-of-hand tactics to further his own ambitions.

"Now this man Jenner had never passed a medical examination in his life. He belonged to the good old times when George III was King—when medical examinations were not compulsory. Jenner looked upon the whole thing as a superfluity, and he hung up "Surgeon, apothecary," over his door without any of the qualifications that warranted the assumption. It was not until twenty years after he was in practice that he thought it advisable to get a few letters after his name. Consequently he then communicated with a Scotch University and obtained the degree of Doctor of Medicine for the sum of £15 and nothing more. It is true that a little while before, he had obtained a Fellowship of the Royal Society, but his latest biographer and apologist, Dr. Norman Moore, had to confess that it was obtained by little less than a fraud. It was obtained by writing a most extraordinary paper about a fabulous cuckoo, for the most part composed of arrant absurdities and imaginative freaks such as no ornithologist of the present day would pay

the slightest heed to. A few years after this, rather dissatisfied with the only medical qualification he had obtained, Jenner communicated with the University of Oxford and asked them to grant him their honorary degree of M.D., and after a good many fruitless attempts he got it. Then he sent to the Royal College of Physicians in London to get their diploma, and even presented his Oxford degree as an argument in his favour. But they considered he had had quite enough on the cheap already, and told him distinctly that until he passed the usual examinations they were not going to give him any more" [57].

Indeed, Jenner was inducted into the Royal Society in 1788, before his vaccination experiments began, on the basis of his writing about cuckoos [58].

Edward Jenner was a high-level Freemason, and he was inducted into the Royal Society while Sir Joseph Banks – a fellow Freemason - was president [59].

Jenner *"maintained an active correspondence with other eminent Freemasons of the period who shared his theories and ideas; Freemasons such as Sir Joseph Banks…and Erasmus Darwin"* (grandfather of Charles Darwin) [59].

In 1812, Jenner became Worshipful Master of the Royal Lodge of Faith and Friendship, based in Berkeley, Gloucestershire. That particular Lodge was frequented by the Prince of Wales – later to become King George IV [59].

Despite being inducted into the Royal Society, Jenner's first attempt to promote his vaccine experiment to them, in 1796, was rejected. His manuscript provided short details of ten patients who had resisted inoculation several years after having cowpox, but Phipps was the only patient inoculated with cowpox [60]. Jenner must have realized that one example was not enough to convince scientific minds, so he expanded his experiment. He had to wait until 1798, a couple of years later, for another outbreak of cowpox. He then began a complicated set of experiments where he inoculated the first person, and then waited for a pustule to develop, of which the contents (pus) were used to inoculate a second person, and so on.

Sometime later, he arranged for smallpox matter (pus from smallpox pustules) to be taken from his nephew, and inoculate his experimental patients. When there was no reaction, he was satisfied that he had proven his theories, and wasted no time in self-publishing a pamphlet on his discoveries that same year, titled "*An Inquiry Into the Causes and Effects of Variolae Vaccinae, or Cowpox*" [61].

His paper outlined 16 case histories of people who appeared to be immune to smallpox, after suffering from cowpox, and he had 'cowpoxed' ten others, but only three of those had been rechallenged with smallpox.

Two doctors at the Hospital for Smallpox and Inoculation, who had been using Lady Worley's method for many years, decided to test Jenner's method...with less-than-promising results. Many of the patients ended up with pustules on their bodies (as might be expected with smallpox), and one patient died [62].

Jenner sprung to the defence of his work, stating that none of his patients had ever developed more than a single pustule at the inoculation site. The problem, Jenner declared, was not his method of vaccination, but the Inoculation Hospital, where the *"atmosphere, fixtures, and even Woodville himself (one of the doctors who carried out the trial), were so marinated in small-pox that he had accidentally contaminated his vaccine"* [63].

(Ouch!)

In 1802, supporters of Jenner then petitioned Parliament to give him an honorarium payment of 10,000 pounds, for income lost while developing his method of vaccination. Parliament voted in his favour, and Jenner found himself a wealthy man [63].

Ten thousand pounds was a huge sum for the time, and, according to online calculators, the rough equivalent of 840,000 pounds today, or $1.3 million US dollars. (Four years later, Parliament would give Jenner an even bigger windfall – a payment of 20,000 English pounds, 'in recognition of his services'. That equates to roughly $2.5 million US dollars today)

The following year, 1803, Jenner and his supporters founded the Jennerian Society in London, to promote vaccination amongst the poor, with Jenner as director. The Jennerian Society later became The Vaccine Establishment [64], but Jenner felt 'dishonoured' by the men selected to run it, and resigned his directorship [65].

Jenner had become a wealthy and influential man of society – he was presented to the King in 1800, and later, would be appointed physician extraordinary to the King. He was also made Mayor of Berkeley, and a Justice of the Peace [66].

Today, Jenner's work is regarded by many as the 'most important discovery in the history of humanity', but did Jenner's method really rid the world of smallpox?

Smallpox: 7 Forgotten Facts

1. Vaccination did not prevent smallpox.

When Jenner first struck upon his solution, which was to inoculate a cow with 'horse-grease', and then collect the lymph pus from the cow, to be introduced into humans via scratches on the arm, he declared the recipient would be "*forever after secure from the infection of the smallpox*" [67].

Unfortunately, his fervent zeal proved to be a bit premature. When it became obvious that this did not, in fact, confer lifelong immunity, the recommendations were updated to *two* vaccinations - which would then surely protect for life.

But still, vaccinated individuals continued to fall victim to smallpox, so it was decided that immunity only lasted fourteen years, after all [68]. When the error of that calculation became evident, it was then reduced even further to seven years [69], then five years [70]!

Unfortunately, vaccination every six weeks didn't even seem to be enough to confer immunity for some...

The American Army in the Philippines were some of the most frequently vaccinated individuals, and yet, in the five years from 1898 to 1902, smallpox ravaged the army, with a 35% fatality rate [71-72].

The *Medical Gazette*, November 6th, 1830, contained the extract of a letter to one Dr. Gregory, from J. S. Chapman, Esq., Acting Assistant-Surgeon 11th Light Dragoons, East Indies, May 4, 1830:

"Small-pox has been playing the very deuce at this station. There appears to be no positive security against the disease, either by vaccination, or by small-pox inoculation, and I have seen several cases where the patients have caught small-pox twice, and have each time been very severely marked, and, in two instances, have died of the second attack of small-pox. Certainly by far the greater number of our small-pox cases have occurred in persons vaccinated in India some twelve or fifteen years ago" [73].

When the first Compulsory Vaccination Bill went before parliament in England, in 1853, the Lancet noted *"In the public mind, extensively, and in the profession itself, doubts are known to exist as to the efficacy and eligibility of vaccination—the failures of the operation have been numerous and discouraging"* [73].

Decades rolled on, with increasingly more stringent laws requiring vaccination, and still the practice did not live up to the earlier promise of protection. Speaking before the Medical Freedom Society in 1937, Dr. William Howard Hay declared:

"I know of one epidemic of smallpox comprising nine hundred and some cases in which 95 per cent of the infected had been vaccinated, and most of them recently. I have had in my own experience one very small epidemic comprising 33 cases, of which 29 had vaccination histories a "good" scar, and some of

them vaccinated within the last year. There was no protection there".

"Among these was one girl who was not vaccinated, never had been, who had five cases of smallpox in the family, nursed those cases that were ill, a baby...the worst case of small-pox among them, refused vaccination and was never infected at all" [74].

2. The vaccine caused serious side-effects, including death.

One of the side effects of the smallpox vaccine, as admitted by doctors, was convulsions. In The New York Medical and Surgical Journal, a Dr. Shaw wrote regarding smallpox vaccination, *"I have known most fearful convulsions brought on by it, and that in children apparently in the firmest health"* [73].

One man had a child vaccinated in 1848, who died fourteen days later, from the effects of vaccination. *"He was summoned by the registrar in January last. He told the magistrate that he had had one child killed by vaccination; and he feared that, if forced to have another vaccinated, it also would be killed. He was forced to comply; and in less than three weeks, the child, though previously perfectly healthy, died of fits, similar to attacks to which some of the family of the child from whom the vaccine matter was taken were subject"* [73].

And this: *"...a poor woman, with tears in her eyes, came to the Author, anxiously enquiring whether the Bill now before Parliament was likely to pass. She stated that she had three children, all very healthy, born of healthy parents. One was vaccinated: its health was so affected by the vaccination that it became the subject of a loathsome disease, and died. The other two are living and healthy; they have not been vaccinated. The mother said that she would rather die than submit her children to vaccination"* [73].

In the Weekly Return, May 1854: "*At the 'Cock and Castle,' Kingsland, on the 1st May, the son of a licensed victualler, aged four months died of 'vaccination; inflammation of the cellular tissue of arm and thorax.' In Haggerston East, at 54, Union Street, on the 1st of May, the son of a hotpresser, aged four months, died of gangrene after vaccination"* [73].

3. Smallpox outbreaks became more deadly after widespread vaccination was implemented.

During the late 1800's, Japan enforced a strict vaccination program for all infants, children, and adolescents with additional vaccines during outbreaks, or upon entry into the armed forces. The scourge of smallpox was declared "all but unknown"...

Alas and alack, several years later, smallpox returned, with more vengeance than ever before. Between 1889 and 1908, there are 171,500 cases, with 48,000 deaths - a mortality rate of 28% [75-78].

Following the Philippine-American war (a bloody conflict, lasting from 1899, through to 1902 - and beyond, in some areas), the US Army embarked on an ambitious vaccination program beginning from around 1905, conducting 30 million vaccinations on a population of just 10 million over the course of 6 years. Many of those living in urban areas were vaccinated 5 or

6 times, while many in mountainous rural areas were not vaccinated at all.

Several years afterwards, in 1918, the Philippines suffered their worst ever epidemic of smallpox, with a mortality rate as high as 65% in some areas. The highest incidence and mortality rates were in urban areas, which were the most highly-vaccinated areas [79-80].

4. Vaccination spread other diseases.

In 1861, the Lancet, published an account of 46 children who were infected with syphilis, via contaminated smallpox vaccine. These cases were all 'well authenticated' [81].

Several years later, in 1866, the Lancet contained an account of deaths caused by syphilitic inoculation with vaccine lymph. Thirty children were vaccinated from a little girl, six punctures being made on each arm, and the little girl had been operated on from another child, who had been vaccinated with lymph preserved between two plates of glass, which had been obtained from the medical authorities. All these children were inoculated with syphilis [82].

Syphilis may not have been the only scourge shared around by smallpox vaccination.

Medical practitioners in many parts of the world began to suspect that vaccination was also spreading another fearful scourge: leprosy.

Dr Roger S. Chew spent six years in the Medical Department of the British Army in India, and fourteen years studying leprosy. Of the leprosy cases treated under his care, he attributed 105 cases to insanitation, 148 cases to vaccination, and 72 cases due to other forms of inoculation.

Extracts from his case book contain examples such as:

"Jahoorie, aged twenty - eight. Married; no children. Duration of leprosy, twenty years".

"There is no history of syphilis, either with himself or his relatives. - When he was about seven years old, he was vaccinated on his right arm. About six months after he- noticed a white patch over vaccine site; a similar patch appeared on his right buttock, and he soon after lost sensation in his left foot. The marks gradually faded away, broke out afresh in - other portions of his body, and again disappeared to reappear, et seq.; but wherever these marks appeared, they were accompanied by loss of sensation, which remained permanent throughout. About sixteen years ago he suffered from enlarged spleen, for which he was fired (i.e., burned with hot iron). Ten years ago the fingers of both hands began to be flexed on themselves" [83].

Discussion amongst the medical fraternity regarding the probability of vaccination spreading leprosy appeared in the British Medical Journal, on several occasions during the 1880's, with medical men reporting cases of leprosy, which they deemed could have come from no other source but vaccination [83].

In 1908, an outbreak of foot and mouth disease amongst animals in the United States, was traced back to the culture used in vaccines. The culture, thought to be cowpox, had been imported from Japan, and upon further investigation, turned out to be a culture of foot and mouth disease [84-85].

In 1901 in Philadelphia, 36 cases of tetanus were believed to be the result of vaccination - nearly all were fatal [86].

5. Mortality from other diseases increased, after introduction of widespread vaccination.

The Registrar General's Report from 1865 shows mortality from measles and scarlet fever increased in the decade following the introduction of widespread vaccination in England [87].

Average annual mortality from tuberculosis (then called phthisis) and bronchitis (in round numbers):

1838 - 1842: 61,000
1847-1851: 65,750
1852-1856: 69,250 (Smallpox vaccination made compulsory in 1853)
1857-61: 79,530
1861-65: 86,336.

In 1865 the highest mortality in England was due to tuberculosis. Combined mortality from all chest diseases—including phthisis (tuberculosis), bronchitis, pneumonia, and whooping-cough— amounted to 5,840 per one million persons living. With mortality from all causes being 23,387 per one million living; chest diseases account for about a quarter of the mortality rate [87].

Charles Pearce's 'Essay on Vaccination' recounts the following story: "*I am 40 years of age. I have a brother living who is 44. My brother and I are the only survivors of a family of ten children. Five of the eight who are dead, died in childhood, two at puberty, and one, at eighteen years of age, of consumption. My brother and I had small-pox; we had neither of us been vaccinated, for it was not much in fashion in the country when we were children, but the eight younger ones born after me were all vaccinated, and my poor mother always attributed their deaths to vaccination; there had been no consumption in the family until then*" [87].

A decrease in mortality from smallpox coincided with an increase in mortality from whooping cough, over and above the decrease for smallpox. Similarly, when smallpox deaths increased, mortality from whooping cough decreased at a greater rate than the increase in smallpox deaths.

Overall, mortality from the two diseases was lower, when smallpox was more severe [87].

6. The statistics on smallpox are unreliable.

The field of statistics developed in Britain during the late 1700's and, by 1830, was being used extensively by different statistical societies to collect data.

In her book 'Bodily Matters: The Anti-Vaccination Movement in England, 1853 – 1907', Nadja Durbach writes: "*Statistics quickly became a tool of public policy, for numbers had the appearance of objectivity, and added scientific weight to otherwise subjective opinion. The state thus frequently mobilized 'facts' to counter anti-vaccination rhetoric. These data, the government maintained, clearly demonstrated that the unvaccinated died more frequently of smallpox than the vaccinated. Government administrators gathered the statistics at isolation hospitals, which treated only a fraction of the cases. There, doctors routinely classified those with no visible vaccination marks as "unvaccinated". A patient pitted with smallpox rarely had vaccination scars that could actually be seen. Those who did have such scars and caught smallpox nevertheless often were classed as "imperfectly vaccinated", which in some cases was incorporated into the "unvaccinated" category. Vaccination statistics are therefore highly unreliable"* [88].

Writing in 1941, Dr. Herbert Shelton says *"Just as before the time of Sydenham (Thomas Sydenham was an eminent English physician who lived in the 1600's), all cases of measles, chickenpox and scarlet fever were diagnosed as smallpox. Today if a case of chickenpox has no vaccination scar, it is smallpox; if a case of smallpox has a vaccination scar, it is chickenpox"* [89].

The famous Irish playwright, George Bernard Shaw, writing in the British Medical Journal in 1931, had this to say: *"I was vaccinated in infancy and had 'good marks' of it. In the great epidemic of 1881 (I was born in 1856) I caught smallpox".*

"During the last considerable epidemic at the turn of the century, I was a member of the Health Committee of London Borough Council, and I learned how the credit of vaccination is kept up statistically by diagnosing all the re-vaccinated cases as pustular eczema, varioloid, or what-not,

except smallpox" [90].

7. Smallpox was made deadly because of improper medical practices.

Writing in the 1600's, Dr Thomas Sydenham wrote: *"As it is palpable to all the world how fatal smallpox proves to many of all ages, so it is clear to me from all the observations that I can possibly make, that if no mischief is done, either by physician or nurse , it is the most safe and slight of all diseases"* [91].

Smallpox treatment in the 1600's included purgatives, and blood-letting, even letting blood from the tongue [92].

Three hundred years later, medical treatment of smallpox, hadn't improved much. Some would argue, it had become even more dangerous. Take the following information from a 1937 medical textbook:

*"The eruption is usually treated by applying gauze immersed in various antiseptic solutions such as **phenol or bichloride of mercury**. The face is sometimes covered with gauze, and oiled silk. The formation of vesicles is sometimes hastened by exposing the patient to sunlight or artificial sunlight. When the odor is particularly bad, continuous warm baths of antiseptic solutions are used. Scratching should be prevented as it often causes deep pitting. When the rash occurs in the throat, various antiseptic gargles are used. It is especially important to keep the eyes clean by frequent irrigations with normal salt solution or with boric acid solution, to prevent extensive inflammation. The fever is treated by coal-tar drugs and by cold sponges. The diet is the usual light diet of fever with plenty of*

water. When the patient is delirious, morphine or <u>*bromides*</u> *are given. During convalescence oil, glycerin or antiseptic ointments are applied to soften the crusts"* [93].

Phenol, also known as carbolic acid, is highly corrosive, and skin contact results in *inflammation and blistering*, according to the MSDS [94].

The side effects of bromides include nausea, fever, skin rashes - usually starting on the face, pustular eruptions on the skin, lethargy, musculoskeletal pain, anorexia, muscular weakness and central nervous system problems [95].

Compare that with symptoms of 'smallpox'...Fever, abdominal pain, nausea and vomiting, rash starting on face then spreading to the rest of the body, which would blister up and fill with pus, then eventually dry up and scab over [96], and one must ask: How many smallpox deaths were really attributable to the standard medical care given during those years?

Stranger Than Fiction: Polio History

Besides smallpox, the other argument most used in defence of the vaccination program, is how efficiently vaccines eradicated polio (from most of the world, at least). In order to gain some perspective on polio, it's critical that we go back in time, to a period where many heavy metals were used excessively, and considered wonder-products.

What's that got to do with polio?

Read on, and I think you'll agree it's got a lot to do with polio...

During the 1800's, arsenic was used to make Paris Green, which added colour to paints, wallpaper and fabrics. Throughout the 19th century, there were reports of people becoming ill from living in homes that were decorated with the poisoned wallpaper. Arsenic was also used in adhesive envelopes, fire-works, medicated soaps designed to enhance complexion.

In the 1890's, the unexplained deaths of over a thousand children in Italy, prompted investigations, and the subsequent discovery that the arsenic in the wallpaper reacted with dampness to form toxic by-product, called arsine [97].

Arsenic, in Victorian times, became the poison of choice for would-be murderers, because it was easy to hide in food and, if dosed correctly, could kill a person without being too obvious about it.

"*Arsenic poisoning was difficult to detect as the symptoms initially mimicked food poisoning, but a single dose could produce severe diarrhoea and vomiting, **paralysis, and death**. Because of its potency, the ease with which it could be obtained, and the discreteness with which it could be administered, it was a favoured poison of the ruling classes to kill off their rivals and adversaries and so became known as the "Poison of Kings and the King of Poisons*" [98].

It is generally agreed that the first clinical description of poliomyelitis was provided by English physician Michael Underwood, in 1799. He attributed these paralysis cases to several causes - one being teething in infants.

During the 17th and 18th centuries there were also sporadic cases of paralysis in young children, referred to as 'dental paralysis', 'teething paralysis' or 'paralysis in dentition', due to its propensity to strike while a baby was teething. It may seem strange to us now, but teething was once a dreaded time of childhood, as it was believed to cause all kinds of health problems including *paralysis, convulsions and deaths.* For example, Michigan registry death reports attributed to teething averaged 68 per year, from 1868 – 1895 [99-109].

George Colmer, an American doctor, published a report on paralysis in teething infants, in 1843. He noted: "*Whilst on a visit to the parish of West Feliciana, La, in the fall of 1841, my attention was called to a child about a year old, then slowly recovering from an attack of hemiplegia (paralysis of one side of the body). The parents (who were people of intelligence and unquestionable veracity), told me that eight or ten other cases of either hemiplegia or paraplegia, had occurred during the preceeding three or four months, within a few miles of their residence, all of which had either completely recovered, or were decidedly improving. The little sufferers were invariably under two years of age, and the cause seemed to be the same in all – namely, teething*" [110].

Now we might wonder at their dread of teething, and for their propensity to blame all kinds of maladies, even convulsions and death, on teething...until one discovers the numerous remedies, medicines and concoctions that were then used on teething infants. Many of them contained ingredients that might have left parents and nurse-maids aghast (if they'd known) but, at the time, medicines were largely unregulated, and ingredients were not required to be listed on the label.

Many teething powders contained mercury, while 'soothing' cordials and syrups marketed towards mothers of fretful teething babies, contained laudanum (alcoholic tincture of opium) or morphine (derivative of opium). In fact, during those years, opium was known as "The Poor Child's Nurse" because it made hungry babies stop crying.

According to LiveScience, "Mercury poisoning can result in hearing and vision changes, personality changes, memory problems, *seizures or paralysis*. When children are exposed to mercury, they may have developmental or *muscle coordination problems*" [111].

Although there were sporadic reports of paralysis in infants, they did not gain widespread attention until later. Meanwhile, Paris Green had been used as an insecticide on tobacco and other crops, but it was about to be surpassed by a chemical more convenient. More effective.

And more toxic.

The story of polio in America begins in Massachusetts.

In 1892, Massachusetts became the first state in America to begin spraying lead arsenate, in an effort to control the gypsy moth [112]. Even as far back as 1824, scientists had observed that "*the fumes of these metals, or the receptance of them in solution into the stomach, often cause paralysis*" [113].

It seems hardly surprising then, that the following season, a Massachusetts doctor, James Putnam MD, writing in the

Boston Medical and Surgical Journal, queried whether 'polio' had been more prevalent that season [114]. There had been 26 cases seen in Boston that season - the largest outbreak so far in America.

Massachusetts also happened to be home to the Merrimack Chemical Company, who produced the lead arsenate, along with sulfuric acid, and other chemicals. By 1899, Merrimack (which was later bought out by Monsanto) was the largest producer of lead arsenate in the United States [115].

There were numerous other chemical companies in the area and, at the time, there was very little awareness of, or controls put into place for, pollution. Waste products were commonly disposed of, into nearby ponds and waterways – in this case, the Aberjona River. Between 1888 and 1929, at least 13 tonnes of arsenic were transported down the river, to the Upper Mystic Lake, which were, during those years, a public water supply [115].

Water from the Upper Mystic Lake then empties into the Lower Mystic Lake, which in turn empties into the Mystic River, which then makes its way into Boston Harbour – the very area where those 26 cases had been noted by James Putnam, MD.

In 1894, an even bigger outbreak occurred in Rutland County, Vermont, just over the border from Massachusetts. There were 132 reports of paralysis and eighteen deaths – almost all of those were children, and almost all (94%) occurred in the Otter Creek Valley [116], - a fertile valley nestled between two mountain ranges, sustained at that time by a thriving agriculture industry and marble quarries.

Although this is officially classed as America's first polio out-break, there are a number of curiosities that don't align with today's description of polio.

Reporting on the outbreak, Charles Caverley MD, member of the Vermont Board of Health, said *"The element of contagium does not enter into the etiology either. I find but a single instance in which more than one member of a family had the disease, and as it usually occurred in families of more than one child and as no efforts were made at isolation, it is very certain that it was non-contagious."*

He also says: *"I might state further that there have been many deaths among horses, attended with symptoms of paralysis, and in which at least one veterinarian tells me he found meningitis. There have been, too, some deaths with similar symptoms among dogs and fowls"* [116].

This is a most interesting observation, because, as of writing this, the CDC clearly states on their website that poliovirus *"only infects humans"* [117].

Also of note, the CDC description of polio symptoms include no mention of convulsions or skin rashes, yet a number of Charles Caverley's case descriptions include skin rashes, and convulsions leading to death, and a number of those who died had no symptoms of paralysis (yet the CDC says *"only people with the paralytic infection are considered to have the disease."*)

Over the next six decades, the use of lead arsenate would sky-rocket, as farmers began to use it in apple orchards right across the United States, to control codling moth, an invasive species, highly destructive to apples [118]. It quickly became popular, because it was inexpensive, easy to mix, and a residue adhered to the plant surfaces, making the pesticidal effects last longer. Multiple applications of lead arsenate, at a rate of 2-4 pounds per 100 gallons of water, were applied each season.

Schooley, et al (2008) explain how it was used: *"The spray schedule was divided into three important sprays:*

The dormant spray was preferably applied in the spring before the buds opened as well as in the fall after leaf drop. A nozzle with a fine mist spray was used to coat the entire tree, including all the limbs and the trunk.

The summer spray was applied with a fine mist nozzle to completely coat the leaves and fruit from every angle. Once the water from the spray evaporated, the fruit and foliage were examined for complete or partial coverage.

The petal-fall spray was the most effective single application for the control of the codling moth (Ibid). After petal-fall, the calyx was left open a short time. Because this was where most of the insect pests entered the fruit, it was very important to fill the calyx cups with insecticide" [118].

Over time, however, the three applications per season increased to 5 or 6 applications per season.

It was not until much later (1920's) that researchers realized lead arsenate residues on apples (and other fruit, such as apricots, plums, peaches, and berries) were not properly removed by washing or rubbing. About two-thirds of the residue remained on the fruit.

Researchers also found that if *dry weather* followed a July spraying, excessive residues remained on the fruit at harvest [119]. It was also found that smaller apples on the lower tree limbs (the apples most likely to be eaten by children playing in the orchards?) carried the highest amounts of residue [120].

Herbert C. Emerson MD, the State Inspector for Health put together a very thorough report on an outbreak in Western Massachusetts in 1908. He noted that, like the earlier outbreak in Vermont, many cases were in valley townships, situated near streams and waterways [121].

Emerson visited the homes of all 69 cases, and painstakingly recorded the details of their illness, their living arrangements, their diets, and incidents preceding the illness.

He noted some interesting findings, such as [121]:

a) if the disease was indeed caused by an infectious agent, then it was only mildly contagious, at the most, given the close contact between the 69 patients and at least 250 other children - siblings, cousins and neighbours, etc - of whom only two got sick.

b) The possibility that the outbreak was linked to their food source. There were no cases of polio amongst exclusively breast-fed infants, but 7 cases among infants who were formula-fed. Numerous cases were attributed to eating berries before illness struck.

c) It was a hot, dry summer (this means that not only would residues on fruit be greater, but contamination of water supplies would have been more concentrated).

There were numerous other reports that pointed to poisoning as the cause of the increasing outbreaks of paralysis. In a statement prepared for the House Select Committee, Dr Ralph Scobey referenced the following writings [122]:

- Colton (1850) noted a case of arsenic poisoning that was admitted to hospital and treated (in those days, possibly with mercurial medicine, or other heavy metals), and 7 days later became paralyzed. Colton noted that this delayed reaction corresponded to the 'incubation' period of infectious diseases.

- After producing 'arsenical paralysis' in animals experimentally, Popow (1881) concluded that arsenic could cause acute central myelitis or acute poliomyelitis, even within hours of ingestion.

- Onuff (1900) reported the case of a painter (presumably exposed to arsenic in the paint he was using), who suffered flaccid paralysis of both legs. Autopsy found lesions characteristic of poliomyelitis.

- Obsrastoff (1902) reported a case of acute poliomyelitis caused by arsenic poisoning.

In 1908, however, something happened that would change the focus of polio investigations. Austrian Karl Landsteiner and his assistant Edwin Popper performed an experiment that is still celebrated today, for purportedly proving the viral causation of poliomyelitis.

At the time, Landsteiner was prosector (a person who dissects dead bodies for investigation) at the Wilhelminenspital in Vienna. When a 9-year-old boy died with poliomyelitis symptoms, Landsteiner and Popper filtered the spinal fluid through fine filters known to trap bacteria, and then proceeded to inject it into the abdominal cavity of rabbits, guinea pigs and mice, but failed to produce any polio symptoms [123].

Undeterred, they then injected the spinal cord mixture into two monkeys of differing species. The first monkey became ill on the 6th day, and died two days later. No paralysis was witnessed, but upon dissection, changes in the nervous system similar to those seen in poliomyelitis were noted. The second monkey became paralysed in the hind legs on the 17th day, and upon dissection, also showed lesions consistent with poliomyelitis. However, a spinal cord concoction of those monkeys failed to produce any illness or death when injected into other monkeys (a technique referred to as 'passaging').

Although they were unable to see any pathogen at work (microscopes not yet being advanced enough), they concluded that poliomyelitis is caused by an infectious particle, smaller than bacteria [124].

Others were later able to 'passage' the illness from animal to animal, which further cemented the theory of infectiousness. One of those credited with furthering this line of research was Simon Flexner (1863-1946), who was director of the Rockefeller

Institute for Medical Research, a trustee of the Rockefeller Foundation, and a friend and advisor to John D. Rockefeller Jr.

A read of Flexner's published work, describes how he, and his assistant Hideyo Noguchi (1876-1928) managed to infect a continuous line of monkeys – and it reveals an elaborate method, so highly contrived that one wonders how any conclusions could be extrapolated as relevant to the 'real world' [125].

Flexner advised harvesting the tissue, preferably the brain, *"about two cubic centimetres extending into the white matter is excised"*, as soon as possible after death of the polio victim, and immediately placed in a sterile dish. The specimen is then added to the culture medium – in this case, human ascitic fluid, which is a watery fluid found in the digestive cavity, designed to lubricate the internal organs. In addition, add a fragment of fresh kidney, taken from a 'normal rabbit', then add sterile paraffin oil.

Incubate at 37 degrees (about 98 degrees Fahrenheit) for 7 – 12 days. The supposed presence of 'poliovirus' is proven by an opalescence that begins to gather around the tissue fragments at the bottom, which can be diffused via gentle shaking.

It is possible, to cultivate the virus without the fresh rabbit tissue, Flexner explains, but you need a much larger fragment of poliomyelitic brain, and even then, the growth is slow and inconsistent, that it becomes necessary to transplant into a medium containing fresh rabbit tissue.

It is also possible to cultivate the virus without the human ascitic fluid, if you substitute 'sheep serum water' or an extract prepared by grinding up a portion of rhesus monkey brain "*in a porcelain mill and then afterwards shaking for half an hour in a machine*". But you still need the fresh rabbit tissue to be successful!

The resulting cultures were then injected into monkeys, either directly into the brain, or "*into the sciatic nerve and peritonial cavity simultaneously*".

The sciatic nerve is a very large nerve that supplies sensation to the lower leg muscles. Damage to this nerve, such as "misplaced injections in the buttocks" can result in paralysis of the legs. This is known as 'injection palsy' or 'traumatic injection neuropathy' (a major cause of paralysis, even today) [126].

Predictably enough, monkeys became paralysed. And when their brain/nervous system tissues were removed and processed according to the above description, it also caused paralysis when injected into second generation of monkeys, and so on. The scientific world felt this was proof enough that an infectious (but as yet, invisible) agent was causing poliomyelitis epidemics, and the fact that dead or decomposing brains/tissues of other species were being injected into highly sensitive areas of the monkey nervous system seemed to be largely overlooked.

Scientists still hadn't figured out how this invisible, infectious micro-organism was being spread from person to person and causing outbreaks of paralysis. In their efforts to learn more, all kinds of materials were injected into monkeys to cause paralysis – including faeces and ground-up flies [127].

With the blame squarely placed on an invisible virus, the concerns and investigations of neurologists and toxicologists, and others, were virtually trodden underfoot in the stampede that ensued, to produce an antidote for this viral affliction.

In 1916, New York experienced a deadly outbreak of polio, which claimed the lives of some 2000 people. The *"epidemic caused widespread panic. Thousands fled the city to nearby mountain resorts. Movie theaters were closed, meetings were cancelled, and public gatherings were shunned. Children were warned not to drink from water fountains; amusement parks and bathing beaches were off limits. In some towns, visitors from the New York City area were turned away by armed citizens who feared the spread of contagion"* [128].

Children under 16 were not allowed to enter New York or surrounding towns, unless they carried a health certificate from their own district, 'proving' they had been examined and found to be free of disease. Some towns surrounding New York hired guards and policemen who, brandishing red flags, pulled over passing automobiles and made thorough searches for any concealed children. Some children found suffering from polio were forcibly removed from their homes and placed into the Isolation Hospital [129].

People began to rebel against the harsh quarantine laws, and many people felt that normal children's diseases were being mislabelled as polio "as a matter of safety" [129].

Approximately 72,000 abandoned cats were killed during the epidemic, by (ironically) the Society for the Prevention of Cruelty to Animals. Many were abandoned by their suspicious owners, who feared they were spreading disease [130].

Dingman (1916) noted that a small outbreak, involving eight cases from three separate Jewish boarding homes, in Spring Valley, New York, all used milk from the same source. *"The house mothers of these homes were quite positive, even before the diagnosis of poliomyelitis was made, that the milk was the cause"* [131].

Others made the same connection, linking polio outbreaks to 'milk poisoning', or the eating of dairy products [131]. We now know that arsenic can be passed via cow's milk. (Arsenic can also be transferred readily through the placenta in humans, so the developing foetus has a similar exposure to the mother [132]).

Other reports pointed to common water sources, as the mode of transmission in polio outbreaks. *"Kling (1928) supported the theory that poliomyelitis could be spread by means of water supplies. He observed that the disease first broke out near the water supply in the hills, cases occurring successively as the stream descended. Paul and Trask (1941) found, during an epidemic of poliomyelitis, that the distribution of cases followed a water course"* [131]. It was noted that polio outbreaks increased during dry or drought years.

By now, there was not only lead arsenate being used, but calcium arsenate widely used on cotton crops...and every summer there were polio outbreaks in at least one state of the US. Animals also, continued to fall victim.

In 1920, J.W Kalkus published a report in the American

Journal of Veterinary Medicine, of a disease he termed 'Orchard Horse Disease' – a fatal disease affecting horses and cows fed on hay raised in orchards, where arsenate of lead was sprayed [133].

In 1921, 'infantile paralysis' claimed its most famous victim – Franklin Delano Roosevelt (1885 - 1945), who would later become the 32nd President of the United States. It was a surprising diagnosis for a fit, 39-year old man, since the vast majority of cases were in children [134].

Later, while serving as President, he founded the National Foundation for Infantile Paralysis, which became the most visible and influential force in polio advocacy and the search for a polio vaccine. (In retrospect, though, modern scientists would later conclude that Roosevelt didn't suffer from polio at all, but rather Guillain-Barre Syndrome [135]).

At the time of his illness, Roosevelt was holidaying with his family, at their summer home on Campobello Island, in the Bay of Fundy. Reports suggest that Roosevelt had been swimming several times, shortly before falling ill - at least one of those occasion was in the Bay of Fundy, after accidentally falling overboard while sailing his yacht [136].

At the time, upstream of the Bay of Fundy was heavily industrialised with ship-building, oil-refining, brewing, tanning, and manufacturing of hardware, paints, and engines [137].

At least some of those industries would have been using heavy metals, such as lead, arsenic, cadmium and mercury and, as was common practice at the time, dumping the wastes into the bay.

Is it possible that Roosevelt was paralysed by exposure to neurotoxic heavy metals? Perhaps we will never know...

Meanwhile, by 1929, almost 30 million pounds of calcium and lead arsenate were being sprayed onto the fields and orchards of America, every year. In fact, the government was so enthusiastic about the bug-killing properties of arsenic, that a 1935 radio show, hosted by the FDA suggested the children's rhyme "A is for apple" should be changed to "*A is for arsenate, lead if you please, protector of apples, against arch-enemies*" [138].

Meanwhile, clusters of polio were noted in relation to fruit consumption.

Barber (1939) reported four cases of 'polio' that occurred the same day as strawberries were eaten, in a boarding school house [139].

Chenault (1941) noted the parallels between 'polio' outbreaks and the appearance of fresh fruit and vegetables [139].

Draper (1935) reported a case series of 'polio' which he theorized originated from a Greek fruiterer [139].

Arsenic-based products were also used to control lice and ticks on sheep and cattle. The symptoms of arsenic poisoning in animals are known to be weakness and a staggering gait, before progressing to convulsions and death [140].

In the early 20th century, arsenic was also being widely used in medicine, especially as a treatment for syphilis. Some patients were given more than 100 injections of arsenic-containing Tryparsamide, in the hope of treating the symptoms of advanced syphilis [141].

Gougerot (1935) reported on two patients who developed poliomyelitis after receiving arsenical treatment for syphilis [142].

Arsenical injections were also employed to treat yaws – a tropical skin disease. In 1936, a large campaign to eradicate yaws in Western Samoa using arsenical injections, preceded a polio outbreak. Most of the paralysis cases occurred 1-2 weeks following the injections [142].

But it wasn't just arsenic that could cause the symptoms known as polio...

- Dr. Altman noted that, just prior to Australia's first polio outbreak in 1897, in Port Lincoln, South Australia, phosphorous had recently been used in the area to control a rabbit infestation [143].

- Phillipe and Gauthard (1903) reported a case of poliomyelitis, caused by lead poisoning [142].

- Dr David Edsall (1907) noted that poliomyelitis had been seen as a result of carbon monoxide poisoning [142].

- Collins and Martland (1908) reported on a 38-year-old man who developed poliomyelitis following exposure to cyanide, used as a silver polish. His illness began as diarrhoea, "followed by headache and pain and stiffness in the back of the neck. About eight days after the onset of the illness, he became paralyzed" [142].

The fear of polio, was about to get much worse, as 'epidemics' were reported in increasing number and severity in the 1940's, and early 1950's.

There were three changes that may explain why:

1) Introduction of widespread vaccination for diptheria-tetanus-pertussis.

In the early 1900's, researchers had begun to realize that paralytic poliomyelitis often started at the site of an injection, whether for antibiotics or vaccination [144-145].

It was hardly a wonder that cases of paralytic poliomyelitis soared after widespread introduction of diptheria and pertussis vaccines in the 1940's [146-148].

In 1949, the Medical Research Council in Great Britain set up a committee to investigate the matter and concluded that individuals are at increased risk of paralysis for 30 days following injections [149]. These findings were later confirmed by others [150-153], and it was shown that receiving a single injection within one month of receiving a polio vaccine, increased the risk of poliomyelitis by eight-fold [151].

During a polio epidemic in Australia in 1949, the polio officer for the Victorian Health Department, Dr Bertram McCloskey also noted the incidence of poliomyelitis with paralysis starting in the limb that last received inoculations. Prominent medical men of the time admitted that *'this raised questions of great*

importance from the viewpoint of public-health administra-
tion...but they "feared that immunisation, particularly against
diphtheria, might be prejudiced if the public were informed"
[154].

A recent article (2014) published in the Lancet, noted that *"the*
application of epidemiological surveillance and statistical
methods enabled researchers to trace the steady rise in polio
incidence along with the expansion of immunisation pro-
grammes for diphtheria, pertussis, and tetanus" [155].

It should be noted here, that thousands of cases of paralysis following injections still occur today, but they are no longer referred to as 'polio', rather they are called 'traumatic injection
neuropathy". Strangely enough, in a study of injection neuropathy in Pakistan, it was found to be more common in children
(probably because children receive the bulk of injections, via
vaccinations or antibiotics), and more common during Summer
months [156] – just as in the old 'polio' epidemics.

It is not clear whether this is because more injections are administered during Summer, or some other physiological factor,
in conjunction with hot weather or heat stress, predispose some
people to paralysis.

In 1999, in India, there were 9586 reported cases of paralysis,
but only 1126 were virologically confirmed to involve poliovirus. So, what was causing paralysis in the other 8460 patients? In a study on a subsection of paralytic patients, they concluded there was little difference in vaccination histories (with
oral polio vaccines) between paralytic and control patients,
with the only clear difference being a history of injection within

the last month before symptoms began [157].

It seems odd, if a virus were solely responsible for the disease we know as 'polio', why so many become paralysed during outbreaks, without any poliovirus being isolated, but on the other hand, in populations where many have evidence of poliovirus, so few are paralysed by it – an estimated 0.6 cases of paralysis were estimated for every 100 infections, during the polio years [158].

The astute reader here must, by now, surely be questioning just how relevant a virus was, either to the epidemics that once traumatised parents, or to the ongoing epidemics, labelled by a different name, that are quietly wreaking havoc, away from the media spotlight.

2) Changing use of pesticide chemicals.

Following World War II, DDT and other orgnanophosphate pesticides were introduced, and became even more popular than lead arsenate.

"Before 1940, relatively small amounts of such chemicals as nicotine, rotenone, pyrethrum, and the aresenicals (sic) were used for insect control. During and following World War II a rapid changeover to DDT, heptachlor, dieldrin, TEPP, malathion, and related compounds occurred" [159].

It wasn't just the chemicals that evolved during those years, but the methods of application also evolved. In earlier years, *"the dusting and spraying was done by the shaking of dusts by hand from a flour sack held over plants, or a hand operated sprayer, or an implement mule drawn"*, which, of course, ensured that the application was limited to a smaller area.

"But in the new era of farming…more and more farmers, especially the wealthier ones who lived in town and cultivated their hundreds of acres from afar, treated their fields using aerial crop dusters and sprayers. With any breeze blowing, the sprays and dusts blew into small farmers' homes and onto their vegetables, pastures, chicken yards, and laundry lines" [160].

Front-page articles extolled the benefits of DDT, for use on livestock, around the garden and in the home [161].

DDT was sprayed on children's hair, and inside their clothing, to control head-lice and ticks [162].

Incredible as it sounds, DDT was even used in the fight against polio. Take the polio outbreak in San Angelo, Texas, in 1949: *"Since poliovirus was often found in human feces and on the legs of houseflies, Dr R.E. Elvins, the city health officer, called for a heavy spraying of DDT, singling out the open pit toilets on the "Latin American" and "Negro" side of town….. Blaming the epidemic on the "wetbacks" who migrated north each year, monitoring the health of migrant workers become the target…"*

"San Angelo bought two fogging machines to bathe the city in DDT. Twice each day, flatbed trucks would rumble through the streets, spraying the chemical from large hoses while children danced innocently in the mist that trailed behind. As a goodwill gesture, the local Sherwin-Williams store provided

DDT at no cost, urging customers to drench the walls and furniture in their homes. ("Bring your own container!" it said.) One hardware store advertised it's own brand of insecticide - "Queen City Kill...Five times more powerful than DDT". Another promised an even stronger concoction, called "Super Activated Bug Juice".

"By mid-June more than half of San Angelo's 160 hospital beds were filled by polio patients, almost all of them children under 15" [163].

An estimated 1.34 billion tonnes of DDT were sprayed in America, between 1946 and 1962 [162].

A further link between polio and pesticides was added, when researchers discovered that poliomyelitis symptoms occurred in the presence of increased porphyrins excreted in the urine [164]. Today we know that excessive excretion of porphyrins is an indicator of organochlorine (eg DDT) exposure [165], and is also used as an early indicator of arsenic poisoning [166].

(On an interesting side-note, porphyrin levels are also increased in children with autism, suggesting an environmental/toxicity cause [167]).

Nevertheless, the viral cause of poliomyelitis was still being enthusiastically pursued (by those racing to create the first vaccine, at least), but there were puzzling anomalies that still didn't seem to fit.

Albert Sabin, in an article published by the Journal of the American Medical Association, wrote *"No circumstance in the history of poliomyelitis is so baffling as its change during the past 50 years from a sporadic to an epidemic disease"* and *"Intimate human contact....does not by itself explain the recurrent summer epidemics of paralysis....With the present high incidence of the disease among children of school age in the United States, it is remarkable that, unlike certain other infections of childhood, the epidemics of paralysis occur during the very months when the children are away from school"* [168].

Sabin also pondered why American troops stationed abroad in China, Phillipines, and Japan were suffering polio outbreaks and paralysis, while there were no outbreaks of the sort, amongst the surrounding native populations.

Perhaps Sabin was unaware of the military spraying program, to control dengue fever in the military bases. In 1945, there was a large outbreak of polio among American troops in the Philippines that affected 246 personnel, with 52 deaths. Earlier that year, the military had set up 'malaria units' in each base in the Philippines, with intensive area spraying of DDT [169].

3) Changes in Reporting

Prior to 1945, non-paralytic cases of polio were generally not included in official polio reporting, but were included thereafter. This virtually doubled the number of cases reported [170], which worked in favour of the National Foundation for Infantile Paralysis, who were relentless in their fundraising efforts...

For those who didn't live through the polio years, it is difficult to appreciate the terror that gripped America during the early part of the 20th century – perhaps the more so because none if the tried and trusted remedies for other illnesses seemed to have any effect on polio. It affected mostly middle-class or affluent families, and often struck down seemingly healthy children overnight [171], (perhaps the families most able to afford indoor pesticides, DDT-coated wallpapers, and the like?).

During outbreaks, swimming pools, movie theatres and youth camps closed. Libraries disinfected their collections, homes were 'treated' and windows sealed up, in a seemingly futile effort to stop the spread.

The panic was cleverly exacerbated by a very powerful propaganda strategy, co-ordinated by the National Foundation for Infantile Paralysis (later to become March of Dimes).

Dramatic images of crippled children, and blaring headlines following every small breakthrough in the race for a vaccine, were broadcast in national and local newspapers. Volunteers went door-to-door to collect funds [172].

TV presenters urged people to mail in their dimes to the nearest NFIP headquarters. The fundraising effort was hugely successful, and netted hundreds of thousands of dollars – more than all other US charities combined, excluding the Red Cross [173].

At the time, one dime could buy a quart of milk, a hot dog, or a copy of Esquire magazine [174].

The spotlight on polio made many doctors uneasy, and they questioned why polio was given so much attention, when much more serious killers were virtually ignored. For example, in 1952, considered the worst outbreak of polio, there were just over 3000 deaths from polio, but 34,000 deaths from tuberculosis [175].

"In truth, polio was never the raging epidemic portrayed in the media, not even at its height in the 1940s and 1950s. Ten times as many children would die in accidents in those years, and three times as many would die of cancer. Polio's special status was due, in large part, to the efforts of the National Foundation for Infantile Paralysis, better known as the March of Dimes, which employed the latest techniques in advertising, fund raising and motivational research to turn a horrific but relatively uncommon disease in to the most feared affliction of its time" [173].

In 1953, before the vaccine was even available, the Foundation co-opted both the Red Cross and PTA (National Parent Teacher Association) to plan an *"educational campaign for prevention of polio"*, (preparing children to accept the new vaccine when it later came out) and later in 1957, the PTA was awarded a plaque from the Foundation, for *"unprecedented participation in historic development of a preventive measure against paralytic polio and for outstanding volunteer leadership in achieving record acceptance of the Salk vaccine"* [176]. (The vaccine trials were carried out through schools).

On an interesting side-note, 1953 was the same year a Dr Henry Kumm was appointed Director of Research at the National Foundation for Infantile Paralysis. He had previously worked at the Rockefeller Foundation for Medical Research, and during World War II, served as a civilian consultant to the Surgeon General - directing field studies on the use of DDT to control malarial mosquitos in Italy [177].

It wasn't just the National Foundation for Infantile Paralysis that had an inordinate amount of influence over polio research, and public relations. The Rockefeller Foundation during those years was the front-runner in virology research, and dominated science in America.

We've already noted that Simon Flexner worked at the Rockefeller Foundation. Karl Landsteiner accepted an invitation from him, some years after he 'proved' that polio has a viral cause, and went to work at the Rockefeller Foundation.

Henry Kumm also worked at Rockefeller Foundation, before moving to the National Foundation for Infantile Paralysis.

But they are not the only connections.

Thomas Francis, who also worked for Rockefeller Foundation, helped establish the School of Health at the University of Michigan, and mentored Jonas Salk, teaching him how to formulate vaccines. Thomas Francis was later placed in charge of determining whether his student Salk's vaccine was safe and effective – a blatant conflict of interest, by today's standards [178].

Albert Sabin, who would later develop the oral polio vaccine, worked for the Rockefeller Foundation during the 1930's. Both Salk and Sabin were members of the National Foundation for Infantile Paralysis Committee on Virus Research.

The field trials for the new Salk vaccine, in 1954, involving 1.8 million school-children, are lauded as the 'largest clinical trial in history', and required 300,000 volunteers to carry it out [179]. The National Foundation for Infantile Paralysis funded the field trials from public donations, to the tune of $7.5 million ($66.3 million in today's money) [180].

As already noted, Salk's mentor Thomas Francis not only designed the trials, but was given the responsibility of evaluating and reporting the results. There was some criticism of how the studies were designed, and some pointed out that only those who received two shots were considered 'vaccinated'. This meant that a child diagnosed with polio after receiving one vaccine, was considered to be 'unvaccinated' [181].

Every child who took part in the trial was awarded a 'Polio Pioneer' certificate and presented with a highly-treasured metal pin [180].

Because of the perceived urgency of finding a vaccine for polio, the Salk vaccine was rushed to market in just 6yrs [182]. (The average time-frame to bring a new vaccine to market is 10 − 15 years [183]).

On April 12th 1955 (the 10th anniversary of Franklin Roosevelt's death), the results of the field trials were announced to a captivated audience...

"(Thomas) Francis announced his findings at Rackham Auditorium (University of Michigan) after months of anticipation from the press and medical community. A crowd of close to 500 was present, and 16 cameras lined the back, some broadcasting on closed-circuit to 54,000 physicians watching in movie theaters across the country. The world was listening when Francis declared the vaccine "safe, effective, and potent" [184].

An expectant public waited anxiously for the news – court hearings were halted, department stores set up speakers, and folks at home sat anxiously by their radios. The news quickly went out via radio and television, and a jubilant public went wild with delight. Fire brigade sirens sounded their horns, church bells rang across the nation, while people danced and celebrated in the streets [185].

Just two hours later, the vaccine was licensed by the licensing committee (who had not even read all the information contained in the Francis Report - of which the final version was not published until two years later), and approved by the Secretary of Health, Education and Welfare, Oveta Culp Hobby.

The first vaccine lots were released immediately, and within two weeks, more than 10 million doses had been distributed throughout America, almost all for use in school-children [186-187].

Salk became an overnight hero.

In the minds of the American public, polio was all but defeated...

Eleven days later, a little girl named Susan Pierce, who had received the new Salk vaccine less than a week earlier, "*developed fever and neck stiffness. Six days later, her left arm was paralyzed. Seven days later, she was placed in an iron lung, and nine days later, she was dead*" *[187]*. On April 26, six cases of paralysis following vaccination were reported.

That was just the start of the tragedy that would unfold – now known as the 'Cutter Incident'. It was blamed on Cutter Laboratories failure to fully inactivate the live virus (although a court trial would later exonerate Cutter from any negligence [187]).

The truth was...other laboratories were having the same problems, but only Cutter vaccines were withdrawn, while Salk vaccines produced by other suppliers were still distributed [188].

The children affected were more likely to be paralyzed in their arms, more likely to suffer severe and permanent paralysis, more likely to require breathing assistance in iron lungs, and more likely to die than children naturally infected with polio. Seventy-five percent of victims were left paralyzed for life [187].

While Jonas Salk had been team leader during development of the vaccine, Dr Bernice Eddy was vaccine safety tester. When she realized that the vaccine was causing paralysis in monkeys, she went to her superiors, and urged them to delay the release of the vaccine. She was ignored [187].

Congressman Percy Priest of Tennessee, who chaired an investigation into the tragedy, later admitted: "... *in the previous year (1955) many responsible persons had felt that the public should be spared the ordeal of 'knowledge about controversy.' If word ever got out that the Public Health Service had actually done something damaging to the health of the American people, the consequences would be terrible... We felt that no lasting good could come to science or the public if the Public Health Services were discredited*" [189].

The full extent of the tragedy we may never know, as vaccinated individuals who suffered from paralysis were subjected to more stringent validation criteria than unvaccinated cases, and 'poliomyelitis reporting officers' were warned to be 'extremely cautious' about diagnosing polio in vaccinees [190].

While the tragedy was quietly unfolding, "*promotion of the vaccine continued unabated with mass media daily reiterations*". President Eisenhower went on national TV, to reassure the public that the vaccines remaining on the market were "absolutely safe" [190].

Herbert Ratner, who was an outspoken critic of the Salk vaccine, put his career as public health officer in Oak Park, Illinois, in jeopardy when he delayed introduction of the new vaccine. This was to hold public information sessions for parents, in the interest of informed consent.

Ratner noted that "*during these very rocky months and years, very few medical scientists felt they were in a position to publicly disagree, since virtually all virologists in the field of polio virus research were dependent on the NFIP (National Foundation for Infantile Paralysis) for their research grants. In general they had to be beholden to NFIP policies. Those working for the USPHS (United States Public Health Service) were also under comparable restraints*" [190].

On May 7th, vaccination was suspended, by US Surgeon General Leonard Scheele.

James Shannon, then associate director of the National Institute of Health, recalls the stormy meeting that led to the suspension: "*O'Connor (Basil O'Connor – head of the National Foundation for Infantile Paralysis) and the polio group in general disallowed any possibility of induced infections [as a result of the vaccine]. ... So Basil O'Connor stormed out with dire warning of what he was going to do to the NIH and the Public Health Service. Further vaccination was stopped. I had many sleepless nights"* [191].

That ban was lifted several weeks later, on May 27th, with reassurances of increased safety, and extra manufacturing steps and control measures put into place [190].

The Times Magazine placed the blame firmly on the National Foundation for Infantile Paralysis: *"In retrospect, a good deal of the blame for the vaccine snafu also went to the National foundation (for Infantile Paralysis), which, with years of publicity, had built up the danger of polio out of all proportion to its actual incidence, and had rushed into vaccinations this year with patently insufficient preparation"* [192].

The great celebration and euphoria that followed the April 12th announcement had cooled markedly, and by late 1956, unused vaccine lots had begun to accumulate.

The situation called for a fresh publicity campaign...and who better to spearhead it than a 21-year-old Elvis Presley, whose star was on the rise, after releasing the billboard hit, Heartbreak Hotel.

Before a scheduled appearance on the Ed Sullivan Show, in October 1956, Presley was filmed being vaccinated for polio, in the CBS studio. The resulting pictures were splashed across the nation's newspapers [193].

It was part of a push to increase vaccination rates amongst teenagers. Aided and abetted by the National Foundation for Infantile Paralysis, a group called 'Teens Against Polio' was formed. Teenage volunteers canvassed door to door, and "*set up dances where only vaccinated individuals could get in*" [193].

In the early 1960's, the Salk vaccine was phased out and replaced by Albert Sabin's oral polio vaccine – which proved to be cheaper and more convenient. Sabin's oral vaccine was vastly more preferred by children, being administered originally in a sugary syrup, and later, via a sugar cube – much more pleasant than a series of injections [194].

Sabin had discovered poliovirus lived in the human gut, and believed an oral vaccine would mimic the natural route of infection, and create a more long-lasting immunity.

Hilary Koprowski, from Lederle Laboratories, had previously worked on developing an oral polio vaccine, passaged through the brains of cotton rats. Koprowski and his technician allegedly drank a suspension of cotton rat brain, in order to test for obvious toxicity, before going on to test the oral vaccine on 20 children housed at a New York state facility for intellectually-disabled and epileptic children [195].

After also testing on himself and research colleagues, Sabin's oral vaccine was then given to inmates at Chillicothe Prison [194].

Sabin's oral polio vaccine was then tested on millions of school-children in the USSR during 1959 – an unusual feat during the Cold War years [196].

Paralysis was also noted in some cases following oral polio vaccination (the very criticism that Sabin had levelled at Salk's injectable vaccine – in fact, Sabin had called it "pure kitchen chemistry" [194]). However, it should be noted that oral polio vaccines, at the time, were administered to children together with the (mercury-containing) DTP vaccine [197], that had already been shown, years before, to cause 'provocation polio' in some cases.

Since then, the polio vaccine has again been linked to cases of paralysis – but they are no longer diagnosed as polio. They are diagnosed as Guillain-Barre Syndrome [198], acute flaccid paralysis [199], transverse myelitis [200], or acute disseminated encephalomyelitis (ADEM) [201].

What can I say, the true polio story is stranger than fiction? There are several other issues that also need to be mentioned:

Polio was eradicated - with the stroke of a pen?

According to Herbert Ratner, former director of public health in Oak Park, Illinois, the National Foundation for Infantile Paralysis was so desperate to inflate polio statistics (before a vaccine was available), in order to keep the funds rolling in, that they were paying doctors for every reported case of paralytic polio [202].

In 1954, the first polio vaccination campaign began. Coincidentally (or perhaps not), that same year the U.S government authorities changed the diagnostic criteria for paralytic poliomyelitis [202]. Prior to 1954, a diagnosis of paralytic polio was given for paralytic symptoms lasting 24hrs or more – no laboratory confirmation required.

As per the new classification, the patient had to exhibit paralytic symptoms for *at least 60 days* after onset of disease. This one change immediately ruled out more than 50% of paralytic polio cases [203].

In the years following the introduction of the vaccine, further changes were made to the diagnostic parameters of disease, which included analysis of cerebrospinal fluid and stool testing, along with 'expert analysis' [204].

Another administrative change also helped to give the illusion that the polio vaccine had put an end to polio epidemics – by changing the definition of 'epidemic'.

As summed up by the Ratner Report, the transcript of a 1960 panel meeting, later published in the Illinois Medical Journal: "*Presently [1960], a community is considered to have an epidemic when it has 35 cases of polio per year per 100,000 population. Prior to the introduction of the Salk vaccine the National Foundation defined an epidemic as 20 or more cases of polio per year per 100,000 population. On this basis there were many epidemics throughout the United States yearly. The present higher rate has resulted in not a real, but a semantic elimination of epidemics*" [205].

As Ratner pointed out, these changes completely erased many epidemics: "*The game of the NFIP (National Foundation for Infantile Paralysis) was to maximise the disease in the pre-vaccine era, and following its introduction, to minimise the disease in the post-vaccine era. The former definition helped raise funds, the latter helped portray success"* [206].

"Again through press conferences and releases and an acqui-escent press, the public, including physicians, were gulled into believing that the emergency vaccination program had stopped the epidemic" [206].

The vaccine caused polio.

As previously discussed, provocation polio came to the attention of medical men, in the early part of the 20th century. In recent years, though, health authorities have been reporting a different trend – one they've labelled Vaccine-Associated Paralytic Polio.

According to the CDC, from 1980 to 1994, 133 cases of paralytic poliomyelitis were reported in the US, and of those, 125 were 'vaccine-associated paralytic poliomyelitis' (VAPP) [207].

Although wild poliovirus has been declared eradicated in many parts of the world, there have been at least eight outbreaks of vaccine-associated paralytic poliomyelitis (VAPP). Researchers estimate these outbreaks have likely affected hundreds of thousands of people, if not millions [208].

The discovery of Coxsackie Virus.

In 1948-1949, Gilbert Dalldorf, a laboratory director, and his associate Grace Sickles 'isolated' coxsackie virus from the stool samples of two children *"with signs of paralytic poliomyelitis"* [209-211].

Coxsackie virus is also said to cause limb paralysis, or weakness, that mimics wild poliovirus infections. In 1991, a study reported on 44 African children with singular, or multiple, limb paralysis. Seven of them required assisted ventilation, and of those, six died.

Sounds remarkably like polio, but they were diagnosed with cocksackievirus [212].

During a 'polio' epidemic in Michigan, in 1958, fecal specimens from 869 patients showed no evidence of virus in 401 cases, poliovirus in 292, enteric cytopathogenic human orphan virus (ECHO) in 100, Coxsackie virus in 73, and unidentified virus in 3 cases. So, in this particular outbreak of 'polio', only about a third tested positive for poliovirus [213].

In 2000, the CDC reported an outbreak of poliomyelitis in Dominican Republic and Haiti, however, out of 19 cases, only 6 (less than one-third) tested positive for poliovirus. Predictably enough, the CDC took the opportunity to urge further vaccinations and high vaccination coverage with oral polio vaccine, as the solution [214].

Tonsillectomy made people more susceptible to bulbar poliomyelitis - the most severe kind.

Even in the 1940's, it was known that people who previously had their tonsils removed, were more susceptible to the most severe type of polio [215]. Studies found that the bulbar type was 3-4 times more prevalent amongst people who had previously had their tonsils removed [216].

That was a problem – given that between 1915 and 1960, ton-sillectomy was the most common surgical procedure in America, (despite dubious evidence as to its efficacy in preventing disease, or a proper understanding of the role of tonsils) [217].

Wealthy philanthropists donated large amounts of money to ensure poor children had their tonsils removed – whether the tonsils were causing problems, or not. They even built a dedicated Tonsil Hospital for this very noble cause [218].

By the late 1940's, health authorities were cautioning doctors not to perform tonsillectomies during polio epidemics [219], but their popularity did not begin to decline for at least another decade.

Poliomyelitis and Dietary/Nutrition Factors

In 1951 – at the height of the polio epidemics – a medical doctor named Benjamin Sandler, announced that diet and nutrition played a role in polio. Most notably, he found that high sugar and high starch intake made one more susceptible to polio [220].

When his work was announced through local media, with the public urged to avoid sugary drinks, ice-cream, lollies, cakes, pastries etc, an ongoing polio outbreak began to subside, with the total cases far below what was expected.

It is ironic to note that the standard diet given to children following tonsillectomies was ice-cream…and then more ice-cream. It is also ironic, that Albert Sabin's oral polio vaccine was administered via sugary syrup, or sugar cube, in the early days.

High sugar intake affects Vitamin C status, too – but that wasn't known until later...

It was not until the 1970's that Professor John Ely proposed his 'Glucose-Ascorbate Antagonism' Theory, after his research revealed that blood glucose (sugar) levels compete with Vitamin C, and high blood sugar levels hinder the entry of Vitamin C into the cells [221].

And why does that matter?

Claus Jungeblut, who was a prominent polio researcher in his time, reported in 1935 that Vitamin C was not only a preventative, but a cure for polio [222]. (He would later show that large doses of Vitamin C could also inactivate both diptheria and tetanus toxins too [223-224]).

Albert Sabin then attempted to 'confirm' Jungeblut's findings on polio, but only used about 35% of the dose that Jungeblut had used, and did not follow Jungeblut's methods precisely. When this failed to show a protective effect, he concluded that Vitamin C was not effective against polio after all – and, unfortunately, his conclusion seemed to be accepted as final, by the medical establishment of the time [225-226].

Fred Klenner, an American physician, used high-dose Vitamin C to treat 60 polio patients, during a 1948 epidemic, and though two patients suffering 'bulbar' polio needed oxygen and drainage, all patients recovered [227].

While early researchers focused on the Vitamin C's ability to neutralize poliovirus, we also now know that Vitamin C is a powerful antitoxin, demonstrated to neutralize poisons from both natural causes (venomous snakes etc) [228], chemicals (such as benzene), and heavy metals, including mercury, arsenic and lead [229-230].

Meanwhile, some astute doctors began to note the similarities between polio and beriberi (severe thiamine – or B1 – deficiency, a condition once believed to be 'contagious').

Dr Fred Klenner (mentioned above for his work in pioneering Vitamin C mega-dose therapy), analysed the findings of Dr. William McCormick (another early Vitamin C pioneer), who attended 50 cases of polio in Toronto (1949). Klenner found that many patients who ate white bread developed paralysis, while none of those who ate brown bread developed paralysis. Klenner noted that "*brown bread has 28 times more vitamin B₁ than does white bread*" [231].

Thiamine is a water-soluble vitamin, and only obtained through the diet, so we need regular intake. High sugar diets reduce thiamine levels, which links to Dr Sandler's observations on sugar intake and polio.

It is interesting to note that agricultural authorities agree that 'polio' in animals, is most often caused by thiamine deficiency, and affects mostly the young. It is more common amongst animals fed a high-grain diet [232].

Indeed, a 1992 Merck Manual describes the symptoms of thiamine deficiency as: "*The most advanced neural changes occur* *in the peripheral nerves, particularly of the legs. The distal segments are characteristically affected earliest and most severely. Degeneration of the medullary sheath has been demonstrated in all tracts of the cord, especially in the <u>anterior horn</u> (my emphasis) and posterior ganglion cells. Lesions of hemorrhagic polioencephalitis occur in the brain when deficiency is severe"* [233].

In addition to sugar intake and thiamine deficiency being linked to polio, Canadian doctor J.F. Edwards reported success by treating polio patients with iodine, after noting that polio-endemic areas in Canada coincided with areas known for goiter (severe iodine deficiency) [234].

"I treated in 1952 three Bulbar polio (the most severe form of polio) patients with intravenous sodium iodide. In these three, control of the disease was found to be most rapid, and convalescence was surprisingly brief"

And again in 1953 *"The season finally ended. I had seen some sixty cases. Two were sent to King George Municipal Hospital because of the possibility of respiratory difficulties and lack of nursing care. The remainder were treated at home. Only one on home care developed paralysis—a paralysis that did not advance after oral iodide administration. None of 200 contacts on prophylactic therapy developed polio. There were no deaths."*

Edwards went on to detail the use of iodine by other physicians, from as early as 1825, to treat 'palsies' (paralysis):

"Manson, of England (1825), advocated its use in palsies,

many of which cases must have been polio.

Coplan (1850) reports benefits in palsy derived from potassium iodide in dosages as small as 1 grain in 24 hours.

Brown-Sequard (1861) recommended potassium iodide as the only known remedy that could be used without danger for various forms of paraplegia.

Webber (1885) recommended [potassium iodide] use in polio.

Sir Thomas Horder (1927) reported the use of colloidal iodine intravenously in the treatment of poliomyelitis. He recommended its early use.

Breuil and Dartiguenave (1937), after trial with chemotherapy failed for polio, reported improvement using iodine therapy.

Maberly (1939) reported complete recovery of four cases of polio on iodine therapy."

He noted that veterinarians had also used iodine to successfully treat paralysis in animals [234].

Improper treatment of poliomyelitis made the disease worse.

Much like early smallpox treatments, some of the early treatments for poliomyelitis were cruel and barbaric, and must surely have added, not only to the dread of this disease, but the high mortality rate. Because nobody, at the time, seemed to know what caused the disease and how to treat it, all kinds of dubious methods were trialled.

These included:

- Radium water [235] - after radium was discovered in 1898, it quickly gained popularity, proclaimed as a 'cure-all' elixir that could make one young again, and cure all kinds of ills and ails.

- Tendon cutting and transplantation [236].

- Lumbar punctures, which by itself can cause or exacerbate paralysis, and may also precede respiratory problems. For example, ten patients with clinical signs of polio, but no paralysis, were given lumbar punctures, and within 12-48hrs, all had developed paralysis, and seven had breathing problems. It was also shown that if experimental polio could not be induced in monkeys via injection of poliovirus, then lumbar puncture could significantly increase the odds of inducing paralysis [237].

- Intramuscular injections of strychnine (which can cause paralysis, and nerve damage – if it doesn't kill you first) [237].

- Intraspinal injections of adrenaline (almost half of the recipients died), human serum, or quinine and urea hydrochloride (3 of 6 children given this mixture orally and intramuscularly died) [237]. Even intraspinal injections of horse serum were tried.

  - Injections of tetanus antitoxin – the rationale being that *"tetanus, rabies and poliomyelitis all attacked nerve cells, so perhaps giving the antitoxin would block access to absorption sites on the cells".* Even injections of diphtheria antitoxin were tried, with 3 out of 5 patients dying [237].

- Prolonged splinting - for 3-6mths, but often up to two years [236]. In 1943, researchers demonstrated that completely immobolising an animal's limb resulted in apparent paralysis, even though the motor and sensory nerve pathways were still intact [238]. In other words, the medical practices at the time likely contributed to the rate of permanent disability, otherwise blamed on poliovirus.

- Painful electrical treatments [236].

- Surgical Straightening - Dr. John Pohl, in an interview circa 1940, said *"We'd take the children to the operating room in those days, straighten them out under anaesthetic, and put them in plaster casts. When they woke up, they screamed. The next day they still cried from the pain. That was the accepted and universal treatment virtually all over the world. I saw it in Boston and New York City and London"* [239].

Even laypeople had their 'cures' and remedies. During the deadly 1916 epidemic, the New York Times reported that one Joseph Frooks had been charged with selling 'Infantile Disease Protector', which, upon investigation, was found to contain "a mixture of wood shavings" that were saturated in a mixture smelling remarkably like naphthalene [240].

The first 'iron lung' was unveiled in Boston (Massachusetts, again!) in 1928, known as a 'Drinker Machine' (named after its inventor, Philip Drinker).

These machines helped those with paralysed chest muscles to breath, so they did save or prolong many lives, but they were large, noisy, expensive machines, costing about $1500 – the same price as the average home, at that time [241].

Some patients were dependent upon 'Iron Lungs' for decades – a Mr Barton Hebert from Louisiana was in an iron lung from the late 1950's, until his death in 2003 [242].

An Australian nurse, Elizabeth Kenny had success treating polio with hot packs and physical therapy, but the medical establishment was reluctant to adopt her methods [243].

Meanwhile, it has become abundantly clear that eliminating wild poliovirus from the world, will not eliminate paralysis from the world.

In 2012, Jacob Puliyel, head of Paediatrics at St. Stevens Hospital in Delhi, India, showed that, while India had been 'polio-free' for a year, there were an extra 47,500 cases of non-polio acute flaccid paralysis (NPAFP) – *"clinically indistinguishable from polio paralysis but twice as deadly, the incidence of NFAFP was directly proportional to doses of oral polio received"* [244].

In late 2018, the CDC announced that 62 confirmed cases of 'acute flaccid paralysis' spanning 22 states, had been reported, with a total of 386 confirmed cases since 2014.

The symptoms were reported to *"start with what looks like a respiratory illness, a little bit of a fever. The hallmark is sudden onset of weakness in the arms or the legs. Children can also have trouble swallowing, trouble with their speech, facial droop, trouble with their eye muscles."*

"The scariest and most severe symptom is when the disease affects the diaphragm, the muscle that helps us breathe".

"That's when children can really deteriorate and end up on a ventilator" [245]. These are the very symptoms once attributed to poliomyelitis, except the patient ended up in an iron lung.

So...the multi-billion-dollar question. Did vaccines really eradicate killer diseases – smallpox, polio or any of the other numerous diseases we now have vaccines for?

Although vaccines are often given the credit, the historical evidence for such claims are hard to find. Although it *is* true that the decrease in mortality over the past two centuries is mostly due to decline in infectious diseases - about 86% can be attributed to decline in infection, according to British physician, epidemiologist, and medical historian, Thomas McKeown.

What is not so clear-cut, however, is what exactly caused the decline, or lessening in severity, of infectious diseases?

Overall, crude death rates from infectious diseases had fallen by roughly three quarters from 1900 to the 1940's, when penicillin was discovered, and widespread vaccination for diphtheria and pertussis, began (with polio vaccinations starting the following decade) [246].

Respiratory tuberculosis accounted for approximately 17% of the fall in mortality rates in England and Wales between 1848 – 1971, more than half of the improvement occurred in the 19th century, long before vaccination began [247].

McKinley and McKinley (1977) examined the decline of ten major infectious diseases and concluded:

"In general, medical measures (both chemotherapeutic and prophylactic) appear to have contributed little to the overall decline in mortality in the United States since about 1900 – having in many instances been introduced several decades after a marked decline had already set in and mostly having no detectible influence."

"More specifically, with reference to those five conditions (influenza, pneumonia, diphtheria, whooping cough and poliomyelitis) for which the decline appears substantial after the point of intervention – and in the unlikely assumption that all of this decline is attributable to the intervention – it is estimated that at most 3.5 per cent of the total decline in mortality since 1900 could be ascribed to medical measures introduced for the diseases considered here" [248].

Indeed, United States Vital Statistics 1940-1960, show that between 1900 to 1940 [249]:

- Pneumonia and influenza mortality fell by more than half.
- Tuberculosis mortality fell by approximately two-thirds
- Diarrhoea, enteritis and ulceration of the intestine fell by more than two-thirds, to disappear off the list of Top 10

    leading causes of death.
- Diphtheria mortality fell by more than half, to also disappear off the list of Top 10 leading causes of death.

All before antibiotics and widespread vaccination were introduced...

3.
VACCINE
PRODUCTION

Although many websites claim to explain how vaccines are made, they only provide a very basic, benign version. After countless hours of searching and reading, I managed to piece together how vaccines are really made. For a viral vaccine, it goes something like this:

1) First, you need to isolate the virus in question. To do this, collect the mucus or urine of someone suspected of having the disease [1]. Or, if you were Jonas Salk or Albert Sabin, inventors of first polio vaccines, you collected the faeces of people suspected of having polio [2]. Refrigerate.

2) Next, prepare a separate culture of monkey cells, or mashed chicken embryo cells - by adding chemicals to make them mutate and turn cancerous [3].

3) Now, arrange these cells, single layer, into a lab vessel, and add a digestive enzyme called Trypsin. Take care to use gloves and splash goggles, because pure trypsin is toxic [4].

4) Next, add a nutrient broth, and sugar, to the cells and allow them to marinate for a few days [5].

5) Now take your original specimen (of mucus, urine, faeces) which has also been marinating in the fridge, and
add to the monkey/chicken cells, then place in a warm
incubation chamber.

6) After one hour, inspect the mixture with a microscope,
and if 50% of the cells are now distorted, you can claim
success! Scrape the cells into a growth medium, such as
the blood of an unborn cow (fetal bovine serum [6]),
store at -70C and you now have a 'pure isolate' with
which to make a vaccine!

7) Next, you take cells that have a) descended from a human fetus that was aborted 60 years ago, whose cells
have been kept alive artificially, and replicating ever
since [7], or b) cells that have descended from the kidneys of an African green monkey, and kept alive artificially, and replicating ever since [8], or c) cells from a
cocker-spaniel that were harvested in 1958, and have not
only been kept alive and replicating ever since, but have
been turned cancerous [9], and then infect these cells
with the virus 'isolate'. Give it some time, so all the cells
can get infected [10]. Collect the fluid (cellular waste
products) that runs out while the virus is 'replicating' in
the large tank of cell cultures, and pass it through a sieve
and separator [10].

8) Add some benzonase, which is a genetically engineered
endonuclease produced in e.Coli, which attacks and de-
grades DNA and RNA [11] (to deal with any DNA fragments that may be still floating around).

9) Next, add formaldehyde to 'inactivate' it.

10) Now, time to filter and concentrate it, via ultracentifugion, which spins the fluid at super high speed, to separate tiny particles from larger particles [12].

11) Add some more benzonase to digest any leftover monkey/human DNA fragments that remain. Obviously, this process is not fool-proof, since DNA fragments are still found in the finished product [13].

12) Add some more chemicals to your now 'pure, concentrated product':

-   Stabilisers, such as albumin from the blood of other humans (to be phased out in 2019) [14], or produced by yeast cells that have had the gene for human albumin inserted into them [15].
-   Emulsifiers, such as Polysorbate 80, to stop the vaccine contents from separating [14].
-   Acidity regulators, such as borax (sodium borate), to maintain pH balance [14].
-   Adjuvants, such as aluminium, to stimulate the immune system [14].

13) Your product is now ready to be added to vials, and distributed.

If you're making an egg-based vaccine, such as the influenza vaccine, the process is slightly different. Instead of adding the virus 'isolate' to a cell culture, you inject it into fertilised eggs and let the chicken embryo 'manufacture' the virus for you.

After a few days, a machine slices the tops off the eggs and the contents are removed, mashed up and spun and filtered, and then the manufacturing process continues.

It takes approximately one egg to make one vaccine, so that equals around 500 million eggs used every year, to manufacture flu vaccines [16].

Egg-based vaccines take about 4 months to make one batch of vaccines [17], which is obviously time-consuming - and probably why manufacturers are looking for different methods of manufacturing...

Now, you may be thinking that, surely, today's modern vaccines are not so crudely made? You're almost right! Although vaccine manufacturing facilities today are high-tech, stainless steel and sanitised, a number of vaccines are still made as described above. But newer vaccines, such as the Hepatitis and HPV vaccines are made somewhat differently.

They don't use a virus, they take certain 'key molecules', said to come from the pathogen in question, and then insert them into an insect or yeast culture, to reproduce the desired quantities.

As you can imagine, a few 'key molecules' don't create much of an immune reaction, which is why adjuvants, such as aluminium hydroxide are required.

Now, let's take a closer look at some of the individual components of vaccine manufacturing:

HUMAN CELL LINES

Some viral vaccines are produced through the use of human cell lines, in order to cultivate sufficient quantities of the virus. These cell lines were procured from aborted fetuses.

There are currently two cell lines used in production of widely-available vaccines, although there are others being used in experimental vaccines, and those still in development stages. The two cell-lines most commonly used are WI-38 (Wistar Institute 38) and MRC-5 (Medical Research Council 5) [18-19].

WI-38 was developed from the lung tissue of a 3-month-old female fetus, in 1962 [20]. The reason given for abortion was that the parents felt they already had too many children [19].

MRC-5 was developed in 1966, from lung tissue of a 14-week male fetus, aborted for 'psychiatric reasons' [21].

The term 'psychiatric reasons' raises some interesting questions, as women who were deemed to be 'feeble-minded' were still coerced into being permanently sterilised in the 1960's, when the MRC-5 abortion took place.

Forced sterilization had become legal in the US, through state laws in the early 1900's. These laws were encouraged and promoted by the newly-formed Eugenics Record Office, as part of their Master Race Project. Their goal was to stop so-called 'defective parents' from reproducing [22]. Eugenicists saw abortion and sterilization as the answer to preventing 'degenerate babies' [23].

During the first half of the twentieth century, as the race for a polio vaccine intensified, and other medical research demanded tissue cultures, abortion methods were altered, in order to harvest the foetal tissue immediately following abortion.

One such method was a hysterotomy abortion - major abdominal surgery, much like a caesarean section, wherein the foetus is physically removed from the amniotic sac. This procedure was "*only done in special circumstances such as when sterilization is required in addition to the termination of pregnancy, as in the case of cardiac disease, diabetes, TB or **mental disease***" [24].

It is not known exactly how many aborted fetuses were used to develop the polio vaccine, but at least 80 abortions were involved in production of the WI-38 cell line, and subsequent rubella vaccine [25]. At least two aborted fetuses were used in the procurement of MRC-5 cell line, but it is likely there were more.

What else is unknown is whether the abortions were performed under duress or coercion or if, in fact, the mothers were even aware of what the foetuses would be used for.

"*Remember that at the time in the early 1960's, when organs from aborted fetuses were sent to the Wistar Institute, no-one had as yet invented the concept of informed consent. I am absolutely convinced that there is no remaining documentation about the fetuses used from the Department of Virus Research at the Karolinska Institute at the time. I was head of this department between 1971 and 1997. Thus in case there is no documentation that allows identification of fetal samples at the*

Wistar Institute, there is no way of tracing them. In fact, I do remember the time well, because we as graduate students made the dissections collecting organs" [26]

In 2012, the FDA noted that *"the current repertoire of cell substrates is inadequate to manufacture the next generation of viral vaccines (i.e., certain viruses cannot be propagated or grow poorly in the available cell lines"* [27]. So, in 2015, a new cell line was procured from a female foetus in China, for the purposes of viral vaccine production [28].

This cell line was taken from a 3-month-old female foetus, aborted due to the "presence of a uterine scar" from a previous C-section, in the healthy, 27-year-old mother [28].

There was public backlash in 2015, over the use of aborted foetal tissue in medical science, after release of undercover footage showing Planned Parenthood officials talking about the prices that aborted baby parts are sold for. Despite public criticism, scientists maintained that aborted foetal tissue was necessary for medical research [29].

There are other cell lines from aborted foetuses that are used in vaccines currently in the development and testing stages - HEK-293 and PER C6.

PER C6 is a tumorigenic cell line taken from an 18-week foetus, aborted because *"the woman wanted to get rid of the fetus, and the father was unknown"* [30].

As per the FDA, *"tumorigenic refers to the ability of neoplastic cells growing in tissue culture to multiply and develop into* tumors when injected into animals" [31].

These cells are called 'designer cells', because they were known to be normal originally, but were then purposely transformed into immortal cell lines (so they replicate indefinitely), via known mechanisms, such as introduction of viral oncogenes. These so-called designer cells are _perceived_ to be safer than cell lines which spontaneously immortalized for unknown reasons [31].

Another cell line currently being used to develop influenza vaccines, is HEK-293, which originally came from the kidneys of an aborted baby [32].

At a meeting of the FDA Vaccines and Related Biological Products Advisory Committee in 2001, Dr. Alex van der Eb, who was involved in the production of HEK-293, is quoted as saying [33]:

"So the kidney material, the fetal kidney material was as follows: the kidney of the fetus was, with an unknown family history, obtained in 1972 probably. The precise date is not known anymore. The fetus, as far as I can remember was completely normal. Nothing was wrong. The reasons for the abortion were unknown to me. I probably knew it at that time, but it got lost, all this information."

In his work on the ethics of HEK-293, Wong (2006) refers to comments made by Dr C Ward Kischer Ph.D, a leading authority in the field of human embryology [34]: *"From a clinical standpoint, the abortion must be pre-arranged in order to have researchers available to immediately preserve the* *tissue ... . In order to sustain 95% of the cells, the **live tissue** would need to be preserved within 5 minutes of the abortion. Within an hour the cells would continue to deteriorate, rendering the specimens useless."*

What exactly is meant by 'live tissue'?

Dr Gonzalo Herranz, Professor of Histology and General Embryology, at the University of Navarra, Spain, describes how abortions should be performed when foetal tissue is to be harvested [35]:

*"To obtain embryo cells for culture, a programmed abortion must be adopted, choosing the age of the embryo and dissecting it **while still alive** to remove tissues to be placed in culture media".*

Current vaccines which are cultured on fetal cell lines are Adenovirus, DTaP-IPV/Hib (Pentacel), Hep A (Havrix), Hep A/Hep B (Twinrix), Measles-mumps-rubella (MMRII), Measles-mumps-rubella-varicella (ProQuad), Varicella (Varivax) [36].

Not all viral vaccines use fetal cell lines. Some use animal cell lines, with the main ones being:

Vero Cells: originally derived from the kidney epithelial cells of a female African green monkey, extracted in 1962 by Japanese scientists. It has an abnormal number of chromosomes [37-38].

Madin-Darby Canine Kidney Cells (MDCK): These were taken from an apparently healthy female cocker spaniel and established as a cell line in 1958 [39].

HUMAN & ANIMAL DNA IN VACCINES

It is often claimed that while vaccines may be produced using animal and aborted foetal cells, these are all removed before the finished product.

Not so, according to the FDA: "*Small amounts of residual cell substrate DNA unavoidably occur in all viral vaccines, as well as other biologics produced using cell substrates*" [40].

In 1986, a World Health Organization (WHO) Study Group met in Geneva, to discuss issues regarding the use of continuous cell lines in the production of vaccines and other biological products.

It was decided that the limit for DNA fragments (from both human and animal cell lines) in the finished product should be 100 picograms, or less - a value that was "*considered to represent an insignificant risk*" [41].

100pg remained the limit for a decade, however this limit was raised to 10 nanograms per dose (100x more), in 1997, as manufacturers could not always meet the limit [42]. It was also decided that, since several factors must be present for a cell to become cancerous, it was *unlikely* that this foreign DNA could cause cancers in the recipient.

In 2015, research revealed that DNA fragments from aborted

foetal cell lines in at least two vaccines - Meruvax II (live rubella vaccine) and Havrix (live Hepatitis A vaccine) contained both single-stranded and double-stranded DNA [43].

In 1997, the FDA's advisory committee discussed whether residual DNA fragments in vaccines had the ability to integrate into the recipient's DNA. According to FDA documents "*It was decided that it was unlikely that DNA integration occurred at a high enough frequency to be a concern, **although no data were available at the time**" [44]*

Given the fact that their recommendations would affect some 300 million Americans, and likely be accepted, without further ado, by other countries around the world, this laissez-faire attitude seems quite extraordinary.

One person who has tried to find out, is molecular biologist Theresa Deisher, PhD. Her research showed there was "*spontaneous cellular and nuclear DNA uptake'* in host cells, from the DNA fragments found in vaccines [45].

Deisher states there is potential for 'homologous recombination' to occur – where a segment of cell's DNA is substituted by another segment of similar DNA, during cell division or cell repair.

"*Homologous recombination occurs naturally to create genetic diversity in our offspring, and is also conveniently harnessed by scientists to introduce experimental DNA into cells or animals. We do not yet know if this occurs with the contaminating human DNA found in some of our vaccines, and if so, to what extent*" [46].

TUMOUR CELLS

The Vaccines and Related Biological Products Advisory Committee (VRBPAC) is responsible for analysing the safety and efficacy data for vaccines in the US, and making recommendations to the Commissioner of Food and Drugs.

In 2012, a VRBPAC meeting was held to discuss the merits of using three cell lines from human tumours, to produce vaccines: *"cell lines derived from tumors may be the optimal and in some cases the only cell substrate that can be used to propagate certain vaccine viruses"* [47].

The discussion was held because 'sponsors' (vaccine manufacturers) had proposed their use in new vaccines, intended for clinical trials. These 'sponsors' also requested that *"these cells be viewed as representative of this type of cell substrate so that the recommendations of the advisory committee will be applicable to other tumor-derived cell lines"*.

The three cell lines in question were:

 - CEM T-cell line, taken from an individual with leukemia.
 - A549 cell line, taken from the lungs of an individual with adenocarcinoma of the lung.
 - HeLa cells, taken from the cells of a cervical carcinoma in 1952.

HeLa cells are the oldest, and most commonly used, human cells in scientific research. They were taken from Henrietta Lacks, in 1951, without her knowledge or consent. Henrietta was a poor, black woman who worked in the tobacco fields of

Virginia. She died later that same year, leaving behind five young children [48].

Researcher Dr. George Gey could barely believe his luck, when he took her cells into the lab and discovered they didn't die out, like all his previous samples, but proliferated and multiplied uncontrollably [49].

Since then, scientists have grown an estimated 20 tonnes of HeLa cells, and published more than 60,000 articles on research that involved these cells. There are approximately 11,000 patents involving HeLa cells [49].

These cells have been used in a diverse range of research, including the development of the polio vaccine, gene mapping, toxicology and cancer research. Her cells were even sent into outer space [50].

Her children had no idea about the secret life of their dead mother's cells, until researchers contacted them in the 1970's. In a tragic case of irony, their mother's cells continue to rake in millions of dollars for others, while her own descendants continue to struggle in poverty - some can't even afford health insurance [50-51].

Because HeLa cells are so prolific and adaptable, they have managed to contaminate some 10-20% of cell cultures in laboratories around the world, interfering with biological research and invalidating many results [52].

Christopher Korch, a geneticist at University of Colorado, found that some 7000 research papers, that were subsequently cited more than 200,000 times, may have been inadvertently using HeLa cells, due to two other cell lines becoming contaminated. That was only two cell lines – an estimated 400 different cell lines have been either contaminated, or lack evidence of origin [53].

The problem of cell culture contamination has been known for more than 30 years, yet most scientific journals don't require proof that the cell lines have been identity-checked [53].

From the International Cell Line Authentication Committee website [54]:

"Regrettably, cross-contamination and misidentification are still common within the research community. Many cell lines were cross-contaminated during establishment; this means that all work using those cell lines has incorrectly used the contaminant – which may come from a different species or a different tissue".

"A cell line is considered to be misidentified if it no longer corresponds to the individual from whom it was first established. Many cases of misidentification are caused by cross-contamination, where another, faster growing, cell line is introduced into that culture."

Is it possible that HeLa cells have already contaminated vaccine cultures anyway, long before that 2012 VRBPAC meeting?

The consensus at the meeting seemed to be that DNA integration from these cells would be too low to be a concern, or to cause cancer in the recipient. They felt that testing them in animals for "at least four months", then assess any tumours to determine the origin, would be sufficient to determine safety [55].

The A549 cell line is currently being used in vaccine research [56-57].

ADJUVANTS

There are currently more than 30 licensed vaccines that contain ingredients known as 'adjuvants' [58]. The CDC describes the role of adjuvants, as designed to "promote an earlier, *more potent* response, and *more persistent* immune response to the vaccine" [59].

Given what we now know about antibodies, immune activation and immune system skewing, this potent and persistent action of adjuvants must surely come with unwanted side-effects.

The discovery that adding adjuvant increases the immune response happened by accident in the 1920's, when a French veterinarian, by the name of Gaston Ramon, realized that horses had higher levels of antibodies to tetanus and diptheria, if an abscess developed at the vaccine injection site [60.].

He went on to use breadcrumbs, starch or tapioca to induce abscesses at the injection site of inactivated toxin, and was able to prove the theory that substances which could induce inflammation at the injection site caused higher levels of antibodies.

Around the same time, Alexander Glenny, a British immunologist, discovered that aluminium salts enhanced the immune response, and consequently, aluminum adjuvant was first used in human vaccines in 1932. For 70 years, aluminum was the only adjuvant licensed for use in vaccines, despite lack of understanding about its specific mechanism of action [61].

In the past 20 years, another six adjuvants have been licensed for use in vaccines [62]. These are:

a) Virosomes, which are vesicles with antigen enclosed within a phospholipid cell membrane bi-layer. Found in hepatitis and influenza vaccines.

b) AS04, which is 3-deacyl-monophosphoryl lipid A, derived from lipopolysaccharide from salmonella bacteria and aluminum. Found in Hepatitis B and HPV vaccines.

c) MF59, which is made from squalene. Found in seasonal and pandemic influenza vaccines.

d) AS03, which is made from squalene and polysorbate 80. Found in pandemic influenza vaccines.

e) Thermo-reversible oil-in-water, which is also made from squalene. Found in pandemic influenza vaccines.

f) ISA51, which is made from refined mineral oil. Found in a new vaccine targeted at treating non-small-cell lung cancer.

Studies show that the use of adjuvant means the vaccine ingredients stay at the injection site for longer before dispersal. This is deliberate, in order to provoke a greater response from the immune system. The use of adjuvant also more than doubles the exposure of the antigen in serum, and increases uptake by regional lymph nodes by 25-fold. Adjuvant also increases response by the humoral immune system, and leads to higher antibody counts [63].

ALUMINIUM

The most common adjuvant currently in use is aluminium, without which, the antigenic components of the inactivated vaccines fail to provoke an adequate immune response [64].

Surprisingly, despite widespread use for almost 90 years, and injected into millions of children and adults, its precise mechanism of action is not well-understood [64].

Aluminium is a known neurotoxin, with the ability to cross the blood-brain barrier and instigate, or exacerbate, inflammation and excitotoxicity in the brain [65-67].

Chronic activation of inflammatory responses in the brain is recognized as a factor in many neurodegenerative diseases, including autism [68-69], multiple sclerosis [70], and Alzheimer's disease [71].

In fact, the structure and physiology of the brain makes it particularly susceptible to accumulation of aluminium over time. Aluminium is not an essential metal, but it still participates widely in brain biochemistry, and substitutes itself for essential metals in critical biochemical processes, further adding to its toxicity [72].

Another troubling aspect of aluminium is that it belongs to a group of metals known as 'metalloestrogens' - that is, capable of binding to cellular oestrogen receptors and then mimicking the actions of physiological oestrogens [73].

Aluminium is also suspected of playing a role in the development of breast cancer. A 2011 study found that women affected by breast cancer had double the levels of aluminium in nipple aspirate fluid (a fluid present in the breast duct tree that mimics the breast microenvironment) compared to healthy, cancer-free controls [74].

The mechanisms by which aluminium may affect breast cancer risk appears to be multifactorial, with the following factors having been explored in the medical literature:

i)   Aluminium can cause genomic instability and inappropriate proliferation in human breast epithelial cells [75].

ii)   Aluminium can increase migration and invasion of human breast cancer cells [75].

iii)   Aluminium acts as a metalloestrogen, and estrogen is considered a risk factor, known to influence multiple hallmarks of breast cancer [75].

iv)   Aluminium induces DNA damage due to oxidative stress [76].

v)   Aluminium may alter the breast microenvironment by causing disruption to iron metabolism, inflammatory responses, and alterations in motility of cells [77].

Aluminium also appears to have an affinity for the spleen, with studies showing that after dispersal from injection site, it travels to distant organs, including the spleen [78].

Animal experiments suggest that aluminium may exert an inhibitory effect on immune functions of T and B lymphocytes [79]. Other research suggests that aluminium suppresses growth of the spleen, upsets the balance of trace elements, and inhibits immune regulation of cytokines in the spleen [80].

THIMEROSAL

Thimerosal is the trade name for organomercurial compound sodium ethyl-mercury (Hg) thiosalicate, that is 49.55% mercury by weight [81]. It was first introduced in the 1930's by Eli Lilly, as a preservative in vaccines. Coincidentally (or perhaps, not), autism was first described in 1943, in children born in the 1930's, and the rates have increased exponentially over the past few decades [82-84].

In 1982, an expert panel at the Food and Drug Administration (FDA) reported that thimerosal was *"toxic, caused cell damage, was not effective in killing bacteria or halting their replication"* [85].

However, efforts to remove thimerosal from vaccines did not become a priority until 1999, although thimerosal-containing vaccine stocks continued to be used up until late 2002 [86].

A 2001 review by the IOM concluded that, although there was

not enough evidence available to render an opinion on a possible link between autism and thimerosal-containing vaccines, the relationship was a possibility and should be studied further [87]. By 2004, the IOM seemed to have abandoned their previous recommendations [88] – rather puzzling, given how limited our current knowledge of the toxicokinetics of thimerosal.

There have been over 165 studies that looked at thimerosal and found it to be harmful [89]. Of these studies, sixteen specifically examined the effects of thimerosal on human infants and/or children, with reported outcomes including death [90], poisoning [91], malformations [92], allergic reactions [93], autoimmune reactions [94], developmental delays [95-96], neurodevelopmental disorders, such as tics, language delay, attention deficit disorder and autism [97-99].

A review published in 2015, which focused on the clinical, epidemiological and biological studies of adverse effects in developing humans, concluded that thimerosal *"is a poison at minute levels with a plethora of deleterious consequences, even at the levels currently administered in vaccines"* [100].

Indeed, thimerosal has been reported to induce cell death, at levels 100 times lower than that currently found in multi-dose flu vaccines, while also suppressing proliferation of T-cells at minute levels [101].

Neurological and other deleterious effects of thimerosal may not be noticeable immediately, but may manifest several years later [102-103].

During the highly publicised phase-out of thimerosal-containing vaccines from 1999-2002 [104], the CDC actually *added* thimerosal-containing influenza vaccines to the recommended schedule for babies from 6mths old [105-107].

Shortly after this, authorities expanded this recommendation for influenza vaccination to include pregnant women as well [108-109]. This, despite research showing that mercury crosses the placenta and accumulates in the foetus, at greater levels than in the mother. Furthermore, it is theorized that the foetus acts as a 'mercury sink' for the mother, although the reason for this is unclear [110-111].

Mercury can exert neurotoxic effects on the foetus [112], especially during critical periods of nervous system development and rapid maturation [113], even if the mother displays no symptoms of mercury-poisoning herself [114].

Mercury exposure can exert neurotoxic effects on the foetus and, depending on the dose and timing of exposure during gestation, the effects may be severe and immediately obvious, or more subtle, and delayed until later in childhood. These symptoms include mental retardation, ataxia and cerebral palsy, seizures, vision/hearing loss, delayed developmental milestones, language disorders, and problems with motor function, visual spatial abilities, and memory [115-118].

Long-term cohort studies suggest that the cardiovascular system is also at risk from mercury exposure in the womb [119].

In addition to mercury-laced vaccines added to the recommended schedule during the 'phaseout' of thimerosal-containing vaccines, six doses of new aluminum-containing vaccines were added to the childhood schedule in the US – 4 doses of pneumococcal vaccine [120], and 2 doses of Hepatitis A vaccine [121].

The addition of thimerosal-containing influenza vaccines and the addition of the pneumococcal and Hepatitis A vaccines to the schedule (which resulted in a 20% increase in aluminium exposure) certainly complicates any attempts to ascertain whether the removal of thimerosal affected rates of autism or other disorders.

Currently, vaccines are still allowed to contain 'trace amounts' of thimerosal, which refers to any amount up to 1 microgram per 0.5ml dose, which is the equivalent of 2000ug/litre - or two thousand parts per billion.

For perspective, two thousand parts per billion is 1000 times the 'safe' amount allowed in drinking water, as set by the US Environmental Protection Authority (EPA) [122].

POLYSORBATE 80

A number of vaccines contain the surfactant known as Polysorbate 80, or 'Tween 80'. This ingredient is used in a variety of products, such as milk and ice-cream products, sauces and dressings, personal care products and medications.

Surfactants prevent individual ingredients from separating, so they act as detergents, foaming agents and dispersants.

There are a number of concerns regarding Polysorbate 80. Firstly, Polysorbate 80 is used in pharmacology to enable drugs and other medications to cross the blood-brain barrier, and gain access to the central nervous system [123].

The blood-brain barrier, which is still incomplete in infants, is there specifically to separate the brain and central nervous system, from the circulatory system. This helps to protect the brain from any toxins or poisons that are present in the bloodstream.

Research shows that the presence of Polysorbate 80 with other substances, can increase brain concentrations of those other substances by *20 to 60-fold* [124-125]. Consider the implications, given what we have already learned about aluminium, and its affinity for the brain.

The Material Safety Data Sheet (MSDS) for Polysorbate 80 states that it "*May cause adverse reproductive effects based on animal test data. No human data found. May cause cancer based on animal test data. No human data found. May affect genetic material (mutagenic)*" [126].

In 1984, there was a tragic situation where 38 premature babies died, and many others suffered severe blood disorders, following intravenous infusion of a Vitamin E product, known as E-Ferol [127].

Upon further investigation, it was discovered that it was not the Vitamin E that was causing the issues, it was the 9% Polysorbate 80 that was added to it [128]. Autopsy investigations revealed extensive damage to the blood vessels in the liver [129].

Studies on female baby rats show that injection of Polysorbate 80 induced changes on their reproductive systems, namely decreased weight of the uterus and ovaries, degenerative folli-cles on the ovaries, and pre-cancerous changes on the lining of the uterus, indicative of chronic estrogen stimulation [130].

ANTIBIOTICS

There is no doubt that antibiotics have saved lives, since the discovery of penicillin by Sir Alexander Fleming, in 1928. How-ever, it soon became obvious that these miracle drugs had a down-side, and that was to cause bacteria to mutate, leading to what is now termed 'antibiotic resistance'.

In recent years, health organizations around the globe have termed this worsening problem a 'crisis' or 'nightmare scenario' that may have 'catastrophic consequences [131]. To give you an idea of the scale of antibiotic resistance, here's a few statistics:

- In the past few years, antibiotic-resistant strains of gonorrhoea have begun to emerge in the United States [132].

- Methicilin-resistant Staphylococcus aureus MRSA, (or commonly known as Golden Staph) now kills more peo-ple in the US each year, than HIV/AIDS, Parkinson's dis-ease, emphysema, and homicide combined [132-133].

- In 2012, 170 000 people died worldwide from antibi-otic-resistant tuberculosis infections [133-134].

- About 12,000 healthcare-acquired Acinetobacter infec-tions occur each year in the US. The majority of these are resistant to at least three different classes of antibiotics, resulting in 500 deaths each year [135].

This alarming situation is blamed mostly on over-use, incorrect prescribing, and widespread use in agricultural farming. But there's another source of exposure that affects millions of people world-wide...and nobody seems to be talking about it.

Antibiotics, such as neomycin, kanamycin, and polymyxin are also used in vaccines [136], regularly injected into millions of children and adults alike. They are added to vaccines to prevent bacterial contamination during manufacture.

According to the John Hopkins Bloomberg School of Public Health, there are 18 vaccines licensed in the U.S that contain antibiotics as an ingredient, with neomycin being the most commonly used [137].

There have been no controlled studies as to how this might potentially contribute to antibiotic resistance. On the contrary there is enthusiastic support for *more* vaccines, under the premise that they will reduce antibiotic resistance, by eradicating the diseases that require antibiotics [138].

Studies show that antibiotic use disrupts the body's microbiome, which has wide-ranging consequences for overall health:

"The use of antibiotics heavily disrupts the ecology of the human microbiome (i.e., the collection of cells, genes, and metabolites from the bacteria, eukaryotes, and viruses that inhabit the human body). A dysbiotic microbiome may not perform vital functions such as nutrient supply, vitamin production, and protection from pathogens. Dysbiosis of the

microbiome has been associated with a large number of health problems and causally implicated in metabolic, immunological, and developmental disorders, as well as susceptibility to development of infectious diseases" [139].

Not only that, but antibiotics during particular periods of childhood (when the majority of vaccines are received), can have lifelong consequences for the gut ecosystem:

"Critical developmental milestones for the microbiota (as well as for the child) occur, in particular, during infancy and early childhood, and both medical intervention and lack of such intervention during these periods can have lifelong consequences in the composition and function of the gut ecosystem" [139].

ANIMAL PRODUCTS

Vaccine production also involves the use of animal products. Some of these include [140]:

i) Bovine serum albumin, or fetal bovine serum - serum extracted from the heart of unborn calves, after their mothers have been slaughtered at the meatworks [141].
ii) Insect cell, bacterial and viral protein -genetically-engineered baculoviruses are used to infect fermented insect cells, which are incubated, and then purified, before being added to final product [142].
iii) Embryonated chicken eggs.
iv) DNA from porcine circoviruses (pig viruses), which are unintended contaminants of the rotavirus vaccines [143].

There is some concern over the use of the monkey kidney cells, and the dog kidney cell proteins, due to evidence that they may be tumorigenic (cause tumor growth) [144]. The monkey kidney cell lines were capable of inducing tumor growths in 100% of mice tested, which exhibited some characteristics of kidney cancer, but later spontaneously resolved [145].

The use of animals in vaccines (and other biomedical) research and manufacture raises many moral and ethical issues.

Conservative estimates say that approximately *115 million* vertebrate animals are used every year in biomedical research and production. These animals may be subjected to all kinds of experimentation, including exposed to toxins and poisons, genetic manipulation, food and water deprivation, and surgical procedures [146].

Humane Research Australia describes how fetal bovine serum (a growth medium used in vaccine production) is collected:

"After slaughter and bleeding of the cow at an abattoir, the mother's uterus containing the calf fetus is removed during the evisceration process (removal of the mother's internal organs) and transferred to the blood collection room. A needle is then inserted between the fetus's ribs directly into its heart and the blood is vacuumed into a sterile collection bag. This process is aimed at minimizing the risk of contamination of the serum with micro-organisms from the fetus and its environment. Only fetuses over the age of three months are used otherwise the heart is considered too small to puncture."

"Once collected, the blood is allowed to clot at room

temperature and the serum separated through a process known as refrigerated centrifugation."

"It remains questionable as to whether or not fetuses have already died from anoxia (deprivation of oxygen) prior to serum collection. Nevertheless, no anesthesia is given, despite their possible ability to experience pain and discomfort" [147].

It is estimated that more than 1 million bovine fetuses are harvested annually [148].

One animal, whose blood is used to test vaccines, and other drugs, for bacterial contamination, is the unfortunate horseshoe crab. According to The Atlantic, half a million horseshoe crabs are captured and bled alive, every year, to be used in the biomedical industry [149].

In the 1950's, it was discovered that the blood of horse-shoe crabs contains a unique substance that can detect and immobilize bacteria [150].

The crabs are collected as they come close to the shoreline in order to mate. They are then taken to a laboratory, and the blood from around their pericardium is bled. Afterwards, they are returned to the ocean, although an estimated 10% - 30% of crabs die following the bleeding process [151].

Although, horseshoe crabs have been used in vaccine and biomedical production since the 1970's, the full effects of this practice are just now starting to become apparent, with research suggesting the bleeding process is affecting population growth of the horseshoe crab, and may be disrupting female fertility [151].

One quart of blood from the horseshoe crab now fetches around $15,000USD, which equates to an estimated $50 million per year net income for the industry [152].

Another animal employed in vaccine and biomedical research, is a genetically-engineered mouse, known as an SCID-hu mouse [153]. These mice have been engineered to be severely immunocompromised, and they then have human tissue, or organs (which have been harvested from aborted foetuses) grafted into them. This allows researchers to study disease progression, and therapeutics in human cells, but without the immune system of the host rejecting the graft.

SCID-hu mice are being used in the quest for an HIV vaccine [154].

FORMALDEHYDE

Formaldehyde is a flammable chemical, often used in building materials and furniture, such as particle-board, plywood, glues and adhesives, and insulation materials. It is used as an embalming agent in mortuaries and research laboratories, due to its fungicidal, germicidal and disinfectant properties, which is precisely why it's also used in vaccines.

It is diluted during the manufacturing process, but small amounts may still remain in the finished product [155-156].

The International Agency for Research on Cancer has classified formaldehyde as a human carcinogen [157]. Numerous studies show increased cancer risk, especially leukemia and brain cancers, amongst those who are exposed to higher levels of formaldehyde in their occupation [158].

Animal studies show that formaldehyde is toxic to the central nervous system, and induces age-related memory decline, as seen in dementia [159-160].

It is oft-quoted that 'there is more formaldehyde in a pear, than in a vaccine'. Besides the obvious difference in route of exposure, there's the possibility that pears (and other pro-duce) contain significant levels of formaldehyde because widely-used fertilizers are made with formaldehyde. This has been the case for at least six decades [161]. Formaldehyde may also be used in pesticides – it's mode of action is via denatur-ing proteins [162].

2-PHENOXYETHANOL

Used in perfumes, insect repellents, dyes, inks, cosmetics - it was added to vaccines in place of thimerosal.

The MSDS states that no data is available for carcinogenity (ability to cause cancer), mutagenicity (ability to cause genetic mutations), teratonigenicity (ability to cause birth defects). According to the MSDS, 2-phenoxyethanol is "Toxic to kid-neys, the nervous system, liver. Repeated or prolonged expo-sure to the substance can produce target organs damage" [163].

According to the National Center for Biotechnology Infor-mation, 2-phenoxyethanol is the same as ethylene glycol

[164], which has been shown to cause "wasting of the testicles, reproductive changes, infertility and changes to kidney function" [165].

2-phenoxyethanol is currently used in DTaP (Daptacel), DTaP-IPV/Hib (Pentacel), TDaP (Adacel) vaccines.

GLUTARALDEHYDE

Used to disinfect and sterilize medical instruments, as a hardening agent in developing x-rays, as a tanning agent, and to preserve tissue specimens in laboratories [166].

According to the Material Safety Data Sheet, glutaraldehyde "may be toxic to blood, the reproductive system, liver, mucous membranes, spleen, central nervous system (CNS), Urinary System". It is classified as a reproductive toxin in females, and suspected reproductive toxin in males, capable of inducing DNA damage in mammals [167].

Glutaraldehyde is found in the combination diptheria-tetanus-pertussis vaccines.

CETYLTRIMETHYLAMMONIUM BROMIDE

Is a surfactant often used in hair conditioning products. It is used in some influenza and typhoid vaccines.

No data available on its ability to cause cancer, birth defects or DNA damage, however, animal research suggests it may cause adverse reproductive effects and birth defects. May be toxic to the liver, cardiovascular and nervous systems [168].

MONOSODIUM L-GLUTAMATE

Used as a flavour enhancer in foods possibly due to its ability to stimulate the taste-buds. It is reportedly used in vaccines as a stabilizer. Glutamate is a non-essential excitatory amino acid, which acts as a neurotransmitter - in other words, it has a stimulatory effect on neurons and the central nervous system [169]. It is found in its natural form in some foods, but always in balance with other inhibitory amino acids, which counter the stimulating effects of the glutamate.

Monosodium glutamate is isolated glutamate, which has been linked, not only to 'Chinese Restaurant Syndrome', but pervasive neurological disorders and symptoms, such as epilepsy and multiple sclerosis [170-171].

Dr. Russell Blaylock, former neurosurgeon, published numerous studies implicating excess glutamate levels in autism spectrum disorder [172-174].

Monosodium glutamate is found in the measles-mumps-rubella-varicella combination vaccines, and also the single chickenpox vaccine, however, free glutamic acid is potentially in other vaccines, in ingredients such as hydrolyzed gelatin.

VIRAL CONTAMINANTS

Due to the use of animal products and human blood products in vaccine production, it is possible for viral contamination to occur.

Contamination may occur due to several reasons:

i) Contamination of primary cell cultures.
ii) Contaminated due to the use of raw materials.
iii) Contaminated via an animal passage.
iv) Errors made by the operator [175].

Viral contamination represents a serious concern, as viruses require more complex and sophisticated detection methods, and presence of some viruses can disrupt detection of other viruses, leading to false negatives [175].

Some viruses can infect the cells and integrate as a 'provirus' - Adeno-associated virus (AAV) being one example. The provirus is present in the cell, but does not become active until it comes into contact with another virus, in which case, both viruses activate [176].

In 1970, research conducted on cell lines intended for vaccine production, found that approximately 1% of embryonic kidney cells (human) and 20% of African green monkey kidney cells produced Adeno-associated virus...but only when infected with a 'helper' adenovirus [177].

Perhaps the most infamous incident regarding viral contamination of vaccines is the contamination of the poliovirus vaccine with Simian Virus 40 (SV40).

According to a Sydney Morning Herald article, decades later [178], at least four batches of Australian vaccines were contaminated, totalling almost three million doses between 1956 and 1962.

It was revealed that two of the batches were released *after* testing positive to contamination. One batch, totalling around 700,000 contaminated vaccines was knowingly released, on the premise that previous batches were "probably similarly contaminated" [178].

The SV40 contamination allegedly came from infected monkey kidneys, which were used as cell cultures. Despite the live polio virus then being killed via formaldehyde, the SV40 apparently survived the process [178].

Conservative estimates indicate that up to 30 million people, both children and adults, in the United States may have been exposed to live SV40 from 1955-1963, due to contaminated vaccines [179].

Research later discovered that SV40 caused cancer in animals, and continuing research suggests that SV40 infection significantly increases risk of human primary brain cancers, primary bone cancers, malignant mesothelioma, and non-Hodgkin's lymphoma [180].

Although it is assumed that poliovirus vaccines were free of SV40 by 1961-1962, research reveals that vaccines from one eastern European manufacturer were still contaminated, up until about 1978. These vaccines were used throughout the world [181].

Only a year before the SV40 incident, there was the 'Cutter Incident' that was discussed in the previous chapter. An estimated 200,000 people in the US received polio vaccines in which the live polio virus was not inactivated (as claimed). This resulted in 40, 000 cases of polio, including 200 cases of permanent paralysis and numerous deaths [182].

In 1942, following a yellow-fever vaccination campaign among US servicemen during WWII, there was an epidemic of hepatitis. An estimated 50,000 cases of hepatitis were recorded before the presumably-contaminated vaccines were replaced by a serum-free version [183].

In 2010, the FDA recommended that doctors suspend use of the rotavirus vaccine, after it was discovered contaminated with porcine circovirus 1 (PCV1), however it was later deemed to present no risk to humans [184].

As award-winning author, Janine Roberts points out: "*Virus interaction can't be controlled -- by their very nature they are mutating organisms. There is a well-founded concern that these animal viruses are able to cross species lines and adapt to their new host environment*" [185].

Live-virus vaccines have found to be contaminated with the bird virus Avian leukosis virus (ALV) and monkey virus Simian retrovirus (SRV) [186].

It is sometimes assumed that the 'species barrier' will protect humans from animal viruses and pathogens. Sometimes, this is the case, however, the efficacy of the species barrier relies on a number of protective features of the immune system...which are bypassed when the product in question is injected, rather than ingested [187].

In the beginning chapter, I posed some questions about viruses and bacteria, and were they really the disease-causing pathogens that we have been taught?

There's another possibility about viruses, and that is the potential that they are, in fact, messenger or communication vesicles, produced by cells (perhaps when sickened, or under attack from toxins), that are taken in by other cells who then decipher the message, and orchestrate a protective response. Scientists discovered that plants do something similar, when under attack from pests.

If we consider this particular paradigm for a minute, what might the result of viral contamination in vaccines mean for the receiver of the vaccines? If the viruses were actually messengers, but designed for a different species, how might our own human cells react? Is it possible that these 'foreign messages' could instruct our own cells to behave in a way that is deleterious to our own health, or the future health of the human species?

There are far too many unanswered questions for us to know for sure, but it is fascinating – and disturbing – to think about!

RETROVIRUSES

It is also possible for vaccines to be contaminated with retroviruses – a class of viruses which replicate in a reverse process to normal viral replication. This reverse transcription process results in mutations, which makes retroviruses particularly hard to treat with antiviral drugs.

Like viruses, retroviruses can remain latent for long periods of time, until a change in cell environment (possibly due to stress, illness etc), causes them to activate. Because of the long time-frame involved, sometimes many years, it is unlikely the victim will trace their symptoms back to vaccination [188].

The most common source of contamination appears to come from the cell lines used to culture vaccines. In a paper published in 2009, researchers discovered contamination of cell-lines by a recombinant (genetically-engineered) virus, while at the same time admitting that current screening methods simply cannot detect all possible contaminants [189].

In 2011, Judy Mikovits PhD, a molecular biochemist who has published over 50 peer-reviewed papers, discovered that 30% of vaccines were contaminated with gammaretroviruses. Her employment was subsequently terminated, and she was arrested for allegedly stealing her own data from her workplace, and placed under a 4-year gag order [190].

The retrovirus that Mikovits focused on was Xenotropic Murine Leukemia Virus-related virus (XMRV), a genetically-engineered mouse virus. The virus was propagated on cell lines derived from a mouse tumour, and presumably spread through contamination of laboratory samples during the 1990's [191]. The retrovirus was later implicated in chronic fatigue syndrome, when 68 of 101 CFS patients tested positive for retrovirus DNA (67%) as compared to 8 of 218 (3.7%) of healthy controls [192].

This finding caused quite a furore in the medical science world, and the work was later retracted, however subsequent work also showed similar findings [193].

MYCOPLASMA

It is claimed that vaccines are contaminated with mycoplasmas, which are the smallest known micro-organisms capable of self-replication. They lack cell walls, which means they are unaffected by common antibiotics [194].

Technically, mycoplasmas could be regarded as *parasites*, since they adhere to host cells, fuse together with host cells, invade host cells, and compete for nutrition [195].

Perhaps the most outspoken person claiming vaccines are contaminated is Dr. Garth Nicolson [196], cell biologist and editor of the Journal of Clinical and Experimental Metastasis, and the Journal of Cellular Biochemistry.

Contamination of cell cultures, such as those used in vaccine production, was first discovered in 1956, quite by accident. Scientists infected cell cultures with mycoplasma, in order to study its effects, only to discover the cultures were already infected [197].

Results from different countries have shown that mycoplasmas now contaminate 30%-80% of all cell cultures, with some laboratories having 100% of cell cultures infected [198-199]. More than 20 distinct species of mycoplasma have been identified from contaminated cell cultures [200].

Research revealed that chronic or persistent (often silent) infection with mycoplasmas could gradually affect many biological mechanisms, and even lead to cancerous changes [201-202].

Further investigation revealed that cellular infection by mycoplasma could be treated during early stages with antibiotics, but persistent infection reached an irreversible stage. During this later stage, chromosomal damage was widespread, with hundreds of aberrant gene expressions identified, some being classified as oncogenes [203]. Beyond this point, the cancerous changes continued even after the apparent elimination of mycoplasmas.

Mycoplasmas have been linked as a cofactor in AIDS, Gulf War Disease, chronic fatigue syndrome, Crohns Disease, rheumatoid arthritis, and more [204-208]

MICRO- AND NANO-PARTICLE CONTAMINANTS

In 2017, research was published showing widespread contamination of vaccines with micro and nanoparticles, some of which could not be identified by researchers [209].

Of those micro and nanoparticles that were identified, many are known to be both non-biodegradable and non-biocompatible, meaning they are likely to persist for long periods of time in the human body. Some of the metals identified include stainless steel, tungsten, gold-zinc aggregate, platinum, silver, bismuth, iron, and chromium (alone, or in alloy, with iron and nickel).

Contamination levels up to 2700 particles per 20 microliter drop of vaccine were detected. Varilrix (chickenpox vaccine), Infanrix (6-in-1 vaccine given to infants, starting from 6 weeks of age), and Cerverix (HPV) vaccines had the highest number of contaminants [209].

Researchers theorised the contamination was due to polluted components, or industrial processes used to produce vaccines, previously not detected or investigated by manufacturers.

Nanoparticles are 1 billionth of a meter in size, and the equivalent of seven hydrogen atoms laying side by side. Their size is comparable to typical human cellular components and proteins, making it possible for them to evade some of the bodies usual defence systems. The use of nanoparticles in medicine has led to unexpected problems, giving rise to the emerging field known as nanotoxicology [210].

Because of their miniscule size, nanoparticles may have negative effects, such as crossing the blood-brain barrier, triggering immune reactions and damaging cell membranes [211]. Their size may also facilitate their absorption by the cells in various organs, such as the brain, heart, liver, spleen, kidneys, and bones, leading to deformation, and inhibition of cell growth [212-213].

Nanoparticles tend to agglomerate (clump together) because of their increased surface area to volume ratio, which can lead to blockages in the small blood or lymph vessels [214].

It has already been observed that particles such as those found in vaccines can enter the cell nuclei and interact with the DNA [215].

OTHER CONTAMINANTS

It is possible that other contaminants (also called adventitious agents) may enter a vaccine during the manufacturing process.

In 2013, the Hib vaccine, manufactured by Sanofi Pasteur, and recommended for babies as young as 6 weeks old, was found to be contaminated with glass. Independent laboratory investigations found evidence of delamination, which occurs when vaccine vials shed flakes of glass, known as 'lamellae' [216].

Engineering experts say that because the process of delamination takes time, it may not be discovered until after the product has been packaged and shipped. Despite knowledge of the contamination, neither the manufacturer, or the Food & Drug Administration warned the public, or issued a recall [216].

Approximately 700,000 HPV vaccines were recalled in 2013, due to glass contamination [217].

Between 2009 and 2011, vaccines from Merck's West Point manufacturing facility were found to be contaminated with shrink-wrap plastic, on a dozen different occasions. Merck did not believe *there have been any adverse events associated with the plastic contamination problem* [218].

High performance spectrometry testing shows that plastic polymers from packaging can also leach into vaccines [219].

In 2012, Sanofi suspended production at its Canadian manufacturing facility, and recalled four batches of BCG vaccine in Australia, following the discovery of mould in the production area [220].

A warning letter sent from the FDA, following inspection of the plant, revealed that Sanofi's testing procedures were not only inadequate for detecting mould/fungi, but there had been no less than 58 documented non-conformances relating to mould isolation in the BCG production area, between 2010 and 2012 [221].

The letter also charged that Sanofi had 'failed to maintain buildings in a good state of repair', noting that nesting birds had been observed in the intake grills for the air-handling units [221].

According to Dr Paul Offit, vaccines are *"tested more extensively than any other drugs before they're approved for the public"* [222].

We are constantly reminded of how rigorously they are tested and monitored [223], but the truth is, it's just not possible to test for all potential contaminants [224].

Several new tests - in-vitro and in-vivo detection assays - have been developed for detection of viral contaminants in vaccines, but they are time-consuming, expensive, labour intensive...and incomplete [225]. This limits their ability to meet the growing demands of the biological industry.

Highly sensitive tests such as polymerase chain reaction technology offer an alternative, but they can only be developed for *known* viruses, leaving novel viruses to escape detection [226]. Regulatory agencies issue guidelines to the industry, in the form of 'guidance documents' on how they *should* assess and screen vaccine lots, but these are recommendations only, not enforceable [227].

So, while we are assured that every vaccine lot is tested, there is no guarantee that every vaccine lot is free of contaminants.

4.
THE VACCINE INDUSTRY

The global vaccine market was worth more than $32 billion USD in 2016, expected to reach 48 billion USD by 2021 [1].

The top 5 vaccine manufacturers, according to 2015 revenue, are [2]:

1. Pfizer = $6.4 billion, projected to be $7.4 billion by 2022.
2. Merck & Co = $6.1 billion, projected to be $7.2 billion by 2022.
3. Sanofi = $5.7 billion, projected to be $8.2 billion by 2022.
4. GlaxoSmithKline = $5.5 billion, projected to be $8.5 billion by 2022.
5. CSL = $1.1 billion, projected to be $1.3 billion by 2022.

The global market for influenza vaccines alone, is worth an estimated $4 billion [3]. Of course, that market has been helped along enormously by expanded recommendations in the US, to vaccinate every person over the age of 6 months. From 32 million doses in 1990, to 135 million doses by 2013, flu vaccines are now given in shopping malls, drug stores and even drive-throughs [4].

Prices per influenza vaccine range from around $10, up to $16 per dose, for quadrivalent vaccines (four strains in one vaccine) [5].

Newer, more glamorous, vaccines fetch higher prices. $178 per dose of Gardasil, and $137 per dose of the 13-valent pneumo-coccal vaccine [6].

The decision regarding if, or where, a new vaccine will be introduced into a national schedule is often taken after a cost-benefit analysis is performed.

This takes into account expected cost of purchasing or subsidising the vaccines versus expected savings, based on an estimated (hoped-for) decrease in disease burden, through less working days lost, less hospitalisations etc.

A cost-benefit analysis does *not* take into account:

a) The likelihood of strain shift, due to selective pressure of vaccines.

b) The long-term side-effects of the vaccine, such as dysregulation of the immune system, leading to increased infections, autoimmune diseases, etc.

c) The potential benefits of being exposed to the natural infection.

d) The added societal and financial cost of developmental delays, and neurological disorders. Consider the parents who can no longer work, due to caring for their disabled children full-time.

How about the strain on the educational system and extra resources required for special-needs children? What about the strain on marriages and the increased likelihood of divorce?

What about all the extra support services required, such as speech therapy, transport services, respite services etc – it is estimated that the lifetime cost of supporting an individual with autism spectrum disorder is in the vicinity of $1.4 million in the US, and if there are intellectual disabilities, it can be as much as $2.4 million [7].

What works in one country does not always translate into best practice in other countries. Jacob Puliyel, head paediatrician at St. Stephens Hospital in Delhi, India pointed out that, although the World Health Organisation and other organizations were pushing for India to implement new vaccines, it was hardly in the country's best interests.

Analyses had revealed that 1000 people would need to be vaccinated, in order to prevent 4 cases of pneumonia. Vaccinating those 1000 people would cost $12,750, while treating the four cases of pneumonia using WHO protocol would amount to $1 [8].

How much has actually been saved by the introduction of vaccines, is overshadowed by the fact that health expenditures in Western countries, have done nothing but go up and up.

In 1950, before the vast majority of today's vaccines were in use, health expenditure in the US accounted for 4.6% of gross domestic product. By 2009, that figure had more than tripled to 17%, "*a larger share than all manufacturing, or wholesale and retail trade, or finance and insurance, or the combination of agriculture, mining, and construction*" [9].

"*It is difficult to see how the health sector can continue to expand rapidly at the expense of the rest of the economy, but every past prediction of a sustained slowing of the growth of health expenditures has been proved wrong"* [9].

Over the past 25 years, health expenditure in Australia has tripled, growing faster than inflation, faster than the population, and faster than the rest of the economy [10].

The number of recommended vaccines has more than quadrupled over the past 40 years, in many Western countries.

From 10 in the 1980's, to 32 in the 2000's, the vaccine schedule in Australia now specifies 48 vaccines by the age of 16 years - forty-one of those by the age of 4 years. That figure does not include the recommended annual influenza vaccines, or other vaccines recommended for 'high-risk' groups and travellers. All up, the number may exceed 70 vaccines by the time a child reaches 18 years of age.

In addition to the usual childhood schedule, Australian Aboriginal and Torres Strait Islander children may also receive one dose of BCG (tuberculosis vaccine) in infancy, two doses of Hepatitis A vaccine in the second year of life, influenza vaccine annually from 6mths of age, and an extra dose of 13-valent pneumococcal vaccine [11].

In the US, the minimum cost to vaccinate a child according to schedule, as per government contract prices, rose from $70 per child in 1990, to $1712 in 2012 [12].

There are numerous ways in which drug companies not only defend their market share, but aggressively seek out ways to expand their influence and customer base. Let's explore a few of them.

1.) Drug Companies Influence Education of Future Doctors

In 2008, it was revealed that the prestigious Harvard Medical School had substantial ties to industry. Out of 8900 professors and lecturers, 1600 admitted that they, or a close family member have financial ties to the industry, sometimes to the tune of hundreds of thousands of dollars.

When a group of medical students rallied on campus to protest conflicts of interest, a Pfizer employee was also there, photographing protesters via a cell-phone camera [13].

It was also revealed that the industry had donated more than $11.5 million to Harvard, in one year alone, for 'research and continuing education classes'

In 2008, the American Medical Student's Association (AMSA) decided to grade 150 US medical schools, based on the amount of money and gifts they receive from drug companies - the more goodies, the worse their grade. Out of 150 medical schools, 40 received an F - including Harvard. Only 22 (less than 15%) got an A or a B [13].

The situation in Canada appears to be similar - a study that ranked Canadian medical schools according to the stringency of their conflict-of-interest policies, found that only 4 of 17 schools - *less than a quarter* - scored higher than 50% [14].

The implication here is that many of today's doctors have been trained in a way that has been influenced and shaped by the pharmaceutical industry.

A study of medical students in France reveals that they were aware of potential bias, caused by conflicts of interest, such as gifts, but felt they, personally, were immune to such influence [15].

Although disclosure of conflicts of interest are important, they also 'normalise' industry ties: "*You start to think that's normal, that most of the people you look up to and want to be like in 10 years receive pharmaceutical support*" says Dr Navindra Persaud, a family physician at St Michael's Hospital in Toronto [16].

One wonders if industry influence in medical schools is the reason why the average student receives 5 times more tuition hours on pharmacology - or the study of drugs - than on nutrition [17-18]?

And how much do medical school students learn about vaccines? A study of medical students in France revealed that only one-third felt confident enough to answer questions regarding side-effects, or respond to vaccine hesitancy [19].

A survey of medical students in Canada found that time spent on the subject of vaccinology ranged from as little as 1hr, up to a maximum of 50hrs. Only 21% of students felt they had received adequate training on the subject. According to the authors, '*Important gaps were identified in the knowledge of graduating nursing, medical, & pharmacy trainees regarding vaccine indications/contraindications, adverse events & safety'* [20].

Delving further into the above-mentioned study, we start to get an idea of the kind of education these students have received on the subject of vaccines. For example, those who scored highest on the knowledge test were more likely to:

a) Strongly disagree/disagree to the statement "Vaccines may cause chronic diseases and learning disorders because they contain small amounts of mercury, aluminium, and formaldehyde."

b) Strongly disagree/disagree with the statement "Routine immunization should be delayed in individuals with moderate to severe illness, with or without fever."

c) Strongly disagree/disagree with the statement "parental stress can be reduced by spreading necessary vaccines over several visits".

From the above, we can deduce that the 'education' they received, was emphasising the safety and efficacy of vaccines to prevent disease, while downplaying side-effects, risks and parental concerns.

This conclusion is backed up by doctors too, who realized that if they wanted to really understand vaccines, they would have to educate themselves.

Dr. Larry Palevsky, board certified paediatrician, received his medical degree from New York University School of Medicine, says: "*I was taught in medical school residency that vaccines are safe, and they're effective...that there's absolutely no reason to question it, because we've done all the studies*" [21].

Dr Bob Sears, board certified Paediatrician, received his medical degree from Georgetown University School of Medicine, says: "*Doctors, myself included, learn a lot about diseases in medical school, but we learn very little about vaccines, other than the fact that the FDA and pharmaceutical companies do extensive research on vaccines to make sure they are safe and effective. We don't review the research ourselves. We never learn what goes into making vaccines or how their safety is studied. We trust and take it for granted that the proper researchers are doing their job*".

"*So, when patients want a little more information about shots, all we can really say as doctors is that the diseases are bad and the shots are good. But we don't know enough to answer all of your detailed questions about vaccines, nor do we have the time during a regular health check up to thoroughly discuss and debate the pros and cons of vaccines*" [22].

Despite this, research shows "*The public views health care providers as credible and trusted sources of vaccine recommendations. Many individuals cite the recommendation of their physician or nurse as **the most important factor** governing their decision to either become vaccinated themselves, or have their child vaccinated, and positive attitudes of health professionals have been shown to correlate with higher vaccination coverage rates*" [23].

2. Drug Companies Influence How Doctors Practice Medicine

While the average medical student has a positive attitude towards vaccines, less than a third feel their education on the subject was adequate...so says one study conducted on medical students at the University of Central Florida, College of Medicine [24]. Now, add financial incentives to vaccinate...

In 2015, the 'No Jab, No Pay' legislation was passed in Australia, which saw low-income families financially penalised if their children were not up-to-date with vaccines. Soon after, the federal budget was handed down – in it, $26 million allocated to boost vaccination rates, which includes a $12 bonus to doctors, every time they provide 'catch-up' vaccines [25].

That may not sound like much, but when you add it to the cost of the consultation, plus the extra charge for the vaccine, plus the charge for administering the vaccine, then it starts to seem like an attractive and convenient way to increase income.

The healthcare system in America is vastly different, with the majority of doctors getting paid, not by the patient or the government, but by insurance companies. Over the past decade or more, the healthcare system has been transformed into an increasingly 'performance-based' system, with bonuses offered for meeting certain targets, including vaccination quotas [26-27].

The National Committee for Quality Assurance ranks and accredits insurance companies. High vaccination rates among their providers, earns the insurance company a higher rating

[28]. A higher rating for the insurance company means a greater slice of the federal funds pie, so there is financial incentive at every level of the system.

According to Time magazine, paediatricians and family practitioners are the lowest paid of all the doctors, making an average of $158,000 a year [29]. That's a lot higher than the average income, but could those bonuses, which are rumoured to potentially run into the tens of thousands of dollars, possibly jeopardize a doctor's impartiality?

There may also be financial incentives directly from the pharmaceutical companies themselves, via speaking engagements, public endorsements, and invitations to conferences, meals, or seminars.

I worked in a large University medical centre for several years, which comprised of 6 doctors, 3 nurses and numerous counsellors. Their policy was that pharmaceutical reps could only come by appointment, but it had to be during morning tea, or lunch – and they had to provide the morning tea or lunch. Most days, there was at least one.

I witnessed conversations between doctors and pharmaceutical reps, where doctors would discuss a certain difficult case (without using any identifying details), and the pharmaceutical rep gave advice on what drug to use. Often, they would give free samples of drugs, and other knick-knacks, such as pens, notepads, desk-calendars – it all helped to keep their brand visible and easily remembered when the doctor was next making a prescription.

I also witnessed medical journals being delivered to doctors, which eventually piled up, unopened, on their desks, or in mail containers. They simply didn't have time to read them. Basically, what I witnessed was pharmaceutical companies providing ongoing education to doctors, who were too over-worked to keep up with new information themselves.

One area where a doctor's integrity can be compromised for financial gain is known as 'ghost-writing'. A pharmaceutical company employs a writer to create a piece that contains 'key marketing messages', and then it gets sent to a doctor who agrees to have his/her name attributed to the work in exchange for remuneration, before it is submitted to medical publications. Studies suggest that anywhere from 8% to 75% of journal articles may be ghost-written [30].

Clearly, this might appeal to some doctors who want the prestige of being a published author, quite apart from the financial incentive. The pharmaceutical company has final control over the paper, and if a doctor is not compliant enough, they simply get no further projects [31-32].

Amanda Laine, editor of the Annals of Internal Medicine, says *"If you're an academic researcher, the currency in that world, the thing that gets you promoted, is not just the quality of work but the number of publications, so the lure of being able to get another publication without a lot of personal investment is really tempting"* [33].

In many cases, if not all, the ghost-writer and the honorary author have not even viewed the raw data, they have merely been supplied with a summary from the sponsor company. The honorary author is usually chosen because of their credentials, and their ability to influence other prescribers [34].

In 2000, pharmaceutical giant SmithKline Beecham created a program called CASPPER (get it?) which sought out doctors who had a positive prescribing experience with the anti-depressant drug Paroxetine (sold under the brand name Paxil). These doctors were then teamed up with a professional ghost-writing service, in order to expand the database of published work for their drug. The project budgeted for 50 articles in one year alone, with the aim to *"benefit the sales force by expanding the database of published data to support Paxil"* [35].

Of course, the desired effect of all this published data is three-fold: a) it gives the appearance that the drug is thoroughly re-searched and widely accepted, b) which boosts doctor and pa-tient confidence, c) while providing an edge over rival products.

Organizers of seminars and conferences are often under pres-sure to design a program, and choose speakers, with the end goal of attracting funding from drug companies [36].

Research shows that events with drug company involvement have a smaller range of topics, and more drug-related content, than those without industry involvement [37].

Would it be unreasonable to suppose that these same pressures have not infiltrated the arena of vaccine research?

In 2007, celebrities, doctors and journalists from across Europe and the United States, were flown in to Paris, by PR agencies working for Sanofi, to attend the 'first global summit against cervical cancer'. Sanofi, who markets Gardasil in Europe on behalf of Merck, spent millions on the summit, which 'resembled a political rally', and 'called for country-wide vaccination programs' [38].

Many doctors claim they can discern bias, and are able to objectively judge the information they receive, but the science says otherwise. Doctors who interact the most with industry have poorer prescribing habits, and are more likely to flout guidelines [39].

One stark example of the dangers of industry involvement in doctor's continuing education, was the OxyContin scandal in the late 1990's. At the launch of their product, the drug company created a 'speaker's bureau' that included thousands of doctors, and sponsored more than 20,000 educational programs, which were led by industry-sponsored doctors, and accredited by professional bodies.

In four years, sales of OxyContin grew from US $48 million to $1.1 billion, however, the massive educational campaign misrepresented the risks and, eventually, adverse side effects became too obvious to ignore [40].

Now, what might happen if a doctor somehow makes it through this system with some niggling doubts about the vaccines that he/she is expected to administer? What if that doctor actually had the audacity to voice those concerns?

The last few years have brought up a number of such cases and, unfortunately, ostracism, ridicule and disciplinary measures seem to be the inevitable end.

Research released in 2015 concluded that *"anyone who questions the dominant views about vaccines is subject to abuse, including threats, formal complaints, censorship, and loss of their livelihoods"* [41].

In 2017, Dr. Daniel Neides, then director of the Cleveland Clinic Wellness Institute, published a blog post questioning the logic of giving newborns the Hepatitis B vaccine, and questioning the safety of aluminium adjuvants in vaccines. His blog post was prompted by his having received a 'preservative-free' flu vaccine (thinking he would avoid the thimerosal found in multivial vaccines), after which he missed two days of work, being bedridden with flu-like symptoms [42].

The public outcry over his blog post was so severe, the Cleveland Clinic Board of Directors promised disciplinary action.

Daniel Neides offered an apology the following day, via a hospital spokesperson: *"I apologize and regret publishing a blog that has caused so much concern and confusion for the public and medical community. I fully support vaccinations and my concern was meant to be positive around the safety of them"* [43].

Daniel Neides was ultimately forced out of his leadership position at the Cleveland Clinic, after which he established himself in private practice, where he utilises a number of integrative treatments.

Note, this doctor was merely raising concerns. He was not being so heretical as to claim that vaccines are useless or dangerous. The unspoken message was this: If you're a doctor, follow without question, or else...

Also, in 2017, Australian Dr. John Piesse had his office raided, and was later de-registered, after it was revealed he had helped families gain medical exemptions from vaccination. A conscientious objection is no longer accepted as valid by Australian government authorities [44-45].

New South Wales Health Care Complaints Commission urged members of the public to 'dob in' any doctors suspected of being 'involved with anti-vax practices' [46].

This message was reiterated again, in 2019, when the Australian Health Practitioner Regulation Authority (AHPRA) issued a warning that *"health professionals who spread anti-vaccination messages will be disciplined"* [47].

The message, loud and clear, then, is don't question or criticise vaccines, if you want to keep your career prospects intact.

On the other hand, the rewards for doctors who encourage and promote vaccines are clear – security, safety, and acceptance from your peers.

Take Dr Paul Offit of the Philadelphia Children's Hospital, who famously calculated that a baby could safely receive 10,000 vaccines at one time [48].

Dr. Offit is one of the inventors of the genetically-engineered Rotavirus vaccine, currently on the childhood vaccination schedule. Offit was a member of the CDC's advisory committee, during the same period that a (different) rotavirus vaccine was first added to the Vaccines for Children program, a coincidence that was later noted by a Government Reform Committee, investigating conflicts of interest in vaccine development [49].

That particular vaccine would later be withdrawn (amidst safety concerns over a 30-fold increase in risk of intussusception– a medical emergency that involves blockage of the intestines) and replaced by Offit's vaccine. An increased risk of intussusception from Offit's vaccine has also been noted in some studies, though not as high as the original vaccine [50].

Dr. Offit hasn't publicly disclosed how much he will earn in total from his involvement in developing the rotavirus vaccine, but according the Philadelphia Children's Hospital policy manual, he was entitled to 30% of the net income [51] - which was around $153 million [52].

In 2005, Merck donated $1.5 million towards establishing the "Maurice Hilleman Chair in Vaccinology" [53] – an appointment awarded to Paul Offit in 2015, and which he still holds [54].

It is abundantly clear that if a doctor wants to keep his career and his reputation, he would do well to toe the line, and accept the official line of 'vaccines are safe', without question or fuss - but is that really serving the best interests of the patients?

3) Drug companies fund charities and 'think tanks'

Save The Children is an international aid agency that works in developing countries to promote education and healthcare - part of which includes childhood vaccines.

In 2013, Save The Children announced they had formed a strategic partnership with pharmaceutical giant, GlaxoSmithKline - maker of numerous vaccines [55].

While many hailed it as an exciting step forward, others working in aid were left feeling distinctly uneasy.

It's not the first time the pharmaceutical industry has funded or worked with charities, and it raises questions over whether there could be a profit-driven motive behind it, rather than simply acting from the goodness of their corporate heart.

'Venture philanthropy' is an emerging trend where non-profits team up with drug companies for mutual benefit. The charity, or patient advocacy group, helps to fund research and development, in exchange for a cut of the profits. Once the treatment comes to market, they promote it to their members, and help to develop guidelines for use - which are then used by doctors [56].

Basically, the charity receives donations from the public, which are then used to develop a new drug or treatment, which is then sold back to the public, who either pay for it outright, or indirectly through Medicare programs which are funded by taxes...

Another approach used by the pharmaceutical industry is to fund 'think tanks' with professional-sounding names, to write reports, and make recommendations on policy.

The Global Pertussis Initiative is an 'expert scientific group', and 'leading voice in the global push to eradicate pertussis' [57], which publishes in leading medical journals, and even makes recommendations to the World Health Organization [58].

The group happens to be funded by Sanofi Pasteur, manufacturer of a pertussis vaccine [58].

An investigation by the Watchdog Institute found that the majority of the group's members have received funding from Sanofi Pasteur and/or GlaxoSmithKline - the other manufacturer of a DTaP vaccine [58].

A statement prepared by Sanofi Pasteur said: "Sanofi Pasteur is committed to public health and we routinely review epidemiological data, as well as the safety and effectiveness of all our vaccines to ensure that we are offering high quality vaccines to patients. At the present time, there is *no evidence to suggest current pertussis vaccines lack effectiveness"* [58].

Yet, there *had* been mounting evidence, for at least a decade, that the vaccine *did* lack effectiveness [59-60]. That evidence has only continued to grow in recent years [61-64].

Think about the implications here – the World Health Organization, the dominant force in global health policy for the 7 billion inhabitants of this earth, receives advice from a group that is, for all intents and purposes, a front group for a major drug company...

GlaxoSmithKline, who manufactures the other DTaP vaccine, also founded a group called the International Consensus Group on Pertussis Immunisation. According to one former member, it is no longer operational, but while they were...one of their articles was published in the journal Vaccine, promoting *universal vaccination of all age groups* [65].

Pharma-funded charities are also instrumental in swaying government policy and mustering up public opinion.

In 2015, Britain became the first country in the world to roll out a national Meningitis B vaccination program for babies. This announcement was applauded by the Meningitis Research Foundation:

"MenB has been at the top of this charity's agenda for decades and we are delighted that vaccinating all babies against this devastating disease is now within sight, cementing the UK's position as a world leader in meningitis prevention" [66].

The Meningitis Research Foundation is funded by GlaxoSmithKline and Pfizer – who manufacture meningitis vaccines [67].

A year later, Meningitis Now – a national UK charity – joined calls for the UK government to expand the meningitis B vaccination program for babies, to include *all* children up to 5yrs of age:

"We are using our voice to support the petition to raise the profile of meningitis, keeping it high on the political agenda and increasing awareness among the public to prevent more lives being lost to this devastating disease."

And *"Moving forward, we continue to campaign to see the meningitis B vaccine rolled out, particularly to at-risk groups, to ensure a future where no one in the UK loses their life to meningitis"* [68].

Meningitis Now is also funded by GlaxoSmithKline and Pfizer [69].

Meanwhile, in the US, Women in Government is a national, non-profit group for female state legislators. The group receives funding from various pharmaceutical companies. During the lead-up to licensure of Gardasil vaccine, and thereafter, Merck donated unrestricted 'educational' grants to Women in Government, which paid for dozens of legislators to attend conferences on cervical cancer, also attended by Merck representatives.

For their part, Women in Government members hosted meetings to brief other legislators on HPV and Gardasil, convened a task-force that made policy recommendations, and prepared a legislative 'tool kit' that contained sample school-entry legislation mandates. All while courting media sources to promote vaccination mandates.

Many of the mandate bills that surfaced after approval of Gardasil, were introduced by members of Women in Government [70].

4) Drug companies influence news and media

The pharmaceutical industry spends $5.2 billion per annum on TV advertising - that figure rose by 60% in the four years from 2012 to 2016 [71-72].

Nine out of ten big pharmaceutical companies spend more on marketing than they do on research and development. As an example, in 2013, Johnson and Johnson spent $8.2 billion on research and development, and $17.5 billion – more than double - on marketing [73].

Besides overt advertising, the industry also employs the use of press releases and advertorials. A review of news and current affair items on free-to-air TV in Sydney, Australia, estimated that up to 42% may have "been triggered by press releases and other forms of publicity" [74].

Advertising is not the only way that the pharmaceutical industry can influence the media. Another avenue is through a situation known as an interlocking directorate. This occurs when the director of one company sits on the board of directors of another company.

In 2009, the Fairness and Accuracy in Reporting (FAIR) group conducted a study of nine major media companies: Disney (ABC), Gannett (USA Today), General Electric (NBC), CBS, Time Warner (CNN), News Corporation (Fox), New York Times Co., Washington Post Co. (Newsweek), and Tribune Co. (Chicago Tribune, L.A. Times). Out of those nine corporations, six had directors who also represented the interests of at least one major pharmaceutical company.

They also showed that these interlocking directorates had an influence on how news outlets covered issues such as healthcare reform [75].

Rupert Murdoch, whose vast media empire includes The New York Post and Wall Street Journal in the US, The Australian and

The Daily Telegraph in Australia, The Sunday Times in the UK, and HarperCollins books, has strong links with the pharmaceutical industry.

Murdoch is co-chairman of the prestigious Partnership for New York City, whose Board of Directors reads like a 'Who's Who' of business, and includes Ian C. Reed, the CEO of Pfizer. The partnership is heavily invested in pharmaceutical and biotech ventures [76].

Rupert Murdoch's son, James was a non-executive director of GlaxoSmithKline from 2009 to 2012 [77]. Was it just coincidence that within a week of the announcement that James had joined the board of GSK, the Murdoch-owned Sunday Times began their vendetta against Andrew Wakefield, via journalist Brian Deer [78]?

Rupert Murdoch's daughter-in-law Sarah Murdoch is an ambassador (and a member of the Board of Directors) for the Murdoch Children's Research Institute. According to their website:

"The Vaccine and Immunisation Research Group (VIRGo) at Murdoch Children's Research Institute is an international centre for expertise in vaccine and immunisation research and has been a leading voice on the issue for over 20 years.

*With the largest and longest standing child and adolescent vaccine clinical trials program in Australia, VIRGo **provides evidence to shape Government policy** regarding best use of vaccines in national schedules.Key to VIRGo's work is research centred on **vaccine hesitancy and studying the factors that determine why parents refuse safe***

vaccines *despite the widespread availability of services and information"* [79].

Do Rupert Murdoch's links to the pharmaceutical industry ever shape the way vaccines or other pharmaceuticals are portrayed in the media? Maybe former Australian Prime Minister, Tony Abbot said it best in a 2013 speech: *"His publications have borne his ideals but never his fingerprints"* [80].

According to research, 'the media can play an important role in influencing both the demand and supply of medical treatments, *regardless of evidence of effectiveness* [81].

Media coverage can increase uptake of the seasonal influenza vaccine by as much as 7%, especially if reported in a headline, and includes words such as 'vaccine shortage' [82].

When it comes to the vaccine issue, media articles are more likely to explicitly mention or support the mainstream position towards vaccination, than mention a critical argument against vaccination [83].

The so-called 'swine flu pandemic', which turned out to be more panic than pandemic, featured experts and academics making media appearances, promoting the use of retroviral drugs. It was later found that those who promoted retroviral drugs, were 8 times more likely to have links to industry - via research grants, honorarium payments, advisory roles, employment, board membership, speaker's fees, etc - than those who did not comment on their use [84].

Yet another avenue of industry influence in the media is via cultivating direct relationships with journalists. Much like doctors, journalists seem to believe they are personally immune from being influenced by relationships with drug companies – despite evidence to the contrary [85].

With the rise and rise of social media, the pharmaceutical industry has another avenue to reach consumers directly, and affect consumer behaviour. Official pages and channels of the major drug companies often have tens, or hundreds of thousands, of followers.

Research found that around 40% of drug company posts include content that is consistent with what the FDA defines as 'help-seeking direct-to-consumer advertising' – this is where they 'raise awareness' about certain illnesses or ailments, without giving any particular remedy, and the end result is that people worried about said ailment, seek out their doctor for help...and hopefully the doctor prescribes their product [86].

5) Drug companies influence medical journals...

The birth of the scientific journal, about 300 years ago, took a hodge-podge assortment of formats and research, and turned them into a uniform system with peer review and measures of quality control [87].

Unlike many other centuries-old inventions, the journal has not only survived, but grown in influence over the years. In 1960, there were 2815 journals published. By 2002, that figure had grown to 22,000 scientific journals, each publishing an average of 154 articles [88].

In 1999, researchers analysed the clinical journals of several leading medical organisations, including the Journal of the American College of Cardiology, Annals of Internal Medicine, Journal of the American Medical Association, American Journal of Respiratory and Critical Care Medicine, Clinical Infectious Diseases, and the New England Journal of Medicine.

They found that the estimated revenue from pharmaceutical advertising ranged from $715,000 to $18 million—a total that they said could place the organisations in a position of dependency. Five organisations raised more than 10% of their gross income from a single journal's pharmaceutical advertising, and four organisations raised as much, or more, from pharmaceutical advertising as from members [89].

Could this compromise the contents of a journal? Could research be published or discarded on the basis of whether it pleases corporate sponsors?

As Richard Smith, former editor of the British Medical Journal once said, "*your opinion may not be bought, but it seems rude to say critical things about people who have hosted you so well*" [90].

Besides that, the evidence says that much of pharmaceutical advertising is misleading, either by overstating the benefits, or minimising adverse effects [91-92]. Many times, the promotional claims are not supported by the references they cite [93].

Doctors claim they are not influenced by advertising, but that is probably inaccurate [91], and it seems doubtful that pharmaceutical companies would continue doing it, without return on investment.

A drug company, however, will always prefer favourable editorial coverage over advertising - it lends credibility.

To that end, a medical journal is more useful to a drug company for publishing trials than for advertising. A major randomised trial with favourable results, published in a prestigious journal, is a major win for a drug company, and an essential step in creating a 'blockbuster' product [94-95].

We already mentioned the practice of 'ghost-writing' - an informal poll of freelance medical writers by the American Medical Writers Association, found that 80% had written at least one manuscript that didn't mention their contributions [96].

The industry is aware that readers are sceptical if they know there is pharmaceutical company involvement in the article. Readers reported that they found the research 'less interesting, important, relevant, valid and believable' when they thought the authors were employees of a pharmaceutical company [97].

A 2010 review of six major medical journals found that studies funded by industry are cited more often than those funded by other sources - more than twice as often in some journals [98]. The authors suggested that medical journals should also have to disclose funding from industry, in the same way researchers are meant to.

 If industry-funded studies are not only more likely to find favourable results, but are then cited more often than other studies (whose findings may not be so positive), we can clearly see how industry may influence the general perception that a drug or medical intervention is not only well-researched, but widely accepted.

At the heart of the scientific process is the concept known as peer review - where an author's work is subjected to the scrutiny of other experts in the same field, before being published. The public perception is that the peer review process acts like a stop-gap that upholds the integrity of the scientific process, and filters out errors or fraud, but does it really?

A systematic review undertaken in 2002, of all the available evidence on peer review at that time, concluded that *'the practice of peer review is based on faith in its effects, rather than on facts"* [99].

The British Medical Journal decided to test for themselves how reliable the peer-review process is, by inserting major errors into papers before sending to reviewers. Some reviewers *didn't pick up any of the errors*, while most picked up only about a quarter. Nobody picked up all the errors [100-101].

So far, the evidence suggests that the peer review process is *"slow, expensive, ineffective, something of a lottery, prone to bias and abuse, and hopeless at spotting errors and fraud"* [102].

The New England Journal of Medicine has long been 'the journal to beat' [103], yet two former editors-in-chief left their role in the top job, and went on to publish books exposing the excessive influence of the drug industry [104-105].

One of those, Marcia Angell, wrote: "*It is simply no longer possible to believe much of the clinical research that is published, or to rely on the judgement of trusted physicians or authoritative medical guidelines. I take no pleasure in this conclusion, which I reached slowly and reluctantly over my two decades as an editor of The New England Journal of Medicine* [106].

In 2009, it was revealed that Merck had paid undisclosed amounts to Elsevier (an academic publishing company), to publish eight compilations of scientific articles under the title Australasian Journal of Bone and Joint Medicine [107].

It looked like an independent, peer-reviewed journal, and it was sent out to some 20,000 Australian doctors - with no disclosure that it was entirely funded by Merck.

Many of the articles referred positively to Merck's products, such as Vioxx and Fosamax.

6) Drug companies influence lawmakers and politicians.

In 2016, the pharmaceutical/health industry spent $248 million lobbying politicians in the United States [108], almost a third more than the second biggest spending industry - the insurance industry [109].

The pharmaceutical industry's lobbying efforts are directed towards *"resisting government-run health care, ensuring a quicker approval process for drugs and products entering the market and strengthening intellectual property protections"* [109].

Over the past 20 years, the pharmaceutical/health industry has spent $3.5 billion on lobbying US politicians [109], and Dr

Raeford Brown, chair of FDA Committee on Analgesics and Anesthetics, who has been openly critical of pharmaceutical industry influence on the FDA, goes so far as to say that *"Congress is owned by pharma"* [110].

The two trade groups representing the industry - Pharmaceutical Research and Manufacturers of America, and the Biotechnology Industry Organization - lobbied on approximately 1600 pieces of legislation between 1998 and 2005 [111].

In 2006, before the Gardasil vaccine had even been approved, Merck had begun lobbying and 'educating' state politicians in a bid to make the future vaccine mandatory. Within a year of gaining approval, legislation regarding the vaccine was introduced in 41 states, including bills in 24 states that would make the vaccine mandatory for 6th-grade girls [112].

According to an investigation published in the American Journal of Public Health, *"Merck proactively contacted legislators to discuss strategies to maximize uptake of Gardasil, either directly through company employees or by using local political consultants, prominent physicians, or public relations firms"* [112].

*"Many respondents reported that company representatives proposed specific legislation, often **drafting the bills and searching for a sponsor**. In most states, their efforts focused on a school-entry mandate. Respondents pointed out that Merck's activities were not unusual, although the public seemed to have been unaware that private companies played such a role in the legislative process. One commented, "Just about every vaccine mandate that we have lately has been the*

result, at least partially, of the drug industry's efforts".

In 2007, Texas governor, Rick Perry simply bypassed the legislative process and signed an Executive Order, making the vaccine compulsory for 11-12yr old girls [113]. It was later revealed that Merck had donated $5000 to Rick Perry's campaign fund, and his former chief-of-staff had become a Merck lobbyist [114].

In Australia, the political and healthcare systems are vastly different, and lobbying not quite so overt - but the pharmaceutical industry has still managed to foster a cosy relationship with government, and influence policy decisions.

Australia's Pharmaceutical Benefits Scheme costs $7.7 billion annually, and is world-renowned for giving consumers access to medications at affordable prices. Naturally, having a product listed on the pharmaceutical benefits scheme is a massive win, and coveted position, for pharmaceutical companies, as it can mean hundreds of millions of dollars in sales, funded largely by the tax-payer.

When Wyeth was aiming to get their arthritis drug, Embrel, onto the Pharmaceutical Benefits Scheme, they hired a political lobby group, who wheeled out sick kids during their meetings with politicians. Well, who could refuse? The politicians knew it would be a public relations disaster if the story got taken up by the media, so the drug was rushed onto the PBS scheme...at a cost of $100 million per year [115].

In 2006, CSL, the Australian promotors of Gardasil, who had signed a partnership deal with Merck, attempted to have the

HPV vaccine listed on the Pharmaceutical Benefits Scheme. The Pharmaceutical Benefits Advisory Committee rejected their application for a three-dose national vaccination campaign, because the vaccine was too expensive, and they were not convinced of its efficacy.

Within days, then Prime Minister John Howard had delivered a glowing endorsement of the product, and not only over-rode the PBAC's decision, but implemented a national vaccination campaign six months earlier than CSL had proposed [116]. Only a month prior, his wife Janette Howard had publicly revealed, for the first time, that she had received treatment for cervical cancer a decade earlier [117]. After ten years of silence, was the timing mere coincidence...or part of a much bigger plan? What kind of lobbying was going on behind the scenes?

The pharmaceutical industry, more than any other, takes advantage of the proverbial 'revolving door', between the government and the industry. A disproportionately high number of political staffers move into the lucrative health sector after leaving the political scene – this holds true, both in the US and Australia.

The following are a few brief examples of the close ties between government and the pharmaceutical industry:

i) Nick Campbell:
- NSW Liberal Party president from 2008-2010.
- Executive director of corporate and government affairs for Johnson and Johnson.
- Former staffer for Senator Bill Heffernan.
- Corporate advisor with Capital Hill Advisory, an advisory

and public affairs firm 'that is dedicated to improving the political and public policy process'. Their objective is 'to improve and facilitate the dialogue between both business and government to develop sound public policy, which is supportive of business, economic development and in the national interest [118]

ii) David Miles:
- Served as a political advisor to federal and state ministers, shadow ministers, and other Members of Parliament.
- Political strategist at Pfizer pharmaceutical company.
- Member of the Medicines Australia Government Working Group.
- Founder of Willard Public Affairs firm, who 'will help you to develop and shape your policy and strategy in a way that assists political stakeholders to understand and embrace the outcome you are seeking' [119].

iii) Catherine McGovern:
- Advisor in the Howard government.
- Head of Government Affairs and Policy for GlaxoSmithKline.
- General Manager of Government and Public Affairs at Medibank.
- Associate at the Agenda Group, another corporate PR firm that "*exhausts all possibilities*" to deliver for their clients [120].

iv) Kieran Schneemann:
- Chief of Staff to a former Senator, and also a former Coalition minister.
- Director of Government Affairs for AstraZeneca

pharmaceutical company.
- CEO of Medicines Australia, the drug manufacturers peak body.
- Chief Executive of the Pharmacy Guild of Australia
- Associate Director of CanTeen, a charity for young people living with cancer [121].

As Toby Ralph, a marketing strategist who has worked on more than 40 election campaigns, says: "*The pharmaceutical industry is awash with cash, much of it siphoned from the taxpayer. Approved medicines share $6 billion or $7 billion, so dipping the corporate bucket into that deep well is always a priority. The starting point is to prove medical efficacy and social and economic benefit, but that just secures a seat at the roulette table. Next they hire people with strong connections to the decision makers. There's no shortage of willing employees, as the rewards can far exceed the pittance of political stipends* [122].

The same 'revolving door' system is evident in the United States, too.

For example, in 2015, Assemblyman Henry Perea resigned from the legislature and took up a lucrative job offer with the Pharmaceutical Research and Manufacturers of America, who represent the major pharmaceutical and biotech companies. State law forbids him from lobbying his former colleagues for a period of 12 months following his tenure [123].

Over 300 former Congressional staffers now work for pharmaceutical companies, or their lobbying firms, and at least 12 former pharmaceutical employees now have jobs on Capitol Hill – often on committees that handle health-care policy [124].

In many cases, those who have moved from politics to pharmaceutical companies, are now lobbying their former work colleagues and employees. Diana Zuckerman, president of the National Center for Health Research says *"You'll take the call because you've got a friendly relationship… You'll take the call because these people are going to help you in your future career [and] get you a job making three times as much"* [124].

How much has the drug industry influenced the increasingly draconian vaccine mandates enacted by governments around the world?

In 2015, the Australian government amended social welfare laws, cancelling certain payments to families if their children were not up-to-date with the current vaccination schedule. These laws are known as "No Jab, No Pay". Conscientious objections are no longer allowed, only a medical exemption is accepted, which must be signed by a licensed general practitioner [125].

But what medical conditions warrant a medical exemption, according to the Australian government?

Not many, it seems. Family history of vaccine adverse reactions won't cut it. Neither will past history of convulsions - not good enough! Allergies and asthma won't get you an exemption, neither will neurological disorders. A 'poorly-recorded' vaccine history (as may be the case for some migrants or refugees) is not enough reason for exemption - if you've already had the vaccines, you get to have them again! Infants born prematurely don't get exemptions, or even a gestation-adjusted delayed schedule. Imminent or recent surgery is not a good enough reason, either [126].

There are really only two contraindictions that qualifies for a medical exemption, and only then for a specific vaccine, not for the entire schedule. Those two contraindictions are: anaphylaxis to a prior dose of that vaccine, or anaphylaxis to a component of the vaccine (gelatin, egg etc).

You *may* get a medical exemption, from live virus vaccines only, if you are severely immunocompromised, such as those undergoing chemotherapy, or with active HIV infection [126].

So, basically, prior adverse reactions - even ones that result in life-long damage - are not regarded as serious enough to warrant exemption from future vaccines.

State laws in the United States, such as SB277 which came into effect in California, in 2016, have begun to implement mandates that mean unvaccinated children are excluded from childcare or school, unless they can provide a medical exemption [127].

Medical exemptions in the state of California tripled, and in early 2019, news reports claimed that some medical doctors were 'selling' vaccine exemptions to parents who wanted to avoid vaccinations for their children [128-129].

In response, Senator Richard Pan (who also wrote the SB277 bill) introduced another bill that would require all medical exemptions be vetted by the State Health Department, and "create a database of which doctors are granting the exemptions" [130].

One wonders how government mandates manage to satisfy valid consent requirements [131]:

"For consent to be legally valid, the following elements must be present:

i) It must be given by a person with legal capacity, and of sufficient intellectual capacity to understand the implications of being vaccinated.
ii) It must be given voluntarily **_in the absence of undue pressure, coercion or manipulation_**.
iii) It must cover the specific procedure that is to be performed.
iv) It can only be given after the potential risks and benefits of the relevant vaccine, risks of not having it and any alternative options have been explained to the individual."

7) Drug companies influence the agencies who are meant to regulate them…

It might come as a surprise to discover that, in the United States, United Kingdom, Canada, and Australia, the regulatory authorities that oversee vaccine and drug safety, are 100% *funded by the industry* [132-135]. It's called a 'cost recovery' model, so that governments don't have to fund the agency, but instead, forces the agencies to operate like a business.

Agency employees are forced to police the customers who pay their wages. There's an old saying 'Don't bite the hand that feeds you'. Does that apply here?

According to Dr. Michael Carome, director of the health

research group Public Citizen, an advocacy group in Washington, the US system faces severe shortcomings. He says:

"The FDA's lax oversight is an unintended consequence of the Prescription Drug User Fee Act of 1992, which required pharmaceutical companies to subsidize the FDA's work. The act effectively turned companies into 'customers' of the agency, and the agency has since been inclined to treat them accordingly."

"Too often the FDA is not an effective regulator. They are often too slow to act when there are serious problems. The [pharmaceutical] industry is more like a client or customer of the agency, and less like a regulated entity" [136].

The Centers for Disease Control (CDC) also benefits from vaccines via licensing agreements [137-138]. Can an agency that benefits financially from a product, be trusted to make unbiased recommendations?

A House of Representatives Government Reform Committee which looked into conflicts of interest in the FDA and CDC, following the withdrawal of the Rotashield vaccine, just months after it hit the market, concluded:

"The Committee's investigation has determined that conflict of interest rules employed by the FDA and CDC have been weak, enforcement has been lax, and committee members with substantial ties to the pharmaceutical companies have been given waivers to participate in committee meetings" [139].

In addition to widespread conflicts of interest amongst regulatory agencies and their staff members, numerous reviews have been scathing in their assessment of the FDA.

For example, in 2007, a sub-committee commissioned by the acting FDA commissioner at the time, investigated the FDA and put together its findings in the Science and Mission at Risk Report [140].

Some of the key findings were that the agency suffered from serious scientific deficiencies, was not positioned to meet current or emerging regulatory responsibilities, lacks sufficient controls, reports of product dangers are still handwritten and slow to make their way through the system, inadequate emergency back-up systems in place, which had resulted in lost data.

Their conclusion was: "*There is a long history of excellent reviews of the FDA that have been **followed by little to no action taken to achieve the recommendations**. Our final recommendation is based on our belief that effective resolution of the issues outlined in this report is urgent. In contrast to previous reports that have issued many of the same warnings, **there are now sufficient data proving that failure to act in the past have jeopardized the public's health**"*.

Conflicts of interest are also evident in government advisory panels. Many of those holding positions on government advisory boards are either currently, or were formerly, involved in financial arrangements with pharmaceutical companies.

In the US, the advisory panel that makes recommendations to the CDC Director, regarding vaccines, is the Advisory Committee on Immunization Practices (ACIP). A 1999 report in the Medical Sentinel had this to say about ACIP [141]:

"The Advisory Committee on Immunization Practices (ACIP), a group of individuals hand picked by the Center for Disease Control (CDC), recommends which vaccines are administered to American children. **Working mainly in secret, ACIP members frequently have financial links to vaccine manufacturers**. *Dependent on CDC funding, state vaccination programs follow CDC directives by influencing state legislatures to mandate new vaccines. Federal vaccine funds can be denied to states which do not "rigorously enforce" mandatory vaccination laws. Conversely,* **the CDC offers financial bounties to state health departments for each fully vaccinated child**".

The advisory committee to the Food and Drug Administration (FDA), is the Vaccines and Related Biological Products Advisory Committee (VRBPAC). This committee, too, was found to suffer from conflicts of interests, which included [142]:

- voting members sitting on the committee for long periods of time, despite term limits,
- voting members owning stocks in vaccine companies,
- voting members involved in development and licensing of vaccines,
- voting members being recipients of large sums of research grant money from pharmaceutical companies.

The report concluded that *'the overwhelming majority of members, both voting members and consultants, have substantial ties to the pharmaceutical industry"* [142].

Many FDA assessors go on to lucrative positions within the pharmaceutical industry.

In 2018, Wellington Sun, former director of the Division of Vaccines and Related Products Applications at the FDA, took up a position with biotech company, Moderna – as their new head of 'vaccine strategy and regulatory affairs' [143].

Also, in the past two years [143]:

- Sarah Pope Miksinski, former director of New Drug Products in the FDA Office of Pharmaceutical Quality, left to become senior director of Global Regulatory Affairs at AstraZeneca.

- Patrick Frey, former chief-of-staff at FDA Office of New Drugs, left to become director of global regulatory policy at Amgen.

- John Jenkins, former director of the FDA Office of New Drugs, was appointed to the board of Corbus Pharmaceuticals.

- Niraj Mehta, former associate director for global regulatory policy at the FDA, left to become director of Global Quality Compliance at Merck.

- Thomas Cosgrove, former director of FDA's Office of Manufacturing Quality in the Office of Compliance, left to join law firm Covington & Burling – who claim to be the 'recognized leader in representing clients on FDA and related regulatory matters involving human pharmaceuticals and biotechnology products'. Covington & Burling also represents industry stakeholders in negotiations to change legislation [143-144].

One study published in the British Medical Journal, which looked at the careers of oncology/haematology assessors at the Food and Drug Administration, found that more than half went on to work in the pharmaceutical industry [145].

Dr. Vinay Prasad, senior author of the paper, and Assistant Professor of Medicine at Oregon Health and Science University, wonders if *"reviewers might make more favorable calculations if they are looking ahead to more lucrative industry work in the future"* [146].

The current secretary of the Department of Health and Human Services (HHS), Alex Azar was formerly a pharmaceutical lobbyist, and President of the US division of pharmaceutical giant Eli Lilly and Co. It's not Azar's first stint at the HHS – between 2001 and 2007, he held other influential positions within the department [147].

Britain, it would seem, suffers from the same vested interests. When the UK rolled out the Meningitis C program for infants in 2000, it was discovered that four members on its advisory panel had financial ties to the companies who make meningitis C vaccines [148].

Not only are regulatory agencies in the US, UK, Australia and Canada funded by industry, they also rely on industry to conduct the trials, provide the safety data, and notify them of any issues that may arise post-licensure. The agencies themselves do not conduct clinical trials [149-152].

In an ideal world, such a situation would not pose a problem.

But what about when we are dealing with an industry that has a history of behaving as a law unto themselves?

According to Transparency International, up to $300 million global health expenditure is lost every year to corruption and errors. Tactics include paying doctors to participate in surveys of medicines they have never actually prescribed, and companies secretly ghost-writing clinical trials research before passing it off as the work of impartial academics.

Bribery and corruption, the report says, also allow some companies to get around manufacturing regulations, helping to create a situation where about a quarter of medicines consumed in low and middle-income countries are falsified or sub-standard [153].

And '*since 1991, the industry has paid $30bn in criminal fines in the US for Medicare fraud, unlawful promotion, kickbacks, monopolistic practices and failure to disclose clinical trial data, yet this is less than half of what the industry made in 2009 alone*" [153].

Here's a brief look at a few examples:

2006: Merck releases 25 gallons of cyanide chemical into the sewer, polluting a nearby creek and killing more than 1000 fish. The chemical was being used to scale up an experimental vaccine, but when the scale-up plans were abandoned, employees dumped the cyanide down the drain [154].

Merck was not only found guilty of breaching numerous

environmental laws, they were also accused by officials from the state's Department of Environmental Protection (DEP) of repeatedly delaying or impeding investigations into the incident [155].

2010: Council of Europe hearings into the World Health Organization's handling of the swine flu outbreak. The inquiry hears that pharmaceutical companies pressured the World Health Organization into changing criteria so that the swine flu outbreak qualified as a 'pandemic'. Allegedly, this was so that pharmaceutical companies could recoup the costs incurred by research and development of new vaccines after the avian influenza scare of 2006. The decision led to millions of people being vaccinated against what turned out to be a mild illness [156].

2011: Merck pleads guilty to illegal, off-label promotion of the drug Vioxx [157], a painkiller that killed up to 60,000 Americans, according to some estimates - as many as died in the Vietnam War [158].

2012: GlaxoSmithKline agrees to plead guilty to criminal charges, and pays $3 billion in fines, for unlawful promotion of certain drugs, failure to report safety data, and alleged false price reporting practices [159].

2014: GlaxoSmithKline is found guilty of bribing doctors in China, and fined $490 million [160].

2016: UK's competition watchdog fines GlaxoSmithKline £37 million for allegedly paying off other manufacturers to delay entry of cheaper generic medicines onto the market [161].

2016: A US federal judge finds Merck guilty of lying to a business partner in a patent dispute, and lying to the courts. She referred to the company's behaviour as "systematic and outrageous deception in conjunction with unethical business practices and litigation misconduct", which included lying, misusing confidential information, breaching confidentiality agreements, and lying under oath [162].

2017: European Union threatens to fine Merck for providing misleading data during takeover proceedings [163].

These are just a few of the instances that we know about.

Emmanuel Stamatakis from the University of Sydney's School of Public Health says it's 'entirely irresponsible' to rely on drug companies to fund necessary research. *"The profits involved are just too large and the temptation to manipulate the evidence is difficult to resist, even when this may lead to the loss of lives"*, Dr Stamatakis said.

"Asking corporate sponsors to conduct pivotal trials on their own products is like asking a painter to judge their own painting to receive an award [164].

5.
VACCINE SAFETY STUDIES

In the early 1990's, the Evidence Based Medicine Working Group announced a 'new paradigm' in medicine, that would henceforth guide the way medicine is taught and practiced [1]. Tradition, reasoning and anecdote were cast by the wayside, in favour of evidence from randomised, controlled trials and observational studies.

There were benefits to such an approach, in that treatments now had to be shown to be effective, rather than just blindly followed because 'that's how we've always done it'.

But there was a very real and concerning drawback - the balance of power quickly swung towards those with the financial clout to fund the science. The 'evidence' was soon misappropriated and distorted to suit vested interests, and such an overwhelming volume of it quickly accumulated, as to be unmanageable for the average doctor [2].

This state-of-affairs can be clearly seen in the vaccine issue today. Thousands upon thousands of parents complain of adverse reactions after vaccines, and they are largely overlooked by the medical fraternity, because the clinical trials – often funded by the industry – purportedly showed the vaccine to be 'safe'.

In the last decade, the number of clinical trials funded by the pharmaceutical industry has increased by more than 40%, while government-funded trials have decreased [3].

Almost 75% of U.S. clinical trials in medicine are now funded by the pharmaceutical industry [4]. Naturally, the industry has a huge financial stake in the outcome of these clinical trials - a phase III clinical trial may enrol 1000 - 5000 people over many years, and cost hundreds of millions of dollars to complete. Average cost per trial participant is around $36,000 [5].

In 2013, the biopharmaceutical industry spent almost $10 billion directly on clinical trials in the United States alone [5].

The usual route for new drugs/vaccines follow the following clinical trial pattern:

Phase I: Usually small numbers (20-100) of healthy volunteers, to ascertain safety and dosage.

Phase II: Usually involves up to several hundred people with the disease/condition, or fits the user profile, to ascertain efficacy and side-effects.

Phase III: Involves several hundred to several thousand volunteers with the disease/condition, to monitor efficacy and adverse reactions.

Phase IV: Sometimes referred to as 'post-marketing surveillance'. Collecting data on adverse events, etc, once the drug/vaccine has entered the market.

What effect does this heavily-vested interest have on the outcome of trials, which are then used by regulatory agencies to assist in decision-making?

10 WAYS THAT DRUG COMPANIES CAN MANIPULATE SCIENCE

1) By choosing participants most likely to give the desired results.

According to Wikipedia: "*Selection bias is the bias introduced by the selection of individuals, groups or data for analysis in such a way that proper randomization is not achieved, thereby ensuring that the sample obtained is not representative of the population intended to be analyzed. It is sometimes referred to as the selection effect*" [6].

Basically, what it means is that you can skew the results in the direction you desire, by choosing, or excluding certain participants from your study.

Let's take a closer look at one example:

A phase 4 clinical trial, sponsored by Merck, titled "Hepatitis A Vaccine, Inactivated and Measles, Mumps, Rubella and Varicella Virus Vaccine Live Safety Study" called for children aged 12mths to 17mths [7].

You could be considered for inclusion if:
- You were in the appropriate age-group, and,

- Had a negative clinical history of hepatitis A, measles, mumps, rubella, varicella (chickenpox), and/or zoster.
- Had no other vaccinations scheduled to be administered at the time of the first or second doses of VAQTA(TM) and ProQuad(TM).

You would NOT be considered for inclusion, if:

- You had been previously vaccinated with any hepatitis A vaccine, measles, mumps, rubella, and/or varicella vaccine either alone or in any combination.
- You had a history of allergy to any vaccine component.
- You had a history of seizure disorder.
- You were immunosuppressed (including congenial and acquired conditions and immunosuppressive therapy).
- You had a known severe thrombocytopenia or any other coagulation disorder that would contraindicate intramuscular injections.
- You had a recent (<72 hours) febrile illness (>100.3 degrees F [>37.9 degrees C] oral equivalent) prior to study vaccination.

Excluding those with history of allergies, seizure disorders or recent illnesses seems to be standard procedure for vaccine clinical trials, and understandably so.

The problem is that the results of those clinical trials are extrapolated, and assumed to apply to the rest of the population, which includes those with history of allergies, history of seizure disorders, immunosuppressed, blood disorders and recent illnesses.

2) By following up for inadequate time periods.

Vaccines can cause adverse reactions in two ways - either via direct action on the tissues and organs by a component of the vaccines (such as aluminium), or via the body's own inflammatory response to the vaccine, and this can be either immediate and acute (Type I hypersensitivity), or later, and more chronic (Type III hypersensitivity).

Given that antibodies can take 2 - 4 weeks to reach peak levels on first exposure, and 3 - 10 days on subsequent exposures, one would expect that many adverse reactions (perhaps even the majority), would not become noticeable until those time-frames following vaccination.

And yet, so many safety studies do not even extend to capture side-effects during those time-frames.

Take, for example, the safety studies found on the insert for Infanrix Hexa, a 6-in-1 vaccine recommended for children aged 6 weeks, 4 months, 6 months, and again at 4 years of age in Australia (and other countries).

The insert includes results from five clinical trials. Three of the five studies followed participants for four days following vaccination.

One study followed up participants for only 48 hours following vaccination. The fifth study, which involved diary entries completed by parents, for 30 days following injection, however, adverse reactions were only specifically solicited for 8 days following vaccination. Only *select reactions* within the first 7 days are included in the insert [8].

According to Accord Clinical Research, Phase 4 trials "*are conducted to identify and evaluate the **long-term** effects of new drugs and treatments over a **lengthy** period for a greater number of patients*" [9].

In the case of Merck's study of Hepatitis A and MMR-V vaccines, the 'lengthy period' was 28 days following vaccination, *for minor side-effects*, and only 14 days following vaccination, for serious **vaccine-related** adverse events (why do serious reactions require a shorter time period?) [10]. As we will soon uncover, most adverse events are not deemed to be related to the vaccine anyway.

3) **By comparing one vaccine with another vaccine, or a combination of vaccines against another combination of vaccines, instead of comparing a vaccine with a placebo saline injection.**

To illustrate this point, I went to pubmed and typed in "safety immunogenicity vaccine". The following is a random sample of the search results.

 - "Immunogenicity and safety of an E. coli-produced bivalent human papillomavirus (type 16 and 18) vaccine: A randomized controlled phase 2 clinical trial."

(Compared a human papillomavirus vaccine with a Hepatitis B vaccine as the 'control') [11].

- "Immunogenicity and safety of a quadrivalent inactivated influenza vaccine compared with two trivalent inactivated influenza vaccines containing alternate B strains in adults: A phase 3, randomized noninferiority study."

(*Compared an influenza vaccine with other influenza vaccines*) [12].

- "The Immunogenicity and Safety of a Combined DTaP-IPV//Hib Vaccine Compared with Individual DtaP-IPV and Hib (PRP~T) Vaccines: a Randomized Clinical Trial in South Korean Infants."

(*Compares a combined vaccine with individual vaccines*) [13].

- "Immunogenicity and safety of a CRM-conjugated meningococcal ACWY vaccine administered concomitantly with routine vaccines starting at 2 months of age."

(*Studied a meningococcal vaccine, administered at same time as other vaccines*) [14].

- "Safety and immunogenicity of 13-valent pneumococcal conjugate vaccine in infants: a meta-analysis."

(*Compares a 7-strain vaccine with a 13-strain vaccine*) [15].

4) Use an unsuitable placebo, or simply fail to disclose what placebo was used.

The Collins Dictionary defines placebo as "*an inactive substance or other sham form of therapy administered to a patient usually to compare its effects with those of a real drug or treatment, but sometimes for the psychological benefit to the patient through his believing he is receiving treatment"* [16].

It seems rather odd then, that some scientists would consider an aluminium injection to constitute 'an inactive substance', suitable for use as a control in medical research. This is precisely what happened in the Phase 3 trial for Gardasil - the 'placebo' contained adjuvant, which happened to be aluminium hydroxide [17].

That particular trial was funded by the manufacturer, Merck, and the authors were either Merck employees and/or members of Merck-funded steering committees or advisory boards.

Although randomized, placebo-controlled trials are widely accepted as being the best way to evaluate the safety and efficacy of a treatment, there are many who argue that placebo-controlled trials are unethical, because the control group are denied treatment [18].

According to a World Health Organization Expert panel, there are clearly situations where placebo-controls are acceptable in vaccine trials: "Placebo use in vaccine trials is clearly *acceptable* when (a) no efficacious and safe vaccine exists (as was the case for Gardasil, being a new and unproven vaccine, at the time) and (b) the vaccine under consideration is intended to benefit the population in which the vaccine is to be tested [19].

Of those studies that do use placebo, the vast majority do not disclose the contents of the 'placebo'. One review found that up to 92% of studies do not disclose what placebo is used [20].

5) Dismiss adverse reactions as not being related to the vaccine in question.

Consider the following examples:

Safety study on influenza vaccine - funded, conducted and reported by GlaxoSmithKline, which actually used a saline placebo control group [21]: "*Nine participants reported 17* **serious** *adverse events;* **none were considered causally related to vaccination**."

No reasons are given as to how or why this conclusion was reached.

Note that this study only allowed healthy adults to take part, following medical history and physical examination. Anybody with prior or familial history of narcolepsy or sleep disorders was excluded. Anybody with prior history of known or suspected allergy was excluded. Anybody with a history of cancer within previous three years was excluded. Anybody with a previous history of neurological or psychiatric disorders was excluded. Anybody with previous history of Guillain-Barre syndrome following influenza vaccine in the past was excluded. Anybody whose screening blood tests did not fall within normal range was excluded. Pregnant women were excluded [22].

Note that the people excluded from taking part in the trials are usually not excluded from receiving the end product! In fact, sometimes they are especially targeted to receive the vaccine.

Consider also a clinical trial of rotavirus vaccine, being injected either concomitantly with, or separate from, a meningococcal vaccine:

"Another infant from group 2 had a nonserious allergy (hypersensitivity) of moderate intensity 5 days after the third dose of RotaTeq which was **not considered to be related to the study vaccine**".

"Only two serious adverse events occurred, one in each group. One infant in group 1 had an episode of epilepsy of moderate intensity, starting 13 days after visit 4, and one infant in group 2 had a severe viral infection, starting 9 days after visit 5. The events resolved in 4 and 7 days, respectively, and were **not considered to be related to either study vaccine**. No deaths occurred in either group. There was one withdrawal from the study due to an adverse event, a dark green loose stool that occurred 3 days after the second dose of RotaTeq; this was (naturally!) **not considered to be related to the study vaccine**" [23].

It really begs the question... who was doing the 'considering', and how did they arrive at such considerations? There is no further information published on the matter, to enlighten us, but the conclusion was thus: "The *convenience* of concomitant administration of RotaTeq and MenCC may, however, outweigh the additive effect of mostly mild adverse events reported after the individual administration of each vaccine."

In other words, giving both vaccines at the same time increases adverse reactions, but it's more *convenient* that way.

Now consider a clinical trial for combined tetanus, diptheria and pertussis vaccine, given during pregnancy or post-partum:

"**Serious adverse event**s were reported by 22 participants, including 7 (21.2%) women who received Tdap during pregnancy and 6 (18.1%) of their infants, 2 (13.3%) women given Tdap postpartum and 6 (40%) of their infants, and 1 (3.1%) non-pregnant woman."

By this point, the reader will hardly be surprised to learn that **"none were judged to be attributable to Tdap vaccine** [24].

6) 'Cherry-picking' the data.

A meta-analysis looks at data from multiple studies, and are used as part of systematic review. Naturally, these are useful and important in the interpretation of data, and hold a lot of weight for scientific advisory and review committees.

A systematic review of vaccine meta-analyses, however, found that the methodological quality of all 121 meta-analyses (100%) included in the review, was *unsatisfactory.*

"The most frequent limitations include non-comprehensive bibliographic research; bias in the selection of the studies; lack of quality assessment of individual studies; absence of evaluation of heterogeneity among studies and publication bias" [25].

7) Cut the study short if it doesn't provide favourable outcomes.

Trials can be terminated early for financial reasons (cost-saving), rather than scientific or ethical reasons [26.]. One trial was aborted two years early 'for commercial reasons', after rates of withdrawal from treatment were higher than expected [27].

In 1996, two drug trials were cancelled by the drug company when unexpected risks were identified and toxicity reported. Not only did the drug company, Apotex, terminate the trials, it attempted to 'gag' the principal investigator from discussing the results, or even informing the patients involved [28].

In this situation, the research or educational institution can also apply pressure on the researcher to acquiesce to drug company demands, in an attempt to protect future research grants [29].

8) Relying on assumptions.

When you hear that a vaccine is '95% effective', what it often means is that 95% of people in clinical trials developed the required measure of antibodies.

It's called *immunogenicity*. Unfortunately, as we have already seen, immunogenicity does not necessarily equate to immunity.

Take Infanrix, for example - the combined diptheria-tetanus-pertussis vaccine - only the pertussis component has been tested in a real-world scenario. The diptheria and tetanus components were assessed and approved based solely on the antibody response of participants [30].

The meningococcal vaccine for A, C, Y and W strains, manufactured by Sanofi Pasteur was assessed and approved based on serum antibody levels in clinical trial participants [31].

According to the World Health Organization, "*if the aim of the clinical study is to evaluate the ability of the vaccine to provide protection against infection, often large numbers of patients must be enrolled in the study to generate sufficient data to be statistically meaningful. When protection against disease is not a suitable outcome of the clinical study, measurement of immune responses to the vaccine could be an alternative approach. However, this must be defined based on scientific **assumptions** and require confirmation of clinical efficacy **after its approval***" [32].

A closer investigation reveals that, surprisingly, assumptions and beliefs are widespread in the field of vaccinology.

For example, this startling admission came from a 2002 FDA workshop on non-clinical safety of vaccines [33]:

"*Historically, the non-clinical safety assessment for preventative vaccines has often not included toxicity studies in animal models. This is because vaccines **have not been viewed as inherently toxic***" (my emphasis).

(Hardly what you'd call evidence-based.)

And this, from the World Health Organization (WHO) special committee on the Safety of Vaccines, in 2005 [34]:

"The Committee considered the safety of adjuvants used in vaccines. This hitherto neglected subject is becoming increasingly important given modern advances in vaccine development and manufacture".

At that point, adjuvants had been used for some 90 years, injected into millions of people, yet it had received little scientific scrutiny.

In 2006, Zinka et al met with criticism after publishing research on unexplained cases of Sudden Infant Death following hexavalent vaccination. They rebutted with this [35]:

"The main problem is that vaccination specialists have failed for decades to establish any tests or other criteria to find out if adverse events are linked to vaccinations or not".

Similarly, a case report of Sudden Infant Death cases following hexavalent vaccination referenced a review conducted by the European Medicines Agency Pathologists panel, which found no explanation for cause of death. The authors noted [36]:

"...to the best of our knowledge, during the mentioned postmortem investigations, little, if any, attention was paid to examination of the brainstem and the cardiac conduction systems on serial sections, nor was the possibility of a triggering role of the vaccine in the lethal outcome considered".

Also, from the European Medicines Agency: "*Vaccines for pandemic or bioterrorism risk are given even less consideration: Special consideration is needed for the clinical development of vaccines when protective efficacy studies are not feasible and when there is no established immunological correlate of protection. For example, vaccines intended to prevent rare infections that carry considerable morbidity and mortality including some pathogens that have the potential to cause widespread disruption to mankind in case of an epidemic or deliberate release. Applicants seeking a marketing authorisation for such a vaccine should discuss considerations for the basis on which authorisation might be possible with EU Competent Authorities at the earliest stages of development*" [37].

And..."*If authorisation has had to be based on such limited data, it may not be possible to estimate vaccine effectiveness in the post-authorisation period unless a substantial natural epidemic or deliberate release occurs. In any case it is likely that reliable data can only be obtained from national surveillance programmes operated by public health authorities*" [37].

9) Fail to publish unfavourable results.

Failing all that, a drug company may simply decide not to publish unfavourable trial results, even though doing so is considered to be scientific malpractice [38].

Research reveals that, less than half of government-funded clinical trial results are published in peer-reviewed medical journals within 30 months of trial completion [39].

One pharmaceutical company managed to suppress trial results for seven years, when they revealed that the drug in question was no more effective than cheaper generic formulations [40].

Drug companies withholding trial data cost governments around the world an estimated *$20 billion*, when they made the decision to purchase and stock-pile supplies of Tamiflu, which turned out to be based on 'slim and skewed representation of the total evidence base' [41]. In other words, the company - Roche - had neglected to publish or share data that would have raised serious concerns about their product.

The full clinical trial data was finally released after a 5-year campaign by the Cochrane Review Collaboration, and the conclusion must have made governments squirm, when they realized they had spent $20 billion of public funds, on a treatment of dubious efficacy and considerable side-effects [42].

10)   Fail to consider those who discontinue the study

Those who discontinue the study due to side effects are often not included in the end results. How might this affect the end results? In one vaccine trial, as many as 20% of participants failed to complete the trial [43].

Pharmaceutical companies have also designed other ways of manipulating 'science' [44]. These include:

i) Seeding trials: Where a drug company induces a doctor to prescribe a certain medication to their patients, in order to gain feedback on the product. These are usually scientifically meaningless, have no clear end-points, but they are large-scale so represent considerable sales for the company. The doctor usually gets paid to enter patients in the trial.

ii) Switching trials: This is a variant of the seeding trial. Doctors are recruited to switch their patients from their usual treatment, to a new treatment. Again, the drug companies know that this will often lead to long-term customers.

iii) Post-marketing surveillance: This is yet another variant of the seeding and switching trials, although with more scientific justification, as they are often published, and can provide important data on adverse effects. Again, doctors are paid substantial sums, and the patients may believe they are getting new and 'better' treatments.

iv) Dosage: The dose can be manipulated in order to give the desired results. For example, a competitor drug may be given at less-than-optimal dosage, to make the studied drug look more effective. Or the competitor drug may be given at higher-than-optimal dosages, to make the studied drug look safer.

v) Economic evaluations: These can be easy to manipulate, because they are too complex for the average journal editor or reader to fully understand.

Analysis shows that trials funded by the industry are 5x more likely to recommend the experimental drug as treatment of choice, *regardless of whether the results justify it, or not* [45].

The scientists who design, conduct, analyze and report on clinical trials may also receive financial reimbursement from drug companies, in the form of salaries, consulting fees, or speaking engagements [46].

Despite the vast amount of 'evidence' produced by drug companies claiming vaccine safety, anecdotal evidence continues to tell a different story.

Online forums and social media comments sections are awash with victims, and guilt-ridden parents, who followed medical advice, and then paid the price. I posed the question about vaccine reactions to my social media followers, and these were some of comments I received:

"My daughter was left severely brain injured after her 4-month vaccine ... she could no longer roll over or lift her head and had severe seizures for many years. That was in 1979."

"In 1970 my brother died within 24 hours of receiving this [the Tdap shot] at his 4-month visit."

"It [the tdap vaccine] gave me psoriasis that covers 90% of my body. Destroyed my immune system."

"My son is adopted and was in foster care. We were told that we didn't have a choice but to vaccinate him. With his 4-month vaccines, he developed a respiratory infection. At his 12-month vaccines he developed asthma. I just got it cleared up and at his 18-month vaccines, the asthma came back and he also lost his speech, coordination, awareness of his surroundings and so on."

"[The vaccine] Gave my son eczema and food allergies. Also behaviour changes which turned into an autism diagnosis."

"My daughter developed tics after her dtap at her 6-month checkup (we were actually behind, she was 7 months when I took her in for the 6 months appointment). She stopped babbling, stopped eye contact, the list goes on."

"My daughter reacted seriously to the DTaP but we kept vaccinating. She ended up with serious asthma, allergies, brain injury and eventually died last year of an asthma attack."

"Back in the 1970's in Australia I was given the DTP vaccine. My parents said I began screaming uncontrollably for 24 hours, I began convulsing, hallucinating, high temperature. Of course the doctors brushed it off. It was later discovered I had permanent one-sided deafness."

"My son was developing normally up until the age of 23 months. He was vaccinated up until 6 months of age, I decided to delay the 12-month shots and had them at 23 months instead ... Big mistake ... my son was given all the catch-up vaccines and two other new ones all at once, That was seven shots at once!! My poor son was inconsolable but I managed to put him on my breast to calm him. From that day, everything changed ... he became absent, no eye contact, couldn't stand being touched, started obsessing over one subject, started spinning, having meltdowns, couldn't sleep through the night, no longer engaged in two-way conversations, became anxious, had bowel problems, became fussy with food and would only eat the same foods, same colour, began routines. Couldn't stand baths anymore or water on his

face..didn't like shoes on his feet anymore, certain clothes, I couldn't use the vacuum cleaner anymore or loud sounds, the dark etc ... .. I am totally convinced this was due to the multiple vaccine shots. He was later diagnosed with High Functioning Autism".

"At my child's 4-month series she got para infectious encephalitis. We now have a medical exemption and no longer vaccinate."

"At her 6-months vaccines I took her in on schedule to be vaccinated. Only a few minutes later she started seizing. The doctors called for an ambulance to bring her to the hospital, on route she stopped breathing. At the hospital they decided she needed to be airlifted to the nearest children's hospital. Once at Children's hospital she was put on full life support. Then a shunt was placed to stop the pressure on her brain due to excess fluid. Then a few days later she developed sepsis due to bacteria in her blood. She spent 3 months fighting for her life. She survived but her life has been destroyed. She has up 15 seizures a day, autistic, brain damage and many other health issues. She has so many seizures even on medication that most of the time she is bed ridden."

"My daughter suffered hives around the ears, face, neck and diaper area for weeks. At all hours of the day. The hives have gone but she now deals with itchy eczema. This was at 4 months old after just one vaccination - the infanrix hexa."

"My son is now 15, had horrible speech delays, lost speech and eye contact after his MMR."

Over the last several years, I have seen, and heard, thousands of stories like these. What are the chances, that:

a) All of them (or even most of them) are making it up?
b) All of them (or even most of them) have faulty memory?
c) All of them (or even most of them) are just coincidental?

At what point does anecdotal evidence bear any weight in the world of science? Apparently, anecdote counts when it comes to other drugs and medications – a patient's verbal declaration of adverse effects occurring after the use of a drug is sufficient to change or withdraw the drug from treatment.

Sadly, a patient's verbal declaration of adverse effects occurring after vaccination is likely to be met with scorn or disbelief – I have experienced that first-hand.

Despite our zeal for 'evidence'-based medicine, there are some glaring gaps in vaccine science...

What is NOT Studied:

LONG-TERM SIDE EFFECTS

Vaccines are not required to be tested for long-term side-effects, such as carcinogenicity (ability to cause cancer), mutagenicity (ability to alter or damage DNA), and ability to impair fertility.

This is clearly admitted in vaccine inserts from the manufacturers [47-48]. With increasing rates of childhood cancers, adult cancers occurring in epidemic proportion, and global fertility rates plummeting, why is this vital research area being over-looked? If a certain cancer takes decades to develop, how can we be sure it wasn't triggered, or affected, by childhood vac-cines, given many decades ago?

Cancer

The most common age for childhood cancer in Australia, is in the 0-4 years age group - the same time period where the aver-age child receives more than 40 doses of vaccines. The second most common age is in the 10-14 years age group, which coin-cides with the scheduled booster shots, and HPV vaccines, for secondary school.

The least represented age group in childhood cancer statistics, is the 5-9 years, which happens to coincide with a period where the average Australian child receives no vaccines, or a yearly flu vaccine, at the most [49].

It is also interesting to note that the most common type of can-cer in Australian children is acute lymphoblastic leukemia [49]. This occurs when there is an overproduction of immature white blood cells in the bone marrow, which prevents the production of red blood cells [50]. It seems plausible that chronic activa-tion of the immune system could potentially cause such a state of affairs – a theory that has already been explored in the scien-tific literature [51-52].

We have already seen that excessive stimulation of humoral im-munity (antibody production) results in suppression of cell-mediated immunity. This exact imbalance has already been shown to play a central role in facilitating tumour growth, invasion, and metastasis [51].

In 2001, a letter published in the Daily Mail, went as follows *"My daughter had the MMR booster at four and her arm immediately swelled up and she started to feel unwell. Within six weeks, she was diagnosed as having leukaemia, and the doctors we spoke to accepted that the MMR jab was probably the trigger for the disease by overloading her immune system — though they believe she may have been already susceptible to the illness"* [53].

In 1965, Dr. Michael Innis, an Australian pathologist and haematologist, wrote to The Lancet, and outlined how rates of leukemia in children at Brisbane Children's Hospital between 1958 to 1964 showed a statistically significant association with diptheria-tetanus-pertussis vaccination [54].

In 1994, researchers found that MMR vaccination (among other things) increased the odds ratio of childhood acute lymphocytic leukemia [55].

Researchers in 2007 proposed a correlation between childhood leukemia and the introduction of widespread diptheria vaccination – *"the significant peak-age (2–5 years) first appeared after 1940 in Great Britain. Since then, childhood leukemia has almost unchangeable incidence. In 1940 the introduction of immunization against diphtheria on a national scale was begun in Great Britain"* [56].

In a study of oral cancer patients in Nigeria, those with cancer were found to have significantly higher levels of antibodies, than healthy controls [57]. Did the cancer cause a shift towards antibody production, or did the immune imbalance cause the cancer?

It was demonstrated as early as 1907, that an inappropriate immune response enhances tumour growth [58-59]. In the 1950's, the phenomena of antibodies promoting tumour growth was labelled 'immunological enhancement' [60].

Several years ago, researchers stimulated blood cultures from BCG-vaccinated and unvaccinated infants, with tuberculosis bacterium for 6 days, then measured cytokine levels. Some pro-inflammatory cytokines were as much as 1000 times greater in vaccinated cultures, than unvaccinated [61]. One of the elevated cytokines was Interleukin-6 (IL-6), which has been shown to promote growth of cervical cancer cells [62], prostate cancer [63], and colorectal cancer [64].

Infertility

In 2012, the British Medical Journal published a case report of a 16-year-old girl who received a cervical cancer vaccine towards the end of 2008. Following that, her menstrual periods became irregular and scant, and by 2011, her menstrual cycle had ceased altogether. Upon further inspection, it was discovered that all of her remaining eggs were dead – she was totally and irreversibly infertile, at just 16 years of age [65].

Other cases of premature ovarian failure in young women following vaccination for cervical cancer have since come before the courts [66].

A recent study (2018) analysed information representing 8 million 25-to-29-year-old US women between 2007 and 2014. Approximately 60% of women who did not receive the HPV vaccine had been pregnant at least once, whereas only 35% of women who were exposed to the vaccine had conceived [67]. It is not just the HPV vaccine raising questions about possibly fertility effects. Research also shows increased risk of miscarriage after influenza vaccination during pregnancy [68].

Note also, that multi-dose vials of influenza vaccine still contain mercury in the form of thimerosal – the Chinese were using mercury as an abortifacient up to 5000 years ago [69].

Globally, the fertility rate has more than halved since 1960 [70].

Fifty-nine countries, representing 46% of the global population, now have fertility rates below replacement level [70]. Of course, much of that has been by choice, through women's rights movements, access to contraceptives, changing religious beliefs, along with increased living standards and higher education, but clearly not all of the plummeting fertility rate has been by choice...

An international team of scientists analysed data from nearly 43,000 men, in dozens of industrialized countries, and found that sperm counts have dropped by more than half over the past four decades [71]. Peter Schlegal, Professor and Chairman of Urology at Weill Cornell Medicine in New York, and Vice President of the American Society for Reproductive Medicine, says *"Since this is the best study that's ever been done, it is concerning that it suggests such a progressive and dramatic decrease in sperm counts over time."*

"Since we don't know what could be causing it, it's worrisome" [72].

Numerous studies also reveal that testosterone levels in men have declined substantially over the past decades [73-75].

Over the past decades, girls in Western countries have also been reaching puberty at younger and younger ages... [76]. There is evidence to suggest that earlier puberty, coupled with no children, doubles a woman's risk of early menopause [77].

 Is there a *possibility* that vaccines could somehow contribute to lower sperm counts, earlier puberty and menopause, not to mention the growing numbers of women suffering hormonal issues such as polycystic ovarian syndrome (PCOS), estrogen dominance etc?

Given that no vaccine on the market has been tested long-term, for ability to damage or impair fertility, we are left to theorize about potentials and correlations. Certainly, there are a number of ingredients used in vaccines that are a possible 'red flag'.

These include aluminium and mercury (metalloestrogens), glutaraldehyde (reproductive toxin in females and possibly males) and Cetyltrimethylammonium bromide (possibly causes reproductive and birth defects, based on animal studies).

Those are the ingredients we know about. What about vaccine contaminants?

In 2003, three states in Northern Nigeria boycotted the oral polio vaccine, due to the alleged discovery of contaminants, including trace amounts of estrogen. The boycott lasted for 15 months [78].

In 2015, Catholic Bishops in Kenya announced that they had tested vials of the tetanus vaccine, then being used to vaccinate women of child-bearing age, and found them laced with beta-HCG, a pregnancy hormone [79].

The Catholic Church operates about 30% of health clinics in Kenya, and is not opposed to vaccination, per se [80], but suspicions began to arise over the secrecy surrounding the WHO/UNICEF vaccination campaign (vials were delivered to health clinics under police guard, and empty vials returned to Nairobi, also under police guard), and the unusual policy of 5 doses of tetanus toxoid vaccine, administered every 6 months [81].

One of the laboratories used to test the vaccines for contaminants, Agriq-Quest, later had their license suspended by the Kenyan government. Agriq-Quest, however, claimed it was because they refused to doctor the samples to show the vaccines were clean [82].

As Oller et al (2017) noted [81]: *"...WHO biomedical researchers have been working to engineer such an "anti-fertility" vaccine for "birth-control" at least since 1972. Research published in 1976 confirmed that recipients of a vaccine containing βhCG chemically conjugated with TT (tetanus toxoid) develop antibodies not only against TT but also against βhCG. The result, first reported by WHO researchers at a meeting of the US*

National Academy of Sciences, is a "birth-control" vaccine that diminishes the βhCG essential to a successful pregnancy and causes at least temporary "infertility". Subsequent research showed that repeated doses can extend infertility indefinitely".

During the 1990's, numerous reports surfaced that millions of women in Nicaragua, Mexico and Phillipines had been targeted by WHO 'anti-fertility' vaccination campaigns, under the guise of 'eliminating neonatal tetanus' [81].

More recently, in December, 2018, Italian research group, Corvelva, announced that they had received a donation from the Italian National Order of Biologists, and intended to test the contents of every vaccine currently on the market.

Their results, so far, have been disturbing. For instance, their testing of Hexyon 6-in-1 infant vaccine (recently approved for use in the US, beginning in 2020, under a different trade name) not only revealed a conspicuous absence of some antigens meant to be in there, they also noted the presence of many contaminants *not* meant to be in there [83].

These include pesticides diethylatrazine and sulfluramid, both linked to adverse reproductive effects [84-85]. Diethylatrazine, it was discovered in one study, emasculated 75% of male frogs, and turned 10% of them into female.

Despite the calls for long-term vaccine studies, the CDC it seems, remains unmoved, stating on their website that "*Observing vaccinated children for many years to look for long-term health conditions would not be practical, and withholding an effective vaccine from children while long-term studies are being done wouldn't be ethical"* [86].

PHARMACOKINETICS

Pharmacokinetics refers to the study of the time course of drug absorption, distribution, metabolism, localisation in tissues, biotransformation, and excretion. Basically, such research would tell us what the ingredients of a vaccine do, after they are injected into the body - where they go after leaving injection site, for how long, and where they eventually end up.

Under current guidelines issued to industry, pharmacokinetic studies for vaccines are not mandatory.

According to the European Medicines Agency, pharmacokinetic studies *"are generally not required for vaccines because the kinetic properties of antigens do not provide useful information for determining dose recommendations. However, such studies might be applicable when new delivery systems are employed or when the vaccine contains novel adjuvants or excipients"* [87].

The lack of such studies is precisely why, after some 90 years in use, the mechanism of action of vaccine adjuvants and ingredients is still poorly understood. In fact, researchers concluded that there was a *"concerning scarcity of data on toxicology and pharmacokinetics of these compounds"* [88].

A study of the pharmacokinetics of a DNA vaccine found that the proteins therein *"could be distributed into all tissues of the body after injection"* [89].

The relatively few studies that have been conducted on individual ingredients are not always methodologically sound. For example, a study on the pharmacokinetics of thimerosal, at levels currently found in annual multi-dose flu vaccines, compared *injected* thimerosal (ethylmercury), with dietary (*ingested*) methylmercury, based on experiments with baby monkeys [90].

Despite the obvious differences between injection and ingestion, the authors conclude that their analysis "*supports the acknowledged safety of thimerosal when used as a preservative at current levels in certain multidose infant vaccines in the United States*".

INDIVIDUAL SUSCEPTIBILITY TO ADVERSE REACTIONS

Pharmaceutical drugs are carefully calculated and administered according to body weight. Wrong dosages are one of the most common errors in medical administration, which authorities admit is putting patient lives at risk [91].

Compare this with the blasé approach to vaccination, which follows a one-size-fits-all approach - unheard of, for other pharmaceutical products. When it comes to vaccines, a 2kg newborn can receive the same dose as a 25kg pre-schooler.

Mass vaccination practices also disregard genetic profile, or potential immune response based on age, weight or overall health profile. There is no routine testing done before vaccination.

Several tests that could determine whether a child may be at increased risk of adverse reaction, so the parents/recipient could be better informed on potential risks versus benefits, are neither offered nor performed. These tests include MTHFR gene mutation, Vitamin C status, presence of auto-antibodies, and allergy testing.

In 2012, the Institute of Medicine (IOM) published a report that stated [92]:

"Both epidemiologic and mechanistic research suggests that most individuals who experience an adverse reaction to vaccines have a pre-existing susceptibility. These predispositions can exist for a number of reasons – genetic variants (in human or microbiome DNA), environmental exposures, behaviors, intervening illness or developmental stage, to name just a few, all of which can interact. Some of these adverse reactions are specific to the particular vaccine, while others may not be. Some of these predispositions may be detectable prior to the administration of vaccine; others, at least with current technology and practice, are not."

And then again, in 2013, from the Institute of Medicine [93]:

"The committee found that evidence assessing outcomes in subpopulations of children, who may be potentially susceptible to adverse reactions to vaccines (such as children with a family history of autoimmune disease or allergies or children born prematurely), was limited and is characterized by uncertainty about the definition of populations of interest and definitions of exposures or outcomes".

So here we have a situation where nobody has any way of knowing whether a child will react badly, and potentially suffer lifelong complications, before administering a vaccine. Yet governments are making it increasingly harder to opt out of them.

One issue that has started to receive a lot of attention – amongst parents of vaccine-injured children, anyway – is MTHFR genetic mutations.

Contrary to first appearance, MTHFR is not an abbreviated version of a curse word, but stands for methylenetetrahydrofolate reductase.

According to the Genetics Home Reference, "*The MTHFR gene provides instructions for making an enzyme called methylenetetrahydrofolate reductase. This enzyme plays a role in processing amino acids, the building blocks of proteins. Methylenetetrahydrofolate reductase is important for a chemical reaction involving forms of the vitamin folate (also called vitamin B9). Specifically, this enzyme converts a molecule called 5,10-methylenetetrahydrofolate to a molecule called 5-methyltetrahydrofolate. This reaction is required for the multistep process that converts the amino acid homocysteine to another amino acid, methionine. The body uses methionine to make proteins and other important compound*" [94].

Those who have a mutation on the MTHFR gene have up to 70% reduced ability to convert folate into its usable form.

 Folate, also known as Vitamin B9, is essential for [95]:

a) synthesis of DNA, RNA and hence, optimal cellular health

b) metabolism of amino acids, which involves production of neurotransmitters, seratonin, and *detoxification* mechanisms (potential implications for vaccination)
c) formation and maturation of red blood cells, white blood cells and production of platelets
d) methylation, which is critical for various vital reactions in the body
e) detoxifying homocysteine.

As you can see, an inability to utilise folate could result in some catastrophic changes in the body, including an inability to excrete toxins or heavy metals effectively, or repair DNA. This situation could conceivably put someone at higher risk of vaccine injury.

There is some debate over what percentage of the population carry a MTHFR gene mutation, and race plays a role in risk, with African Americans having the lowest rates, and Hispanics having the highest [96].

Over the course of two years, one paediatric doctor tested nearly all her young patients for the mutation, and says around 75% have at least a single mutation, and around 40% have a double mutation [97].

Many genetic combinations are possible, but only two mutations have really been studied, and are tested for. These are C677T and A1298C, and various combinations of these genes can be passed on from each parent [98-99].

Homozygous: C677T or A1298C genetic mutation is passed on from BOTH parents. This results in 40% - 70% loss of function.

Heterozygous: C677T or A1298C genetic mutation is passed on from ONE parent. Results in an estimated 40% loss of function.

Compound Heterozygous: C677T mutation is passed on from one parent, and A1298C mutation passed on from the other parent. Results in approximately 50% loss of function.

A meta-analysis conducted in 2013 concluded that MTHFR gene mutation is associated with autism spectrum disorder [100], which may be the result of folate deficiency for normal growth and brain development, as well as inability to excrete harmful neurotoxins.

Given that MTHFR gene mutations are linked with increased risk of drug adverse reactions [101], we could surmise that the same also holds true for vaccines.

Unfortunately, doctors are generally not well-versed on this genetic mutation, testing is not offered prior to vaccination, and indeed, not usually offered afterwards when the adverse reaction becomes apparent. Having MTHFR genetic mutation is also not considered sufficient to warrant a medical exemption from vaccines.

NON-SPECIFIC EFFECTS OF VACCINATION

In the 1980's, Peter Aaby, a Danish doctor and anthropologist, head of the Bandim Health Project in Guinea-Bissau, West Africa, realized that vaccines had effects that went beyond the disease being vaccinated against.

When DTP and oral polio vaccines were introduced for children aged 6 – 35 months in 1981, they noted during weigh-in sessions, that vaccinated children had significantly better weight-for-age scores than unvaccinated. They fully expected that this would translate into better health outcomes in vaccinated children.

To their surprise, what they found was that, over time, the vaccinated children had double the mortality of unvaccinated children [102].

Given that many of the unvaccinated children had received no vaccines because nurses and mothers had deemed them too sick or weak, it's likely that the negative effects of DTP vaccine were even greater.

It wasn't just the DTP vaccine, either. In 1989, the World Health Organization recommended vaccination of babies under 9mths, in measles-endemic areas, with a new, high-titer measles vaccine. Reports of increased mortality in females came from Guinea-Bissau, Senegal and Haiti, forcing the WHO to rescind their recommendations in 1992 [103].

After four decades of gathering and analysing data in Africa, Professor Aarby recently commented in a presentation "*I guess most of you think we know what our vaccines are doing...We don't".*

Aarby went on to explain how the World Health Organization originally reacted to his findings (they thanked him for his concern, and then proceeded to ignore those concerns). He managed to convince them to convene an expert panel to look at the data – they still were not convinced, saying the numbers were too small, and the results were simply not 'plausible'.

When others reported the same findings in Haiti, and elsewhere, the World Health Organization withdrew the vaccine, with no explanation, and without any further investigation into why it had caused a higher death rate.

"You can have a vaccine that is fully protective against a specific disease but associated with higher mortality. How is that possible? That's nowhere in the textbooks..." [104].

All-cause mortality data is not required for new vaccines. Now this raises some disturbing issues, when we consider how many deaths and/or serious health problems occur in clinical trials, and are deemed to be 'unrelated' to the vaccine. Clearly, there is a great deal about the immune system, and the non-specific effects of vaccines, still to be learnt, and in a future time, we may well realize that these conclusions were, in fact, erroneous.

The 'gold standard' of scientific research is the double-blind, randomized, placebo-controlled trial [105]. This type of trial involves two groups of people, assigned at random, to receive either a treatment or a placebo control. 'Double-blind' means neither the researcher, or the participant, knows whether they are receiving a treatment or a placebo. This removes, as much as possible, potential biases, such as placebo effect, or the potential for healthier people to be put into the treatment group, and the less healthy to be put into the control group, or vice versa.

There has never been such a study performed for the entire vaccine schedule, to provide data on possible differences between completely unvaccinated and fully vaccinated. This would further our understanding of potential cumulative effects or synergistic toxicity.

In 2013, the Institute of Medicine (IOM) pointed out that the current vaccination schedule for infants and children had not been adequately tested for safety [106].

They concluded that studies were needed to investigate the long-term, cumulative effects, the timing of vaccine doses in relation to the age, weight and health of the child, synergistic effects of vaccines given simultaneously, and the biological mechanisms of vaccine injury.

In the absence of such studies, we are left to rely on the data collected by individual organizations, in an attempt to assess the difference in health outcomes between vaccinated and unvaccinated children. None were double-blinded or randomized, but nevertheless, they do give some valuable clues that back up the anecdotal evidence of many parents...

In 1992, the New Zealand Immunisation Awareness Society distributed a questionnaire amongst their members, plus member's friends and associates. Two-hundred-and-forty-five families responded, with a total of 495 children surveyed. Two-hundred-and-twenty-six children were vaccinated, and 269 were unvaccinated, with an age range of 2 weeks to 46 years.

Eighty-one families had both vaccinated and unvaccinated children, with the vast majority having elder children vaccinated and younger ones unvaccinated, suggesting that parents had developed an awareness of vaccination issues over time [107].

The results showed that asthma was three times more prevalent in vaccinated than unvaccinated. Eczema was more than double. There were three times as many ear infections in vaccinated children as unvaccinated children. Tonsilitis was 10x more prevalent in the vaccinated than the unvaccinated. Hyperactivity was 3x more common in vaccinated than unvaccinated.

Of the eleven health conditions surveyed, the unvaccinated fared better in every category except diabetes - there were zero cases of diabetes in both groups.

In 2004, the Dutch Association for Conscientious Vaccination surveyed the parents of 635 children, including both members and non-members. Only children that were fully vaccinated as per the Dutch Vaccination program, and those that were entirely unvaccinated, were included in the results. Those that were partially vaccinated were excluded from the study [108].

Three hundred and twelve children were fully vaccinated, compared with 231 children never vaccinated.

Instances of aggressive behaviour was more than double in vaccinated than unvaccinated. The incidence of febrile convulsions, ear infections, and throat inflammation in vaccinated children was also more than double that of unvaccinated children. Episodes of lengthy crying, greater than 3 hours, were more than double in vaccinated children, than unvaccinated.

Doctor visits and hospital admissions were also higher in vaccinated children, despite whooping cough and German measles being more common in unvaccinated children. However, incidence of heart rhythm disorders was slightly higher in unvaccinated children. It's possible this underlying health issue was the original reason for vaccine exemption.

The highly-anticipated Kiggs Study, conducted by the Robert Koch Institute in Germany, between 2003 and 2006, included over 17,000 children between 0 and 17 years. The researchers removed all immigrant families from the results, which further decreased the small pool of unvaccinated children. Any child who had received even one vaccine was classified as vaccinated, which also may have affected the results [109].

Even so, their results showed that despite unvaccinated children having higher incidence of 'vaccine-preventable' diseases, vaccinated children had more infections overall, which emphasises the information provided in this book, regarding the effects of vaccination on the immune system.

A German homeopath started a website on vaccine injuries, after hearing numerous personal accounts of adverse reactions following vaccines. At the request of his readers, he began collecting data on unvaccinated children, and comparing it with Kiggs and other data. So far, more than 11,000 unvaccinated children from all parts of the globe have been surveyed, and the project is still ongoing [110]

Compared with the unvaccinated children surveyed, the average rate in the highly-vaccinated paediatric population is:

- 10 times more epilepsy/seizures
- Almost 20 times more autoimmune disorders.
- More than 10 times the rate of scoliosis.
- More than double the incidence of allergies.
- More than 3 times as much hayfever.
- More than 15 times the rate of sinusitis.
- More than 7 times the rate of asthma or chronic bronchitis.
- 10 times more middle-ear infections.
- More than 3 times the rate of hyperactivity.
- More than double the rate of autism.

In 2017, a study was published comparing health outcomes in vaccinated and unvaccinated children who are home-schooled. They found that diagnoses of chickenpox and pertussis were more common amongst unvaccinated children, but diagnoses of pneumonia, otitis media (ear infection), allergies and neuro-developmental disorders were more common among the vaccinated [111].

After controlling for other factors, vaccination, together with preterm birth was associated with 6-fold greater odds of neuro-developmental disorders.

Of course, surveys are not the most reliable method of data collection - there's always room for memory lapses and personal biases. This is precisely why - in the minds of sceptics, at least - the question will never be settled until a double-blind, randomized, controlled trial is conducted.

It appears that won't be any time soon, because ... ethics [112]. It is considered unethical to offer a placebo to somebody if there is an effective treatment available. Vaccines are considered effective, so we are left with a Catch-22 situation.

Meanwhile, one hardly knows how much 'science' can be trusted, when so much has been corrupted by vested interests and industry connections. The question is, what percentage of scientific work has been corrupted, and is therefore unreliable?

A study published in 2005, found that 'overall, 33% of scientists funded by the NIH (National Institute of Health) *admitted* that they had engaged in questionable scientific behaviour during the previous 3 years" [113].

Other research from 2005, concluded that '*about 70% of clinical trials published in major journals are funded by the drug industry. Studies funded by the industry are 4 times more likely than studies funded from other sources to have findings favourable to the company*" [114].

Richard Horton, editor of The Lancet wrote "*The case against science is straightforward: much of the scientific literature, perhaps half, may simply be untrue. Afflicted by studies with small sample sizes, tiny effects, invalid exploratory analyses, and flagrant conflicts of interest, together with an obsession for pursuing fashionable trends of dubious importance, science has taken a turn towards darkness*" [115].

Even more shocking though, is the work of John Ioannidis, professor at Stanford University, and one of the world's foremost experts on the credibility of medical research. He contends that as much as **90%** of the medical research relied upon by doctors is '*misleading, exaggerated, and often flat-out wrong*" [116].

"*At every step in the process, there is room to distort results, a way to make a stronger claim or to select what is going to be concluded,*" says Ioannidis. "*There is an intellectual conflict of interest that pressures researchers to find whatever it is that is most likely to get them funded*" [116].

"*To get funding and tenured positions, and often merely to stay afloat, researchers have to get their work published in well-regarded journals, where rejection rates can climb above 90 percent. Not surprisingly, the studies that tend to make the grade are those with eye-catching findings. But while coming up with eye-catching theories is relatively easy, getting reality to bear them out is another matter*".

"*The great majority collapse under the weight of contradictory data when studied rigorously. Imagine, though, that five different research teams test an interesting theory that's making the rounds, and four of the groups correctly prove the idea false, while the one less cautious group incorrectly "proves" it true through some combination of error, fluke, and clever selection of data. Guess whose findings your doctor ends up reading about in the journal, and you end up hearing about on the evening news*" [116].

6.
PREGNANCY, INFANTS & THE ELDERLY

PREGNANT WOMEN

Pregnancy represents a unique scenario for the mother's immune system. It must tread a delicate balance between being active enough to protect the mother from illness, but not so active that the mother's body begins to attack the foetus, via pro-inflammatory reactions.

Despite this, vaccines are increasingly promoted to pregnant women, namely the influenza and whooping cough (pertussis) containing vaccines - even though it is known that toxins found in vaccines can cross the placenta and affect the unborn child.

Since 1997, the Advisory Committee on Immunization Practices (ACIP) has recommended the trivalent inactivated influenza vaccine (TIV) for pregnant women, after the first trimester. In 2004, this recommendation expanded to include all trimesters of pregnancy [1].

In 2009, pregnant women were also urged to get the H1N1 (swine flu) vaccine. Research later concluded that vaccination for H1N1 during pregnancy could break the immune tolerance against the fetus, which *"could theoretically result in pregnancy loss, restricted growth of fetus and/or placenta, or in the development of pre-eclampsia"* [2].

Another study released in 2012 discovered a 116-fold increase in reports of fetal loss during the 2009/2010 influenza season, suggesting that concomitant administration of both seasonal influenza vaccine and H1N1 vaccine may have resulted in synergistic toxicity [3].

Since 2005, the 'cocooning' method has been promoted to minimise risk of pertussis (whooping cough) in neonates who are too young to be vaccinated. This strategy meant vaccinating the mother and all other close contacts during the post-partum period.

It was deemed to be inefficient and difficult to execute, however, so in 2011, the CDC updated its recommendations. TDaP (tetanus-diptheria-acellular pertussis vaccine) is now recommended during the second or third trimester of pregnancy [4].

Somehow, the fact that the pertussis portion of the vaccine has a rather dubious record, when it comes to efficacy, has never entered the conversation. Studies show that some 80% of pertussis cases are now caused by strains not covered by the vaccine [5], and what's more, those who are *vaccinated* for pertussis are more susceptible to the new strains [6].

Research published in 2015, also suggests that the current resurgence of pertussis is likely caused by vaccinated individuals who are asymptomatic (show no clinical symptoms) [7].

Naturally, one of the most concerning aspects of maternal vaccination during pregnancy, is the unintended consequences on the unborn child.

Study after study, in animals, show that immune activation during pregnancy causes deleterious effects in the unborn, particularly relating to the brain and central nervous system. Many of these studies show brain changes that are strikingly similar to those found in autism, and other neurological or psychiatric disorders [8-14].

Conclusions from some of these studies, were as follows: "*We find that activation of the maternal immune system yields offspring with cardinal symptoms of autism: highly repetitive behaviour and deficits in communication and sociability*"[9].

"*Maternal immune activation yields offspring with abnormal repetitive behaviours, communication, and social interactions*" [10].

"*These data indicate the maternal immune activation leads to long-lasting, region-specific changes in brain cytokines in offspring - similar to those reported for autism spectrum disorder and schizophrenia - that may alter central nervous system development and behaviour*" [13].

In addition, animal studies also show that maternal immune activation may have long-term consequences in the offspring that are not manifest until adulthood, including behavioural and pharmacological changes related to schizophrenia [15-17].

Incredibly enough, some research suggests that maternal immune activation may even cause the development of Alzheimer and Parkinson diseases in the offspring, many decades later [18]. Meanwhile we have safety studies that declare the influenza vaccine to be 'safe' during pregnancy, after only following the infant up to 6 months of age [19].

Many of these studies are viewed via the aspect of maternal immune activation from viral infection, with seemingly little attention given to the inevitable immune activation that comes via injection of adjuvants and antigens in vaccines.

Many of the above studies induced immune activation by injection of Polyl:C, a synthetic cytokine releaser. Aluminium adjuvant (found in the pertussis vaccine recommended for pregnant women) can also cause cytokine release. According to research published in 2013 [20]:

"Injection of vaccines containing alum elicits profound broad local effects on the immune system. Within a few hours after injection, pro-inflammatory cytokines are released and there is an influx of inflammatory monocytes followed by dendritic cells (DCs), natural killer (NK) cells, neutrophils, and eosinophils by 24h".

And then*: "In summary, the immunostimulatory effects of alum are broad, rapid, and seem to involve multiple pathways, both direct and indirect. More investigation will be required to fully elucidate these pathways."*

Here we have a situation where, on the one hand, immune activation during pregnancy is well-documented to cause adverse reactions in the unborn, some which may not manifest until teenage years or even late adulthood, but on the other hand, we have health authorities promoting a product to pregnant women, that does exactly that - activates the immune system.

If vaccination during pregnancy did, indeed, cause or exacerbate similar problems to those seen in animal studies, could we expect to see a marked increase in not only children being diagnosed with autistic disorders, but also young adults suffering mental health disorders?

One recent study did, in fact, look at autism rates of children born to mothers vaccinated during pregnancy. They concluded that there was no increased risk – however, a closer look reveals that influenza vaccination during the first trimester, did correlate to an increased risk of autism [21].

Another study in the 1970's looked at cancer rates of children born to mothers vaccinated for polio or influenza during pregnancy. Children born to mothers vaccinated while pregnant had double the rate of cancers...incredibly, researchers concluded there was no increased risk [22].

Could these potential risks actually be worth it, if vaccination during pregnancy was found to protect your newborn child after birth? Unfortunately, that may not be the case, either. Several reviews of the available literature on influenza vaccination during pregnancy have failed to find any benefit to either the mother, or the unborn child/newborn [23-24].

At the time of writing, at least another two vaccines are currently in the later stages of development and 'expected to be licensed', for use on pregnant women. One is for Respiratory Syncytial Virus (RSV) [25], and the other for Group B Streptococcus (GBS) [26].

Respiratory Syncytial Virus (RSV) is a common cold-like illness that is usually mild in healthy people. Nearly all children will have had an infection by their second birthday – according to the CDC, and of those who have an infection before 6mths of age, around 1-2% will be hospitalised, due to complications such as bronchiolitis or pneumonia [27].

The quest for an RSV vaccine began decades ago - and it had disastrous beginnings.

In the early 1960's, an RSV vaccine, propagated on human embryonic kidney cells, and passaged through monkey cells, before being inactivated with formalin, and adjuvanted with aluminium, was trialled on infants, with disastrous results. Up to 80% of vaccinated infants were hospitalized with severe lower-respiratory infections, and two babies died [28].

It took scientists nearly four decades to figure out why the vaccine had such tragic results – which just goes to show how little is understood about the very system they seek to modify. It was due to *"Lack of antibody affinity maturation followed poor Toll-like receptor stimulation"*, according to the paper, published in Nature journal, in 2009 [29].

With this new knowledge in hand, the quest for an RSV vaccine resumed.

At the forefront of the current charge for an RSV vaccine, is Novavax, a biotechnology company with several products currently in the clinical testing stages. Following the announcement of positive results of Phase 2 clinical trials in older adults, in 2015, CEO of Novavax, Stanley Erck declared their RSV vaccine could be *"the largest selling vaccine in the history of vaccines in terms of revenue"* [30].

Unfortunately, the following Phase 3 trial in older adults failed to show efficacy, and the company lost more than $1.5 billion in market value, within hours, as disappointed investors pulled their money [31].

This gives us some idea of the pressure faced by companies to come up with a new 'blockbuster' vaccine. For a company like Novavax, with no products on the market yet, (just the potential of new products), investor confidence is crucial to financing the lengthy clinical trial and regulatory approval process.

Novavax then turned their focus to pregnant women, and in February 2019, announced favourable results from a Phase 3 clinical trial on pregnant women. The vaccine, is not only aluminium adjuvanted, it is also genetically-engineered with nano-particles. The press release announced *"Our next steps include meeting with U.S. and European regulators to review these data and to discuss the path forward for licensure"* [32].

The trials on pregnant women were funded, in part, by an $89 million grant from the Bill and Melinda Gates Foundation, with the stated purpose *"to advance to WHO Pre-Qualification the development of a respiratory syncytial virus (RSV) vaccine for maternal immunization to reduce the burden of RSV disease in infants less than six months of age in developing countries"* [33-34].

Obviously, the burden of RSV disease falls mainly on developing nations, however, it's likely that a new RSV vaccine will also be targeted at pregnant women in western countries.

One of the main ways to prevent respiratory disease in infants is via breastfeeding. A study published in *British Medical Journal* found that among 115 babies who had been hospitalized for RSV infection, only 8 were breastfed [35].

Given that breastfeeding rates are vastly lower in developing countries, one wonders why $89 million (and more) wasn't spent to increase maternal nutrition and breastfeeding rates? In West/Central Africa, only a mere 20% of infants are exclusively breastfed for the first six months of their life [36].

One of the main groups behind the current drive for an RSV vaccine during pregnancy, is the Oxford Vaccine Group, who admit that almost all infant deaths due to RSV are in developing countries [37].

The director of Oxford Vaccine Group is Andrew Pollard, who holds several patents relating to vaccines [38-39], and is Chair of the UK Department of Health's Joint Committee on Vaccination and Immunisation and the European Medicine Agency's scientific advisory group.

Another member of the Oxford Vaccine Group, Matthew Snape, has been Principal Investigator in clinical trials of numerous RSV vaccine candidates. He is also the Director of the National Immunization Schedule Evaluation Consortium (NISEC) [40].

It is also interesting to note that, since 2010, the CDC has held a patent for an RSV vaccine [41].

Group B streptococcus

According to the World Health Organization, between 20-25% adult women carry Group B strep bacteria vaginally, though it doesn't appear to cause illness or symptoms. Approximately 50% of babies born to affected mothers will also be colonized, but only 2% will be infected [42].

Of those 2% of infected babies, around 2 – 3% will die from complications [43]. Ninety-eight percent of neonatal deaths attributed to GBS disease occur in developing countries [44].

INFANTS

In terms of medical science, infants and children are often viewed as 'small adults', with concessions made only for their smaller body-weight, but not for their unique physiology that makes them more susceptible to toxic insults.

The nervous system undergoes rapid development during childhood, and there are critical periods of neurodevelopment that occur in the first few years of life, when a child may be ultra-susceptible to central nervous system damage, via exposure to toxins [45-46].

For example, after birth, the human brain does not grow at a steady pace, but rather goes through 'growth spurts', specifically between the age of 3-10 months [47], which happens to correspond to a period when numerous vaccines are given. The human brain continues to develop right up until early adulthood [48].

Potential damage to the central nervous system may not become evident until a later stage of development [48].

In addition, the blood-brain barrier in infancy is more permeable to toxic substances than in adulthood [48], which means that toxins have easier access to the brain and therefore, more likely to affect the nervous system.

In a 2015 EPA report on the magnitude of neurodevelopmental disorders in US children, this issue was also raised [49]:

"A child's brain and nervous system are vulnerable to adverse impacts from pollutants because they go through a long developmental process beginning shortly after conception and continuing through adolescence. This complex developmental process requires the precise coordination of cell growth and movement, and may be disrupted by even short-term exposures to environmental contaminants if they occur at critical stages of development. This disruption can lead to neurodevelopmental deficits that may have an effect on the child's achievements and behavior even when they do not result in a diagnosable disorder. "

The infant immune system is also undeveloped and limited in function [50]. This seeming anomaly was once considered a 'defect' and 'dysregulation' in the infant immune system [51]. However, three years later, in the same medical journal, researchers had started to gain some respect for this supposed defect, referring to it as "an important developmental program" [52].

They concluded that *"this anti-inflammatory phenotype may be beneficial to the neonate at a time when tissue growth and remodelling events are taking place at a rapid pace"* [52].

An infant goes through incredible growth and development in the first years of life – in the gut, the brain, the musculoskeletal and immune systems – activation of the immune system (which inevitably results in inflammation) could have serious long-term consequences.

Prior to the introduction of mass vaccination programs for children, the immune system gradually built up to capacity via sporadic challenges, usually in the form of relatively minor childhood illnesses.

Vaccines are designed to stimulate antibody production, which leaves the innate immune system unchallenged. A prolonged stimulation of the humoral immune system, due to repeat vaccinations, may result in a prematurely stunted innate immune system (the first-line-of-defence immune system) [53], which would leave the child vulnerable to infections and result in a less robust immune system overall.

Another aspect of human physiology that is undergoing rapid development in the first years of life is the microbiome, which has been shown to affect behaviour and central nervous system development [54].

In 2014, researchers noted: *"The microbiome is a dynamic entity that is under continuous evolution throughout the host's lifetime, in particular during the first three years of life, during which time a stable microbiome is established. It is sensitive to a whole array of manipulations such as diet, stress, infection, pharmacological interventions and thus is it clear that the composition of the microbiota is distinct at different milestones of life"* [55].

Although scientists acknowledge that the microbiome can affect vaccination response [56], research is clearly lacking on just how vaccination might affect the microbiome.

In 2010, researchers were investigating why rotavirus vaccine has been less effective in developing countries, and suggested that the neutralizing antibodies found in breastmilk were responsible. Although other research shows that breastfeeding actually protects infants from rotavirus infection [57], these researchers concluded that strategies such as "delaying breastfeeding at the time of immunization" may be necessary to overcome the 'negative' effect of breastfeeding [58].

THE ELDERLY

According to the Alzheimer's Association, deaths from Alzheimer's disease have increased by 89% since the year 2000. There are currently more than 5 million Americans living with the disease, the vast majority of them over the age of 65, with a national cost of $259 billion. At current rates, that figure could be as high as $1.1 trillion by 2050 [59].

And what exactly does that have to do with vaccines?

Quite a bit, according to some scientists. One of those was Hugh Fudenberg, who was a neuroimmunologist and one of the world's most cited scholars, having published more than 600 articles in medical and scientific journals before his death in 2014.

Fudenberg sat on the World Health Organization's expert committee on immunology for 20 years.

Fudenberg claimed that having the flu vaccine three or more times over a five-year period, increased your chances of Alzheimers by ten-fold [60].

In 2001, research - which was partially funded by the pharmaceutical giant Pfizer - not only refuted his claims but concluded that vaccination actually *protects* from Alzheimers [61].

One wonders how such a finding is possible, given the wealth of evidence now showing that exposure to mercury and aluminium, both of which are found in various vaccines, has neurotoxic effects that induce changes in the brain, such as those seen in Alzheimer's disease [62-65].

Meanwhile, those over 65 are being increasingly targeted for vaccines. It is now recommended that they receive a yearly flu jab, despite evidence that it has little benefit for them [66-67], as well as a shingles vaccine, diptheria-tetanus-pertussis booster, and pneumococcal vaccine [68].

The reason for this focus on the over-65 age group, is due to a less robust immune system as people age, therefore, in theory, they need help from vaccines. Ironically, this less robust immune system is the very same reason that vaccines often don't elicit the required antibody response in the elderly - their immune system doesn't respond with the same vigour as a younger person. This is known as immunosenescence.

According to some researchers, the solution to this problem requires new approaches, which included "*high-dose vaccines, booster vaccinations, different immunisation routs and use of new adjuvants*" [69].

This is obviously the reason why the shingles vaccine for older adults contains the same varicella virus as the chickenpox vaccine for children...except 14x more of it [70].

The 'high dose' influenza vaccine is formulated especially for those over 65 - it contains 4x the amount of antigen, as the normal flu vaccine [71].

In order to be 'protected' against meningitis and pneumonia, older adults are urged to get, not one pneumococcal vaccine, but two vaccines - both the 13-strain, and the 23-strain vaccine [72].

Thirty-two states in the US have laws expressly relating to flu vaccination in long-term care facilities. For example, Alabama law requires that "a *long-term care facility shall document the*

*annual immunization against influenza virus and the immun-
ization against pneumococcal disease for each resident*" [73].

North Carolina law regarding nursing homes "*shall require residents and employees to be immunized against influenza virus
and shall require residents to also be immunized against pneumococcal disease.*" [74].

Nursing facilities in Delaware must "*have on file evidence of
annual vaccination against influenza for all residents*" [75].

Given that many of those patients are likely suffering from dementia and memory-loss, there is a potential that adverse reactions are being overlooked and unreported.

In 2017, an outbreak of influenza in a nursing home in Tasmania, Australia, sickened 31 residents, of whom 6 died. Management of the nursing home were quick to point out that "All precautions to prevent an outbreak ahead of the flu season were
taken, with 95 per cent of Strathdevon's 37 residents receiving
a flu vaccination" [76].

What this tells us, is that, despite 95% of residents being vaccinated, 84% were still affected by influenza...

Also, in 2017, an influenza outbreak at a nursing home in Victoria, Australia, affected 123 residents and staff, and at least 8
elderly residents died of complications. Experts were careful
not to blame an ineffective flu vaccine, but instead reminded
people they can get a second booster shot towards the end of
'flu season' to stay protected. Due to the death toll amongst the
elderly during the winter of 2017, the Australian government

then moved to mandate yearly flu vaccines for those working in aged-care settings [77].

7.
OTHER VACCINATION ISSUES

The vaccination issue is far from black and white. Here's an example of other vaccination issues, that are rarely, if ever, discussed in the mainstream media.

VACCINES SUPPRESS THE IMMUNE SYSTEM

Scientists have known for several decades that vaccines suppress normal function of the immune system, via numerous mechanisms.

For example, research published in the Journal of Infectious Diseases in 1988 found that one-year-old infants, vaccinated with measles vaccine, experienced a significant decrease in the level of alpha-interferon produced by lymphocytes. This marked reduction was still evident when the study ended a year later [1]. Researchers concluded that "*the study showed that the measles vaccine produced a significant, long-term immune suppression*".

Interferons are a group of signalling proteins that belong to a class of immune cells known as cytokines. These molecules communicate between cells to co-ordinate immune responses that help to expel pathogens and interfere with viral replication. Interestingly enough, interferon therapy is now being used as a cancer treatment [2].

A study from 1996, also using the measles vaccine, found that vaccination decreased production of lymphocytes, with the most marked decreases found in children with the highest antibody counts [3].

What are lymphocytes? Lymphocytes are a class of white blood cells, necessary for fighting off infections and protecting against cancer [4].

In 1984, researchers tested levels of T-lymphocytes in 11 healthy adults, before and after vaccination with a tetanus booster and found a significant, though temporary, drop in T-helper lymphocytes in all subjects. In four of the subjects, T-helper cells fell to levels found in active AIDS patients [5].

One has to wonder...if a single vaccine can do that in a healthy adult, what about multiple vaccines administered concomitantly to an infant child?

There were a number of studies during the 1980's and 1990's, showing the immunosuppressive action of vaccines [6-8], which have since been largely forgotten, in the increasingly hostile climate of vaccine mandates, and disease fears.

VACCINATION MAKES PEOPLE MORE SUSCEPTIBLE TO OTHER ILLNESSES

There have been numerous reports in the medical literature of vaccination making people more susceptible to other illnesses not covered by the vaccine.

i) Annual influenza vaccinations have been shown to increase risk (by more than 4-fold) of non-influenza respiratory virus infections, such as coxsackievirus or rhinovirus [9].

ii) Annual influenza vaccination has also been shown to reduce immunity against potentially pandemic strains of influenza [10].

iii) MMR vaccine has been found to increase incidence of aseptic meningitis [11-13].

iv) Widespread vaccination against chickenpox (varicella zoster) is expected to cause an epidemic of shingles (herpes zoster) over the coming years [14], thought to be due to less exposure during adulthood to boost cell-mediated immunity. Goldman and King [15] concluded that *"When the costs of the booster dose for varicella and the increased shingles recurrences are included, the universal varicella vaccination program is neither effective nor cost-effective."*

Cost-benefit analysis of universal varicella vaccination in infants were highly optimistic, but when the increasing disease burden, and possibly higher fatality of shingles, is taken into account, the numbers don't look so promising [16-18].

SHEDDING FROM LIVE VIRUS VACCINES

Some vaccines contain live viruses, which may 'shed' following vaccination, even though the person may display no symptoms themselves. This information is not widely known, nor are recently vaccinated individuals advised to avoid the very old, the very young, or the immunocompromised.

Similar to wild viruses, live-virus vaccines can shed via saliva [19], breastmilk [20], urine and blood [21], stool [22], and skin lesions [23].

It is generally accepted that live virus vaccines may shed for up to 6 weeks, however, if the vaccine recipient is immune-compromised themselves, shedding can continue for a lot longer. Take the case of a British man who was still excreting (via stool) highly virulent poliovirus *28 years* after vaccination [24].

Over the past five decades, there have been at least 73 other individuals found to be 'chronic excreters' of poliovirus [25].

Mutated poliovirus has also been identified from sewage samples in Slovakia, Finland, Estonia and Israel, suggesting there may be 'chronic excreters' in other parts of the world, too [26].

Rotavirus vaccine – which is genetically-engineered from human and bovine (cow) retroviruses – is given at 2, 4 and 6 months of age, and can also shed and infect others, even in the absence of symptoms [27].

VACCINES CAUSE PATHOGENS TO MUTATE

Much like the widespread use of antibiotics has resulted in antibiotic-resistant superbugs, so the widespread use of vaccines has resulted in some diseases mutating into more virulent, deadly forms.

This is known as 'selective pressure', a phenomenon that causes a pathogen to mutate, in order to survive and thrive. In fact, research shows that not only do mutated versions of disease seem to favour the vaccinated, the mutated pathogens become even more virulent when they evolve in vaccinated hosts [28-30].

This has been the case with whooping cough (pertussis), pneumococcal and Haemophilus Influenzae type B (Hib) vaccines.

Before widespread pertussis vaccination, b.parapertussis infection (a strain not covered by the vaccine, but with identical symptoms to the usual pertussis infection) accounted for 1% - 35% of whooping cough cases [31-32].

However, after decades of vaccination programs, b.parapertussis has now become the most common strain of pertussis, accounting for up to 84% of new cases in Australia [33]. B.parapertussis is also known to affect children at a younger age than pertussis [34].

 Ironically, studies also show that vaccination for b.pertussis *increases* risk of b.parapertussis infection [35-37], although researchers do not know exactly why this is.

The pneumococcal vaccine has been in use for some years now in the US (and Australia), and numerous studies confirm there has been a strain shift. Those strains covered in the vaccine are being replaced by other strains which are highly multi-drug resistant [38-40].

In a study published in 2008, one hospital reported a five-fold increase in pediatric parapneumonic empyema (build-up of pus, much like an abscess, in the pleural cavities), since the introduction of the pneumococcal conjugate vaccine in 2001.

Researchers noted that serotypes not covered by the vaccine had become more prevalent since introduction of the vaccine [41].

The same scenario is also being played out for the Haemophilus Influenzae Type B (Hib) vaccine, with studies in Brazil showing that while Hib infections had decreased, other strains of haemophilus had increased by 8-fold [42]. Similar findings were reported in Alaska, where the incidence of Hib declined, but the incidence of infection via other serotypes doubled [43].

Research conducted in Utah found that Hib infection had remained steady since the introduction of infant vaccination, but Haemophilus influenzae type A (HIA) had more than doubled, so overall haemophilus infections had increased since widespread vaccinations began [44].

Italian researchers managed to identify 78 strains of haemophilus influenzae, with non-type B strains having quadrupled since introduction of Hib vaccines. In addition, haemophilus infections had become more common amongst the elderly, and had affected trends in antibiotic resistance [45].

Canadian data suggests that Haemophilus non-type B infections caused hospitalization, neonatal intensive care admission, or mortality at similar rates to Hib [46].

The more we try to vaccinate diseases into oblivion, the more they spring up in different forms. Maybe there's a lesson to be learnt here? Maybe it's time we thought about exploring different solutions?

No, the solution always seems to be more vaccines. Predictably enough, while admitting that Hib vaccination had caused a strain shift, and that non-type B strains were a cause of serious mortality and morbidity, these researchers proposed that a new bivalent (two-strain) vaccine might offer protection against both A and B strains [47].

The meningococcal C vaccine was introduced into the Australian schedule in 2003, and there are now clues that a strain shift is taking place [48].

One wonders why the powers-that-be felt it necessary to add the meningococcal vaccine to an already over-crowded schedule, for a disease that, although serious, was 'rare', and was already declining - probably due to less smoking, and less over-crowding [49].

Research in 2007 noted that *"the vaccine is expensive and its long-term impact on the emergence of non-vaccine strains and on nasopharyngeal microecology is unknown" [50].* A decade later we are starting to find out: Strain W, with twice the mortality rate of other strains, has almost tripled within the past two years alone, and at the time of writing this book, NSW state government rolled out a $9 million vaccination program for all secondary students, against Meningococcal W [51].

An article in the Sydney Morning Herald noted that [51]: *"W strain has become the most prevalent strain nationally and in NSW. Though the total number of cases is low, NSW notifications have almost tripled since 2015, from nine to 26 cases in 2016. Two more cases have been confirmed in 2017."*

"The hypervirulent strain has an increased propensity to spread and tends to cause more severe disease. W strain has twice the mortality rate of other strains. Some eight per cent of people who contracted the strain have died in the last decade, compared to a four per cent mortality rate for other meningococcal strains, according to NSW health".

"Federal Health Department officials have been having discussions with pharmaceutical companies regarding options for managing meningococcal W disease."

I don't suppose the admission that widespread vaccination has contributed to this state of affairs will be on the agenda...

BENEFITS OF CHILDHOOD ILLNESSES

Several decades ago, many mothers welcomed the onset of common childhood diseases [52], such as measles and chickenpox, knowing they were usually mild, and often preceded a quantum leap in development of the child.

Indeed, the evidence shows that naturally-acquired childhood diseases provide life-long benefits to the child. These include:

i) Proper development of T-cell mediated immunity [53].
ii) Protection against development of asthma [54-55].
iii) Protection against some neurodegenerative diseases [56].
iv) Protection against ovarian cancer [57-58].

v)   Protection against glioblastoma multiforme (the most common and most aggressive type of primary brain tumour in humans) [59].

vi)   Protection against influenza pandemics [60].

In 1973, the British Medical Journal published a case study, describing remission of infantile Hodgkin's disease after natural measles infection [61]. The 23-month-old child developed measles, before radiotherapy could be started, and the researchers noted, *"much to our surprise, the large cervical mass vanished without further therapy"*.

In fact, vaccine-strain measles is currently being investigated as a potential treatment for cancer, with early results deemed as 'promising', with open trials still being conducted [62]. Earlier research stated that attenuated live measles virus demonstrated "propensity to preferentially infect, propagate in, and destroy cancerous tissue" [63].

It was explained that the reason for using modified viruses was *"concerns regarding the potential of wild-type-viruses to cause serious side effects, technical limitations in manufacturing viral lots of high purity for clinical use, as well as the overwhelming excitement and fervent support the, at the time, newly emerging chemotherapy approaches that slowed down research on alternative strategies"* [63].

It is possible that political factors were also taken into account. If the public realized that natural measles infection could be used to treat cancer, they would inevitably start to ask questions about the logic of trying to prevent children from getting measles, and whether the long-term benefits really outweighed the long-term risks.

MASS GENETIC ENGINEERING OF THE HUMAN RACE?

Contrary to earlier beliefs that genetics were set in stone, science is becoming increasingly aware, via the field of 'epigenetics', how fluid the genome actually is, and how many internal/external influences affect how, or when, certain genes will activate.

This was obvious from as early as the 1960's, when a letter published in the journal Science, pointed out that "*In point of fact, we are practicing biological engineering on a rather large scale by use of live viruses in mass immunization campaigns...Crude virus preparations, such as some in common use at the present time, are also vulnerable to frightful mishaps of contamination and misidentification*" [64].

Of course, vaccine manufacturing and detection methods may have become more sophisticated since then, but as we have already seen, it hasn't eliminated contamination or mishaps.

Factors shown to influence, and be influenced by genetics, include diet (including diet of our ancestors) [65], exposure to environmental toxins (in ourselves, or our ancestors) [66], viral infections (in ourselves, or our ancestors) [67], and *use of pharmaceutical drugs* [68].

Science still has many knowledge gaps about how viruses interact with the human genome, with researchers in 2012 admitting that *"the mechanisms of epigenetic control of gene expression continues to baffle scholars"* and *"It is a great challenge for future scientists to unravel the nuances of viral epigenetics. Most of the discovered mechanisms are still incomplete"* [69].

In 2015, researchers at Stanford University School of Medicine announced their discovery that, within days of conception, the human embryo begins to produce what appears to be viral proteins [70]:

"These viral proteins could manipulate some of the earliest steps in human development, affecting gene expression and even possibly protecting the cells from further viral infection."

Lead author of the study, Edward Grow elaborates, by saying:

"Does the virus selfishly benefit by switching itself on in these early embryonic cells? Or is the embryo instead commandeering the viral proteins to protect itself? Can they both benefit? That's possible, but we don't really know."

What *is* abundantly clear, however, is that after more than half a century of using live-virus vaccines, scientists are still not clear about how genes and viruses interact. It is also clear that nobody can confidently say what the long-term effects of injecting live-viruses, or genetically-engineered viruses, on a mass scale will ultimately be...

THE MICROBIOME

Over the last few years, research into what we now call the 'microbiome' has exploded, as we realize that we are inhabited by trillions of bacteria [71], and that's a good thing (mostly). In fact, we have so many viral and bacterial species living in, and on, us (skin, nose, throat, digestive tract, body orifices etc) that we carry far more viral and bacterial genes, than we do human genes.

There are thousands of strains of different viruses and bacteria living in symbiosis together in, and on, our bodies. The balance of these microbiota is critical for health and well-being, although we are still learning just how much. Many things can upset the balance, and these include diet, stress, emotions, medications and vaccines, environment, and even the microbiome of people around us.

Since this is a relatively new area of research, there is not a lot of science regarding the relationship between vaccines and microbiota, however, we are starting to see hints of the effect that widespread vaccination has on the personal, and communal, microbiome.

It has become well-established that an individual's microbiome affects their response to vaccines and medication, which has some clear ramifications for the current one-size-fits-all vaccination paradigm [72].

But how do vaccines affect a person's microbiome?

One area that has been looked at, is the change in nasopharyngeal (nose and throat) microbiota in children vaccinated with pneumococcal vaccine, versus unvaccinated children.

It was found that vaccinated children had a decreased amount of bacteria covered by the vaccine, but an increase in strains not covered by the vaccines. In other words, other strains had proliferated to fill the niche vacated by vaccine pneumococcal strains [73]. This was termed "replacement invasive pneumococcal disease with serotypes not covered by heptavalent pneumococcal conjugate".

Funnily enough, (or perhaps, predictably enough), the authors suggested that this problem could simply be fixed by producing new vaccines to cover the other strains that were now proliferating, due to perturbation of the microbial balance.

Other research has also found that the decrease in vaccine-types of pneumococcal had resulted in an increase in S. aureus (commonly known as 'Golden Staph') [74], and H. influenzae (Hib) colonization [75].

(It is interesting to note that 'Golden Staph' has become a major problem, with increasing antibiotic resistance, and attempts to develop an effective vaccine over the past 40-odd years, all coming up short [76]).

Long-term follow-up revealed that this microbial change had not only become more marked over time, but the parents of vaccinated children had also experienced a change in microbial balance, presumably via the close contact with their vaccinated children [77].

What this suggests is that widespread vaccination is not only changing our microflora on a personal level, but possibly even on a communal level, as we have relationships and contact with vaccinated individuals.

How this might be affecting us is anybody's guess, given our limited understanding of the vital roles that bacteria and 'pathogens' play in human health and development. Research shows that mice, born and raised in a strictly sterile environment, have abnormal, weak immune systems, decreased sociability, and other behaviours that correlate to autistic-like behaviours seen in humans [78].

Very little is known about why or how microorganisms affect physiology, neural development and behaviour, but clearly, any attempts to artificially change the pathogenic landscape (such as through widespread vaccination) could potentially have long-reaching consequences for society, and attempts should be made to study and quantify such effects.

POST-VACCINATION CARE

I remember, thirteen years ago, taking my eldest son to have his vaccinations. I was encouraged to give him panadol, if he became unsettled or feverish.

Nothing much has changed. The official advice is still the same...

From the New Zealand Ministry of Health: "*If your child is unsettled, miserable because of the fever, or seems to be in pain, you might consider giving them paracetamol or ibuprofen to make them feel more comfortable. You must follow the dosage instructions on the bottle. It is dangerous to give more than the recommended dose".*

"Routinely giving babies and children paracetamol before and repeatedly after immunisation just in case they feel unwell is not recommended. There is some evidence that paracetamol may reduce the effectiveness of childhood vaccinations" [79].

Unfortunately, there's some other evidence that they completely overlooked...

i) Paracetamol reduces the body's ability to detoxify vaccine ingredients, due to depletion of glutathione - the body's most important endogenous (produced in the body) antioxidant [80-86].

ii) Paracetamol use is linked to autism spectrum disorder [87-91].

iii) Paracetamol disrupts hormones, especially in males [92-93], which in turn, affects behaviour and neurodevelopment [94-95].

One study found that the children of mothers who used paracetamol during pregnancy had greater likelihood of being diagnosed with ADHD, and being medicated for ADHD - the longer the duration of usage, the greater the likelihood of behavioural disorders [96].

Another birth cohort study found similar results, most notably a greater likelihood of autism in male offspring [97].

One study from 2008 found that children under five who received paracetamol following measles-mumps-rubella vaccination were 6x more likely to be diagnosed with autism, than children who received ibuprofen after the same vaccine [98].

Acetaminophen was first sold in 1955, under the name of Tylenol Elixir for Children. Approximately 52 million Americans now use an acetaminophen-containing medication every week [99].

Acetaminophen is used in more than 600 over-the-counter and prescription products, and accounts for "*more than 100,000 calls to poison centers, roughly 60,000 emergency-room visits and hundreds of deaths each year in the U.S*" [99].

Patients taking paracetamol are almost four times more likely to have abnormal results on liver function tests. In fact, paracetamol is the number one cause of acute liver failure in children [99].

Another effect of acetaminophen is that it inhibits the user's ability to feel empathy for others - a finding that should raise concerns, given the vast numbers using this medication on a regular basis [100].

WHISTLEBLOWERS

In July of 2015, Representative Bill Posey addressed the House of Representatives of the US federal government, revealing that a whistle-blower from the Centers for Disease Control had come forward with explosive claims of a cover-up. The documents obtained by Rep. Posey were provided by a Dr. William Thompson, senior scientist at the CDC [101].

Dr. Thompson had worked in the Immunization Safety Branch of the CDC from 2000 to 2006. During that time, he led, or co-led, three major vaccine safety studies, investigating a possible link between the MMR vaccine and autism [101].

According to Dr. Thompson, when the data revealed a strong correlation between the vaccine and autism in African-American boys, the decision was made to avoid reporting any race effects, and co-authors *'scheduled a meeting to destroy documents related to the study"* [101].

In 2014, Dr. Thompson released a statement, saying "*I regret that my coauthors and I omitted statistically significant information in our 2004 article published in the Journal of Pediatrics.*"

Rep. Posey concluded by saying "*Considering the nature of the whistleblower's documents, as well as the involvement of the CDC, a hearing and a thorough investigation is warranted. I ask, Mr. Speaker, I beg, I implore my colleagues on the Committee on Appropriations to please, please take such action.*"

To date, Congress has failed to take any action, or subpoena Dr. Thompson.

Lawyers for a 16-year-old boy, who allegedly regressed into autism following vaccination, attempted to subpoena William Thompson to testify in the Tennessee State Circuit Court. This request was denied by CDC director, Thomas Frieden, stating that *"Dr. William Thompson's deposition testimony would not substantially promote the objectives of CDC or HHS"* [102].

Although not directly related to vaccines, another CDC whistle-blower came forward in 2016, alleging that researchers under the CDC's autism monitoring network had been *"publishing data under people's names who had not done the work and that the data contained uncorrected errors"* [103].

Dr Judith Pinborough-Zimmerman, former Principal Investigator for the CDC's Autism and Developmental Disabilities Monitoring Network (ADDM) in Utah, filed the whistleblower charges in the U.S District Court [103].

Another whistle-blower suit from two former employees has landed Merck in court, amidst claims it falsified data regarding the efficacy of its mumps vaccine.

According to court documents, Merck *"failed to disclose that its mumps vaccine was not as effective as Merck represented, (ii) used improper testing techniques, (iii) manipulated testing methodology, (iv) abandoned undesirable test results, (v) falsified test data, (vi) failed to adequately investigate and report the diminished efficacy of its mumps vaccine, (vii) falsely verified that each manufacturing lot of mumps vaccine would be as effective as identified in the labeling, (viii) falsely certified the accuracy of applications filed with the FDA, (ix) falsely certified compliance with the terms of the CDC purchase contract, (x) engaged in the fraud and concealment describe herein for the purpose of illegally monopolizing the U.S. market for mumps vaccine, (xi) mislabeled, misbranded, and falsely certified its mumps vaccine, and (xii) engaged in the other acts described herein to conceal the diminished efficacy of the vaccine the government was purchasing"* [104].

The two former employees allege that rabbit antibodies were added to samples, in an effort to achieve the required efficacy rate of 95%. They also allege that they were threatened with jail, if they alerted the FDA to the fraud [105].

Perhaps Dr Peter Fletcher, former Chief Scientific Officer at the Department of Health, UK, said it best, in a 2016 interview: *"There are very powerful people in positions of great authority in Britain and elsewhere who have staked their reputations and careers on the safety of MMR and they are willing to do almost anything to protect themselves"* [106].

COMPENSATION FOR VACCINE INJURIES

In the US, a 'no fault' compensation system was put in place in 1986, following the passage of the National Childhood Vaccine Injury Act [107]. This came about due to increasing pressure and complaints from pharmaceutical companies, due to differing state laws, threats of litigation, increasing costs and insurance issues [108].

The system is funded via an excise tax (surcharge) on each vaccine administered - basically a self-insurance system, paid for by the user. As of 2014, that surcharge was 75c per vaccine [109].

The original aim of the vaccine court was to establish an *alternative* to costly, emotionally-draining, and time-consuming civil court action [110], while also preserving some economic incentive for vaccine manufacturers to ensure their product was as safe as possible [111].

That all changed in 2011, however, with the U.S Supreme Court ruling that vaccines are 'unavoidably unsafe', and effectively made the Vaccine Injury Compensation Program the only legal remedy available to those adversely affected by vaccines licensed and recommended by the government [112].

As the National Vaccine Information Centre NVIC, a non-profit consumer advocacy group rightly points out [113]:

"There is no other for-profit and publicly traded manufacturing industry in America that enjoys this kind of blanket liability protection for products, which not only carry a risk of injury or death, but also are recommended and mandated by government."

To date, approximately $US4.1 billion has been paid out in compensation to victims, or their families, for vaccine injury and death [114]. That may sound like a lot, but it represents only a fraction of vaccine injuries and adverse effects suffered by victims.

For example:

- More than 2 out of 3 petitions are denied compensation by the Court [114].

- There are only a very limited number of adverse effects and conditions outlined in the Vaccine Injury Tables used by the Court to assess cases, and only a limited time-frame within which those symptoms must be experienced and recorded, in order to qualify for compensation. For example, anaphylaxis reactions need to occur within 4hrs of vaccination, in order to qualify [115].

- There is now a very limited definition of what constitutes encephalopathy [114] - one of the more commonly reported serious adverse reactions, which can have life-long implications. The original definition from 1986 was "*any acute or chronic significant acquired abnormality of, or injury to, or impairment of function of, the brain*". In 1995, this definition was rewritten to be "*a significantly decreased level of consciousness lasting for at least 24 hours*", effectively disqualifying many children who displayed classic symptoms of encephalopathy, such as seizures, high-pitched screaming and unusual drowsiness [116].

- Many parents and even healthcare providers are unaware that the National Vaccine Injury Compensation program exists [117].

- In 2002, it was decided that a Special Omnibus Proceeding would be held (even though no such clause was included in the Childhood Vaccine Injury Act), to determine whether MMR vaccine and/or thimerosal-containing vaccines cause autism. More than 5000 petitions were filed in the program, on behalf of children who had regressed into autism following vaccination. In 2009, the US Court of Claims ruled that the biological plausibility of the vaccines cause autism hypothesis had not been proven [118]. Due to this universal ruling, thousands of children with vaccine-induced neuroimmunological disorders, labelled as 'autism' by doctors, were dismissed, or encouraged to withdraw their claims [119].

Although the Vaccine Injury Compensation program was originally designed to provide financial assistance for *children* injured by vaccines, the vast majority - some 80% - of compensation payouts today, are for adults [120]. Given that children are receiving far more vaccines than the average adult (CDC estimates adult vaccination coverage ranges from approximately 9% - 40%, depending on vaccine [121]), we must ask ourselves why children are so under-represented in vaccine compensation?

Could it be at, least partly, due to the fact that a baby, or small child, cannot articulate when they have symptoms that are unseen?

A small child cannot easily verbalise the extent of their pain or discomfort, either to their caregiver, or to medical professionals for documentation purposes. They are solely at the mercy of others, and whether they pick up the cues, and seek further diagnosis or action.

Although symptoms such as extended crying, fever, and lack of appetite may be seen as 'minor' and 'normal' by some, they probably feel anything but minor, to the child – they just don't have the verbal skills to tell you so.

When the Vaccine Injury Compensation program was set up in 1986, the CDC recommended all children receive 23 doses of 7 vaccines, between the ages of 2 months and 6 years [122]. That number has more than doubled, to 49 doses of 14 vaccines, given by age 6.

The American Medical Association's Council on Ethical and Judicial affairs states that "[a] *physician who suspects the occurrence of an adverse reaction to a drug or medical device has an obligation to communicate that information to the broader community, including, in the case of a serious adverse event, the Food and Drug Administration (FDA)*" [123].

But, do doctors actually follow this code? According to the literature, probably not.

Only an estimated 1% - 10% of adverse drug reactions are reported to authorities [124].

The Institute of Medicine (IOM) suggests this may be at least partly due to "time pressures, fear of liability, and lack of perceived benefits", which then results in "significant underreporting of adverse outcomes, and thus the inability to calculate true rates of such events" [125].

During hearings in 2001, Dr Thomas Bradstreet, testified before Congress [126]:

"At a recent autism conference in Chicago, and prior to either my own presentation or that of Dr. Wakefield, I asked the audience of 500 parents if they felt their child regressed following a vaccine. In that obviously non-scientific survey, approximately 90 percent the parents raised their hands to affirm vaccines were what they suspected had caused their child's symptoms."

"When I asked for how many had reported the event under the VAERS system, fewer than 15 said they had."

"Then I asked if their pediatrician had offered to report this, they just laughed. I have now conducted this simple survey with over 5000 parents at conferences around the world with similar findings. Yes, media attention creates bias."

"But despite the informal nature of this survey, it does tell us something about this debate we are currently engaged in: (1) parents of children with autism suspect vaccines damaged their child, (2) parents are not reporting this using VAERS forms, (3) pediatricians are not reporting to VAERS either, (4) and despite efforts by policymakers at CDC, FDA, AAP, IOM and elsewhere to reassure parents of the safety of vaccines, they remain unconvinced."

DIAGNOSTIC BIAS IN THE MEDICAL PROFESSION

How much of the 'success' attributed to vaccine programs, is really a self-fulfilling prophecy?

When a vaccine is licensed, and the corresponding disease is then referred to as a 'vaccine-preventable disease', the diagnostic criteria is often strengthened. For example, measles was once diagnosed solely on the presentation of symptoms. If you had the tell-tale rash, with a fever, and maybe conjunctivitis, chances are you would have been diagnosed with measles.

How many of these 'measles' cases were actually measles, though? In 1963, the year the vaccine was introduced, only 11%

of measles diagnoses turned out to be correct, when tested in a laboratory [127].

Now measles, and many other so-called vaccine-preventable diseases, requires laboratory confirmation. But in order to pursue laboratory confirmation, a doctor must be suitably convinced as to the likelihood that the patient has that disease - and this is where issues arise. Due to the belief that 'vaccines work', a doctor may be less inclined to test their vaccinated patients, even if they show symptoms of the disease they were vaccinated against.

This obviously skews the data in favour of vaccines - you won't find evidence of disease if you do not test for it!

Yet this 'diagnostic bias' is actively promoted by health authorities.

From the CDC: "*Clinicians are reminded to consider the diagnosis of respiratory diphtheria in patients with membranous pharyngitis **and who are not up-to-date with vaccination against diphtheria**" [128].

What about those who *are* up to date, though? Obviously, you need to find another explanation for the symptoms. In the case of diptheria, the differential diagnosis may be viral myocarditis, pharyngitis, or mononucleosis.

When it comes to measles, the CDC recommends "*To minimize the problem of false positive laboratory results, it is important to restrict case investigation and laboratory tests to patients most likely to have measles*" [129]. Those who are 'most likely' to have measles include the unvaccinated.

In other words, refrain from testing those who are up-to-date with measles vaccination, because it might come back positive, which (naturally!) would be an error. Instead, those who are up-to-date with vaccination, might get a diagnosis of Epstein-Barr Virus, Meningitis, Roseola, or Kawasaki Disease.

By 1998, only a mere 14% of measles diagnoses turned out to be correct in Australia [130]. Even today, 1 in 10 of all medical diagnoses are incorrect, according to the Society to Improve Diagnosis in Medicine [131].

Given this information, we must ask ourselves two important questions:

a) How many cases of diptheria, polio, pertussis, influenza, etc, were actually something else, in the era before laboratory testing was required? If only a very small minority of 'measles' cases were actually measles, then the pre-vaccine statistics are grossly over-inflated.

b) How many cases of 'vaccine-preventable disease' are now being overlooked amongst fully vaccinated individuals, in favour of other differential diagnoses? If fully vaccinated people are not being tested for those diseases, even if they present with the classical symptoms, then this has over-inflated the efficacy of the vaccines.

8.
VACCINE
SIDE EFFECTS

"Chronic illnesses are now so common, having a sick child seems to be the 'new normal'. Children are supposed to be vibrant, healthy, free of disease."
- Janet Levatin MD, Pediatrician.

FOOD ALLERGIES

Over 100 years ago, Nobel Laureate Charles Richet demonstrated that injecting proteins (even those considered to be well-tolerated) into humans or animals causes immune system sensitisation to that protein, and subsequent exposure can result in anaphylaxis [1].

His findings were repeated in numerous studies over the century that followed [2-5].

In 1964, the New York Times reported on the first use of peanut oil in vaccines, when it announced that Merck had begun to use a new vaccine ingredient that promised to extend immunity [6].

The use of peanut oil in vaccines became common practice during the 1970's and 1980's [7]. The incidence of peanut allergies began to rise in epic proportions during this same time period. Miranda Waggoner, post-doctoral researcher at the Office of Population Research in Woodrow Wilson School of Public and

International Affairs, says that peanut allergies were rarely mentioned in medical studies, or the media, before 1980 [8].

The use of adjuvants, such as aluminium increases the immunogenicity (ability to provoke an immune reaction) of the food proteins that are also present in the vaccine [9]. In fact, food proteins are injected into mice, with aluminium as adjuvant, with the express purpose of studying food allergies [10].

In 2010, the Institute of Medicine (IOM), in its review of current medical and scientific evidence on vaccines and vaccine adverse events, concluded that food proteins contained in vaccines can induce "*sensitization in some individuals and subsequent hypersensitivity reactions, including anaphylaxis*" [11].

AUTISM SPECTRUM DISORDER (ASD)

When it comes to the vaccination issue, no subject has proven more contentious than the vaccine-autism debate, which was brought to the forefront by the now-infamous Lancet paper by Andrew Wakefield [12]. That paper was later retracted.

Although Wakefield, et al were not specifically looking at a vaccine-autism link, the case series of gastrointestinal issues in 12 children with developmental disorders noted that "*in most cases, onset of symptoms was after measles, mumps and rubella immunisation*" and "*further investigations are needed to examine this syndrome and it's possible relation to this vaccine*" [12].

It was originally suggested, via other studies, that the thimerosal portion of vaccines may have been linked to the growing numbers of children diagnosed with Autism Spectrum Disorder (ASD), a link denied by the US Centers for Disease Control and Prevention (CDC), even going so far as to declare that "thimerosal is not a toxin in vaccines" [13].

At least one of the studies used by the CDC, and also used in Vaccine Injury Court to dismiss autism cases, was co-authored by former visiting CDC scientist Poul Thorsen – who is now a wanted fugitive, after allegedly diverting $1 million in CDC grant money to his own bank account, among other unethical activities [14].

Despite claims that there is no link between thimerosal-containing vaccines and autism disorders, a study conducted by the CDC themselves showed a 7.6-fold increased risk of autism from exposure to thimerosal during infancy [15]. Unfortunately, this earlier data was left out of the final results, published a couple of years later, in 2003 [16].

The claims made by the CDC, that thimerosal-containing vaccines are not linked to autism disorders, seem to be largely based on six published epidemiological studies completed, funded and/or co-sponsored by the CDC, starting from the late 1990's – including one co-authored by a wanted fugitive, and the other which left out vital data from an earlier phase of the study. Indeed, all six studies have been shown to have serious methodological issues which affected the outcomes [17].

Since the 'phase-out' of thimerosal, other vaccine ingredients have been investigated as possible culprits, including aluminium adjuvant, and the use of fetal cell lines in vaccine production.

Despite a number of highly-publicised studies claiming to show no link, there is a large body of circumstantial evidence that vaccines are at least contributing to the current autism epidemic, via a number of mechanisms. Some of this research includes:

a.) Overstimulation of microglia and astrocytes in the brain. Microglia and astrocytes are first-responder immune cells located in the brain that protect against foreign pathogens. Former neurosurgeon Russell Blaylock compiled a mass of evidence that repeated stimulation of microglia and astocytes, via vaccination, can cause inflammation and/or bleeding, synaptic and dendritic loss, and abnormal nerve pathway development [18-19].

In a study published in 2005, researchers examined the brains from autopsies of 11 autistic patients, and found the presence of extensively activated microglia and astrocytes along with pro-inflammatory cytokines [20].

b.) A 2011 study found a positive and statistically significant relationship between vaccination coverage and prevalence of autism or speech or language impairment. They found a 1% increase in vaccination coverage was associated with an additional 680 children having autism, or speech/language impairment [21].

c.) Another study published in 2011 found that *"children from countries with the highest ASD prevalence appear to have the highest exposure to Al from vaccines"* and *"the increase in exposure to Al adjuvants significantly correlates with the increase in ASD prevalence in the United States observed over the last two decades"* [22].

d.) A 2014 paper published in the Journal of Public Health and Epidemiology identified several 'change points' when autism diagnoses seemed to increase exponentially, and all of these change points *"corresponded to introduction of or increased doses of human fetal cell line-manufactured vaccines, while no relationship was found between paternal age or Diagnostic and Statistical Manual (DSM) revisions and autistic disorder diagnosis"* [23].

e.) Those with autism spectrum disorder have been found to have lower endocannabinoid levels [24]. The endocannaboinoid system regulates immune homeostasis in the gut [25].

Animal studies reveal that a fully-functioning endocannabinoid system serves to modulate and restrict immune activation after vaccination or infection, decreasing inflammation [26]. This could potentially help explain a link between autistic disorders and chronic immune activation/inflammation, however, researchers intend to use this information to alter (down-regulate) the endocannabinoid system in order to make vaccines more 'immunogenic'.

It is therefore feasible that vaccines may increase risk of Autism Spectrum Disorder via a number of factors, and may be exacerbated by synergistic or accumulative mechanisms, such as use of acetaminophen to control fever following vaccination (Tylenol etc) [27].

MACROPHAGIC MYOFASCITIS (MMF)

Macrophagic myofascitis is a relatively new condition, first emerging in France in 1993, and appearing in the scientific literature in 1998 [28]. Clinical symptoms include myalgia, arthralgia, muscle tenderness, muscle weakness, fever and fatigue. Neurological symptoms resembling multiple sclerosis have been reported in some patients [29], and also co-existent autoimmune diseases among some patients [30].

It is thought that macrophagic myofascitis is caused by an ongoing local immune reaction to the long-term persistence of aluminium in the muscle [31].

In one study, 50 out of 50 patients with macrophagic myofascitis had received vaccines for Hepatitis B (86%), Hepatitis A (19%) or tetanus toxoid (58%) in the 3-96mths leading up to biopsy. Vaccination preceded the onset of myalgia in 94% of patients. Serological tests were compatible with exposure to vaccines containing aluminium-hydroxide [31].

Israeli, et al (2011) defined macrophagic myofascitis as *"an emerging novel condition that may be triggered by exposure to alum-containing vaccines, in patients with a specific genetic backgraound, and this temporal association may be exhibited from a few months up to 10 years"* [32].

The true importance of the discovery, and subsequent research into macrophagic myofascitis, is that it has furthered our understanding of the pharmacokinetics of aluminium. Up until the last decade or so, aluminium was generally assumed to be well-tolerated, and efficiently excreted by the body, due to its quick withdrawal from interstitial fluid.

In his original work on macrophagic myofascitis, Rhomain Gherardi took biopsies from the patient's deltoid muscle, which revealed lesions up to 1cm in diameter. Upon analysis, it was discovered the lesions consisted mainly of macrophages – large white blood cells whose role is to envelop and digest foreign invaders in the body. Enclosed within the cellular fluid of these macrophages were agglomerates of aluminium nanocrystals [28].

Gherardi and colleagues continued their research by injecting mice with aluminium, the particles of which were engulfed by macrophages, forming lesions similar to MMF, which later dispersed to lymph nodes, spleen, liver and eventually brain. "*This strongly suggests that long-term adjuvant biopersistence within phagocytic cells is a prerequisite of slow brain translocation and delayed neurotoxicity*" [33].

PARALYSIS DISEASES

In the Chapter on Vaccine History, we explored the incredible timeline of polio, which casts doubts on what role a virus played, in the scheme of things. If polio outbreaks were really caused (or exacerbated) by poisons, toxins, or injections, then it stands to reason that we should still have those polio-like illnesses today, since we are still exposed to poisons, toxins - and more injections than ever.

And so we do.

But now they are obfuscated by numerous different labels and diagnoses due to increasingly sophisticated diagnostic equipment and techniques, that are able to measure subtle differences in pathology or function. These diagnoses may include:

a) **Meningitis:** actual incidence is unknown due to under-reporting, but European figures suggest as many as 70 cases per 100,000 children under one year, decreasing to 7.6 per 100,000 adults. The majority of cases are diagnosed as aseptic (viral) meningitis, with as many as 25,000 – 50,000 cases per year in the US alone [34]. Meningitis begins with flu-like symptoms, and in severe cases, progresses to muscle weakness, paralysis, and coma.

   A UK study in the early 90's found that half of all aseptic meningitis cases in children aged 12 – 24 months were vaccine associated [35]. This led to the withdrawal of MMR vaccines containing the Urabe mumps strain, and was replaced by MMR vaccines containing Jeryl-Lynn strain [36].

   Other countries, such as France, Japan, and Brazil also reported outbreaks of aseptic meningitis in the weeks following mass vaccination campaigns with mumps or MMR vaccines [37-39].

   In Bahrain (1995), an outbreak of aseptic meningitis, involving 286 cases, 95% of which occurred among children aged 0 – 12 years, followed in the wake of a national immunization day against polio. The following year, another outbreak occurred, again after a national immunization day against polio – this time involving 169 cases [40].

b) **Acute Flaccid Myelitis (AFM):** In 2018, there were 286 cases of suspected or confirmed acute flaccid myelitis in the United States (though these numbers are likely under-reported, and surveillance only started in 2014) [41].

AFM occurs more commonly in late summer, early autumn, most commonly affects children (some 90% of cases), features lesions on the spinal cord, and usually begins with fever and a cough, about 10 days before onset of paralysis [42-43] - all very similar to poliomyelitis prior to 1960's.

Acute flaccid myelitis is a devastating disease, with only 8% - 18% of patients making a full recovery. At least one astute (retired) paediatrician has pointed out that incidence peaks just happen to coincide with back-to-school vaccination schedules [44]. Acute Flaccid Myelitis is considered to be a sub-type or variant of Transverse Myelitis…

c) **Transverse Myelitis**: caused by inflammation and demyelination in a section of spinal cord, causing muscle weakness in the legs (and possibly the arms), and loss of bowel and bladder control (a feature that occurred in many cases labelled as polio in early 21st century). An estimated 1,400 new cases are diagnosed each year in the US [45]. The onset of transverse myelitis has been linked to vaccinations, specifically influenza, human papillomavirus (HPV), and hepatitis vaccines [46-47]

Joshua Coleman, who became an activist following his son's vaccine injury at 17 months old, tells of his experience [48]:

"My son was vaccine injured at seventeen months old. I have his vaccination cards here. I actually looked at his vaccination records. At seventeen months old, he had received thirty-seven vaccines, which is about three times the amount I got in my entire adult life. He ended up paralyzed with **transverse myelitis***."*

"I was very much under the impression that vaccine injury was extremely rare, that's what they told me at the time. Right off the bat, after the MRI, they were aware that it was in all likelihood a vaccine injury, which of course was later proven at Johns Hopkins, but that it was very, very rare."

"And when something like that happens to your child, you want to be under the impression that okay, if this happened, they were as careful as possible and this couldn't be avoided. Over time, doing my research, I, in fact, saw that the vaccine program is extremely careless, and possibly this could have been prevented had they just done better safety studies."

" ... And nobody told me about VAERS (Vaccine Adverse Event Reporting System), so there was no VAERS report submitted by the doctors who saw him, which

they are obligated by law to do. They didn't tell me about Vaccine Injury Court. I had no idea the kind of expenses that come along when you have a child that's a paraplegic. I very quickly learned how expensive it can be. It makes it very difficult to work or do the types of things to earn money.... It's extremely difficult..."

d) **Neuromyelitis Optica**: also known as Devic's disease, and features inflammation and demyelination of the optic nerve, and lesions on the spinal cord, causing weakness or paralysis in the legs or arms, loss of sensation, and bladder and bowel dysfunction. Onset or relapse of this disorder has been reported following HPV and influenza vaccinations [49-50], and compensation via the National Vaccine Injury Program has been awarded for cases of neuromyelitis optica following both HPV and influenza vaccines [51].

An estimated 4000 people in the US are affected by the disease.

e) **Acute Disseminated Encephalomyelitis (ADEM)**: About three-quarters of ADEM cases are preceded by either symptoms of infection, or a vaccination. Vaccines that have been linked to ADEM are rabies, DTaP, polio, measles, mumps, rubella, influenza, hepatitis B, Japanese Encephalitis, and HPV [52-53].

In October 2015, 9-year-old Breanna Browning received an influenza vaccine at school, and eight hours later, she began vomiting profusely. Two days later, she was blind, and paralyzed from the waist down. She was later diagnosed with Acute Disseminated Encephalomyelitis, and, although the family was convinced it was caused by the flu vaccine, doctors saw fit to remind the public that it was really influenza they needed to fear, and not the flu shot [54].

f) **Amyotrophic Lateral Sclerosis (ALS) also known as Lou Gehrig's Disease, or Motor Neurone Disease**: is a progressive neuromuscular disease, causing weakness in the legs and feet, which eventually effects muscles required to breathe and eat. ALS has an incidence of around 5 people per 100,000 in the US [55].

Approximately 5% - 10% of ALS cases are considered to be inherited, with the other 90% - 95% of cases having unknown origin, however studies have shown that a) smokers are at increased risk b) military personnel have double the incidence of ALS than civilian population [56] c) pesticide exposure has been shown to increase incidence of ALS by five-fold [57], and d) patients have higher glutamate levels than normal, in spinal fluid [58].

Conventional medicine has no cure for ALS, but a new drug came onto the market in 2017, which does not make patients feel any better or stronger, but is claimed to have a 'modest' effect on slowing the disease – with a price-tag of more than $145,000 per year [59].

Readers may remember the 'Ice Bucket Challenge' from several years ago, which challenged people to record themselves dumping a bucket of ice water over their head, in order to raise awareness and funds for the ALS research and support groups. The challenge swept across social and mainstream media, with celebrities, politicians and sports-stars taking part.

All in all, the ALS Association received $115 million in donations from the Ice Bucket Challenge, and almost $90 million was ploughed into research programs – unfortunately, they were overwhelmingly focused on searching for genetic causes, identifying biomarkers for diagnostic and disease progression management purposes, or advances that could be used to produce new pharmaceutical drugs, and only a miniscule amount to studying potential environmental risk factors [60].

Vaccines have been flagged as one potential risk factor, and this may explain the increased incidence of ALS in military personnel, who are required to have extra vaccines [61].

In 2018, a case report was published, describing a 15-year-old girl who developed '*rapid progressive muscle weakness one week after the third injection of a bivalent human papilloma virus (HPV) vaccine. Although immunotherapies were performed for possible vaccine-related disorders, she died of respiratory failure 14 months after the onset of the disease*' [62].

ALS patients have been found to have "*Statistically significant higher concentrations of manganese, aluminium, cadmium, cobalt, copper, zinc, lead, vanadium and uranium*" [63].

g) **Guillain-Barre Syndrome (GBS)**: has an annual incidence of 1 – 3 per 100,000 population, and causes muscle weakness in the limbs (but may include neck and respiratory muscles). It was named after researchers who described the symptoms of motor weakness in two French soldiers in 1916 [64]. (Note that vaccination for typhoid fever was compulsory by law, amongst the French army [65], and smallpox vaccination was likely employed too).

Case reports and epidemiological studies suggest a possible association between GBS, and rabies, oral polio, influenza, MMR, tetanus toxoid-containing, and Hepatitis B vaccines [66].

Following a swine flu vaccination campaign in 1976-1977, reports of Guillain-Barre Syndrome increased. Upon investigation into the matter, The Expert Neurology Group of the CDC concluded there was increased risk of developing Guillain –Barre Syndrome within the first six weeks after vaccination [66] – a finding that bore remarkable similarities to that of the finding reached in 1949, following increase in 'polio' after receipt of diphtheria and pertussis vaccination.

h) **Cerebral Palsy**: In 2001, Angelica Black was almost three months old, when she received four vaccines. She was healthy, and developing normally up to that point, but three days later, she stopped breathing. After being rushed to hospital, she started having seizures, and was later diagnosed with vaccine-related encephalopathy. Today, she is profoundly disabled – cannot speak, requires a feeding tube, a wheelchair, and around-the-clock care. Her condition is labelled as cerebral palsy – a condition caused by damage to the developing brain of a child before, during or after birth, which results in muscle weakness and/or spasticity, and often accompanied by developmental disorders [67].

According to the CDC, some 10% - 15% of cerebral palsy cases occur in the first years of a child's life [68], and usually preceded by an infection (note the possibility that fevers and other side-effects of vaccines may be labelled as 'infections', if they happen to isolate a virus or bacteria from specimens).

It is interesting to note that high rates of 'cerebral palsy' were clustered in Minamata Bay area, Japan, during the 1950's and 1960's. It was later discovered that these children were actually suffering from Congenital Minamata Disease, caused by high levels of methylmercury in Minamata Bay – they had been exposed while still in utero [69].

Could there be a similar risk for the unborn babies of mothers vaccinated with thimerosal-containing vaccines during pregnancy? Or mothers who received Rhogam injections during pregnancy, which also contained mercury, prior to the late 1990's/early 2000's [70]?

i) **Multiple Sclerosis (MS)**: the most common acquired neurological disease affecting young adults, commonly diagnosed between the ages of 20 – 40 years. It occurs when the immune system attacks the myelin sheath – the insulating, protective sheath that covers nerve cells.

Conventional medicine seems to offer little explanation as to why this occurs, and offers no cure, although researchers are hopeful that a (yet another) new vaccine could prevent it, by protecting from Epstein-Barr Virus [71].

One wonders how a vaccine might protect from MS, if said MS was first caused by a vaccine? There are numerous reports of multiple sclerosis occurring after vaccinations, with Hepatitis B vaccine being the main suspect [72-74], although other vaccines have also been implicated.

In 1994, the French health authorities launched a national Hepatitis B vaccination campaign for secondary-school students. The following year, Hepatitis B vaccination was added to the national schedule, for all babies and preteens.

Adults were also encouraged to get vaccinated, which led to an 'unprecedented wave' of vaccinations in adults. Between 1994 and 1997, some 20 million French were vaccinated for Hepatitis B – which correlates to a significant rise in reported cases of MS through the French passive surveillance system. Researchers agreed that even those were likely under-reported [75].

An advocacy group named REVAHB, formed by Hepatitis B vaccine victims, collected more than 2000 reports of injury, and forwarded to authorities. However, not all of these reports were included in the pharmacovigilance registry, due to inability to confirm results with doctors (who failed to respond to requests for information) [75].

SUDDEN INFANT DEATH SYNDROME (SIDS)

In June, 1987, 4-month-old Christopher Blum receives vaccines, and vomits almost immediately afterwards. Later he seems lethargic ... and eight hours later, his father, Steve, finds him dead in his cot.

At the hospital, they conduct investigations, and find evidence of an 'infection', but fail to establish a cause of the infection, so his death is listed as SIDS. His father insists the death was caused by vaccines and refuses to sign the death certificate. The council refuses to allow little Christopher to be buried without a death certificate.

For 21 years, baby Christopher's body lies in the mortuary, on ice. His parents are not allowed to see him or touch him. No further investigations are allowed to be conducted.

Steve is haunted by his son's death, and vows to find answers. It takes him three years and a court order to get access to his son's medical records. He becomes obsessed with poring over medical textbooks, teaching himself basic principles of medicine. Solicitor after solicitor deserts him. The strain eventually destroys both his marriage and his health, and authorities all the while refuse to conduct any further tests or investigations.

Finally, the council rules that they can sign the death certificate themselves, and organize to have baby Christopher buried, in 2008 [76].

One can't begin to imagine the depth of a parent's anguish in such a situation, but the truth of the matter is, even if tests could prove beyond doubt that vaccines caused the death, it would still not be reported as such, on the death certificate.

There are 130 internationally-recognized cause-of-death categories for infants, covering just about every tragic situation imaginable...except death by vaccination [77-78]. If a baby dies following vaccination, the death will *not* be attributed to vaccines, hence, there is no reliable way of knowing how many infant victims there are.

The term 'SIDS' was coined in 1969, after an alarming rise in sudden, inexplicable deaths in infants began to attract the attention of astute doctors [79].

Within just three short years, Sudden Infant Death Syndrome was the leading cause of death among neonates in the United States [80].

The sudden death of an infant after vaccination had been reported in the literature, from as early as the 1930's, when two babies had vaccines for pertussis at birth, and died within 2 hours of their second shots, at 4 and 11 days old, respectively [81].

In 1946, it was reported that 10-month-old twin boys had both passed away within 24 hours of receiving diptheria-tetanus-pertussis (DTP) shots [82]. Again, in 1985, five-month-old twin boys both died within 3 hours of DTP vaccination [83].

Throughout the 1970's and 1980's, DTP vaccination dropped in many countries around the world, including Japan, Australia, Great Britain, and United States, amidst fears of a link between the vaccine and severe side effects [84]. One of the greatest decreases in vaccination rates was seen in the 1970's and 1980's in the UK, which happens to coincide with falling infant mortality rates. Infant mortality rates level out after 1990, which is also when DTP vaccination rates began to increase again [84-85].

In 1975, Japanese authorities raised the age of vaccination from 3 months to 2 years, following the post-vaccinal deaths of 37 infants. Over the following decade, the infant mortality rate dropped by 60%, and sudden unexplained deaths in infants were virtually eliminated [86].

In 1992, the American Academy of Pediatrics (AAP), began to recommend that babies be put to sleep on their back, to lower the risk of Sudden Infant Death Syndrome, and subsequently began the 'safe sleeping' campaign [87]. Any lingering doubts about a link between vaccines and SIDS were apparently put to bed also, when the SIDS rate fell by 8.6% per year [88]. The campaign was hailed a success...

Unfortunately, infant deaths due to 'suffocation in bed' increased at an average rate of 11.2% per annum. Neonatal deaths from 'suffocation other', and 'unknown and unspecified causes' also increased, and the overall infant mortality rate remained fairly stable [89]. What was once diagnosed as SIDS was being diagnosed as something else, after the 'safe sleeping' campaign was introduced.

A review of claims to the Vaccine Injury Compensation program in the US, between 1988 and 1996 found 107 were DTP-related deaths. Of those, 73 were awarded compensation after the Special Masters agreed they were vaccine-related. Out of 73 deaths, fifty of them (68%) were originally diagnosed as 'SIDS' [90].

According to researchers, the current method of post-mortem investigation following a sudden infant death is inadequate to identify if vaccines played a role [91].

In 2006, Zinka et al published a study of six babies who died within 48 hours of vaccination [92], and were subjected to heavy criticism for their work. In their response, they noted [93]:

"The main problem is that vaccination specialists have failed for decades to establish any tests or other criteria to find out if adverse events are linked to vaccinations or not. To our knowledge they did not even try hard - why?!"

"A precise description of the mechanism leading to serious adverse events after hexavalent vaccination is not the task of forensic pathology. This would be the job of vaccination specialists, and actually this job should have been done before phase 1 and phase 2 studies in order to get valid data on drug safety."

Even the CDC felt compelled to address the 'coincidence' of sudden infant death following vaccination [94]:

"Babies receive many vaccines when they are between 2 to 4 months old. This age range is also the peak age for sudden infant death syndrome (SIDS), or infant death that cannot be explained. The timing of the 2 month and 4 month shots and SIDS has led some people to question whether they might be related. However, studies have found that vaccines do not cause and are not linked to SIDS."

Indeed, there *have* been studies that concluded there was no link between vaccines and SIDS.

One of the ways researchers have attempted to investigate a link is by comparing the rate of SIDS after vaccines, with the expected rate of SIDS in the community. Basically, the community acts as the 'control group'.

But if 90% (or more) of children in the community are fully-vaccinated, and vaccines were increasing the rate of SIDS...do you see the problem here? The 'control group' has already been compromised, and therefore, any comparisons are of limited value.

The grieving parents and families may rightly ask why the CDC sees fit to overlook the following studies which *do* suggest a link between vaccines and SIDS:

- 2011: Research on infant mortality and vaccination schedules in developed countries found that those with more intense vaccination schedules had higher infant mortality rates, and those with fewer injections had lower infant mortality rates. Analysis showed a statistically significant correlation between number of vaccines given, and infant mortality rates [95].

- 2011: A case series looking at a relationship between penta- or hexa-valent vaccines, and sudden infant death, found a 16-fold increased risk of sudden death after a fourth dose, and twice the risk of sudden death following vaccines in general [96].

- 2011: A case series in Italy found double the risk of SIDS, 1-7 days after a first dose of hexavalent vaccine [97].

SHAKEN BABY SYNDROME

On December 4, 1998, Lorraine Harris took her 4-month-old son Patrick to have his vaccines. In the early hours of the following morning, she found him lifeless in his bed, and called an ambulance. He was rushed to hospital and placed on life-support, but sadly passed away a day later.

The post-mortem found marked brain swelling, some post-dural haemorrhaging and extensive retinal haemorrhaging (bleeding behind the eyes). The death was recorded as cerebral hypoxia - where the oxygen supply to the brain is cut off due to excessive swelling, intracranial haemorrhaging, and...shaken baby syndrome.

Lorraine was charged with manslaughter and taken into custody. Her baby son was buried without her.

Despite being described as a caring, loving mother, no evidence of bruising or gripping, no history of fractures, Lorraine was convicted on September 7, 2000, and sentenced to three years imprisonment, on the basis of 'expert evidence'.

While on bail, awaiting trial, Lorraine had become pregnant again, and as she was starting to serve her sentence, gave birth to another baby boy. He was removed from her at one day old, given up for adoption and she was never allowed to see him again. Her partner left her, while serving her sentence [98].

One of the experts whose report helped to convict Lorraine Harris was Dr. Waney Squier, one of only two consultant paediatric neuropathologists in England, with more than three decades of experience.

After Lorraine's conviction, however, Dr. Squier began to have a change of heart, due to research by Dr. Jennien Geddes, another neuropathologist. Dr Geddes had become troubled by the number of cases where there was no sign of physical damage to the child's body [99-100].

Dr. Squier then *"began to conduct her own investigations and concluded that shaking as a cause of death in babies could 'virtually be excluded' unless there was also evidence of body trauma, such as serious damage to the neck"* [101].

Dr. Squier later appeared as expert witness at Lorraine Harris' appeal – but this time for the defence.

Lorraine's conviction was overturned, and her name restored, but her life would never be the same again. Despite the clear miscarriage of justice, her application for compensation was denied. She was also denied access to the baby boy who was adopted out.

The story doesn't end there for Dr. Waney Squier...

In 2010, after acting as expert witness in several successful appeals, Dr. Squier was reported to the General Medical Council, by police, for 'deliberately misleading' the courts on Shaken Baby Syndrome. After a long inquiry, she was struck off the medical register. She successfully appealed through the High Court and was reinstated, but was banned from giving evidence in SBS cases for three years.

She says *"We need a public inquiry into how this syndrome is still being used to condemn people in the family and criminal courts. They are being accused on the basis of it, yet it is only an hypothesis with no scientific evidence to support it"* [102].

Sadly, there are more heart-breaking stories like Lorraine Harris...

In 1999, Sally Clark, a solicitor, was sentenced to life imprisonment for killing her two baby sons [103].

First, her 12-week-old son Christopher in 1996. His death was originally thought to be caused by a 'lung infection', but then ...

In 1998, she found her 8-week-old son, Harry, dead. He had received vaccines just five hours earlier [104]. The second death raised the suspicion of authorities.

She was charged, and convicted, for their murders, based on 'expert' witnesses, one of which claimed that the chances of two babies dying, from the one family, were 1 in 73 million. He also assured the jury that the vaccine could not be the cause of death [105].

After serving three years of her sentence, during which time she was assaulted, and detested by fellow inmates as a 'baby killer', her conviction was overturned based on the discovery of medical evidence showing infection in baby Harry's spinal fluid, that was hidden during her trial.

Although she was released, she never did recover from the trauma, and in 2007, she was found dead in her home, aged 42 years [106].

An estimated 250 cases of 'Shaken Baby Syndrome' come before the family and criminal courts every year, in Great Britain alone [107].

In the US, there are an estimated 1000 – 3000 cases of shaken baby syndrome each year, with approximately one-quarter of those babies dying, and survivors often have life-long conditions and brain injury [108].

How many of these cases are violent monsters, and how many are loving parents, just following guidelines to vaccinate their children?

Research shows that cases of 'SBS' peak at around 6-8 weeks of age...when babies apparently cry the most (also when most babies receive numerous vaccines, at the one time) [109].

Some authorities have called for the consideration of homicide in *any* case of sudden death in a child [110].

And yet, a systematic review published in 2017, concluded that nearly all studies in the area of SBS were of very low quality, with a high risk of bias, and that, therefore, *"there is insufficient scientific evidence on which to assess the diagnostic accuracy of the triad in identifying traumatic shaking"* [111].

More than 50 years ago, Australian doctor Archie Kalokerinos discovered that the symptoms of 'Shaken Baby Syndrome' are perfectly identical to scurvy, or Vitamin C deficiency. He was able to halt the epidemic of SIDS and 'Shaken Baby' deaths in the Aboriginal community he worked in, via the use of intravenous Vitamin C [112].

In his book "Shaken Baby Syndrome: An Abusive Diagnosis", he writes "*Crucially for babies, the innate immune system is dependent on Vitamin C, for without that, the neutrophils, lymphocytes, and phagocytes <u>which process toxins in the body</u> come to a halt*".

And "*While the Vitamin C recommended daily allowance might be sufficient to avoid a pre-morbid state called "scurvy', it bears no relationship to the amounts required for the body to effectively manage essential biochemical processes brought into play after **vaccines, toxin exposure, malnutrition, illness or stress***" [113].

He also details how Vitamin C deficiency, or a malfunction in ascorbate transporters, can lead to spontaneous fractures in the bones of small children, and healing deposits - which appear to be old fractures that have healed over - another 'sign' that is regarded as proof of abuse.

Parental smoking is accepted as a strong risk factor for sudden death in infants. Smoking depletes the body of Vitamin C [114].

If the mother smoked during pregnancy or breastfeeding, the child is likely to be depleted of this vitamin, so essential for growth and cellular function.

Also, if a child is raised in a home where she is subjected to second-hand smoke, *even in small amounts*, she is at increased risk of Vitamin C deficiency [115].

Vitamin C - or ascorbic acid - also has a protective effect against heavy metals [116].

Could it be that Vitamin C-deficient infants are simply overwhelmed by the aluminium, and other ingredients, found in vaccines? Or perhaps overwhelmed by the body's histamine response, in the absence of sufficient ascorbic acid to counteract it [117]?

More than 70yrs ago, it was shown that injections are three times more likely to cause death, if the recipient had been on a Vitamin C-deficient diet for 15 days beforehand [118].

BLOOD DISORDERS

Idiopathic thrombocytopenia purpura: is a bleeding disorder that results in low platelet count, and can manifest as easy, or severe, bruising, nosebleeds, and possibly bleeding on the brain (all of which sound similar to 'Shaken Baby Syndrome'). This disorder is very rare in small children, but there is increased risk in older children, above the age of seven, after receiving vaccines - most notably, hepatitis A, chickenpox and combined diptheria-tetanus-pertussis vaccines [119-120].

Neutropenia: involves abnormally low levels of neutrophils, a type of white blood cell that is important for fighting infection, particularly bacterial infection [121].

In a small clinical trial of a genetically-engineered dengue virus vaccine, almost half of vaccinees developed neutropenia following the first dose, 22% of those were classified as severe, and 13% as moderate. Following the second dose, 9% of vaccinees developed neutropenia, but all cases were considered to be mild [122].

Vasculitis: is caused by inflammation and damage to the blood vessels, and the symptoms depend on the location of the blood vessels in question, but may involve skin, eyes, brain or other internal organs.

Vasculitis in general, along with specific forms of vasculitis have been linked to vaccinations [123-124]. The specific forms of vasculitis reported following vaccination include Henoch-Schonlein purpura [125], Kawasaki Disease [126], and polyarteritis nodosa [127].

Kawasaki disease is most common in children under 5 years of age, with symptoms including rash, fever, swelling of the hands and feet, swelling of lymph glands in the neck, and inflammation of the mouth, lips and throat. Serious complications can involve heart problems [128]. It was first described in Japan in 1967, and the incidence has been rising over the past few decades [128-129]. The peak incidence occurs at one year of age.

In 2010, a thirteen-strain pneumococcal vaccine replaced the seven-strain vaccine for use in children. Studies revealed that the incidence of Kawasaki disease within 28 days of vaccination with the new thirteen-strain vaccine was almost double that of the original seven-strain vaccine [130].

Trials of the current rotavirus vaccine showed a five-fold increase in Kawasaki disease compared to placebo [131].

AUTO-IMMUNE CONDITIONS

Yehuda Shoenfeld, also known as the 'Godfather of Autoimmunology', has been studying the human immune system for more than three decades, and authored dozens of textbooks on the subject.

He's highly esteemed among the mainstream medical establishment, and yet...

Over the past few years, Shoenfeld - and others - have begun to point the finger at vaccines, or specifically the adjuvants found in vaccines, as playing a major role in the current epidemic of auto-immune disorders. In fact, he was confronted with so many cases of auto-immune conditions following vaccination, that in 2015 he proposed a new syndrome, named Autoimmune/Inflammatory Syndrome induced by Adjuvants (ASIA) [132].

Autoimmune conditions develop when the body's immune system begins to attack parts of the body it belongs to. That much is easy to understand. The question is *why* does the body start to do this?

One possibility is that vaccinations may disturb immune system homeostasis in some people, causing dysregulation that obscures the fine line between preserving normal immune function against pathogenic invaders, and attacking oneself.

Another possibility is that the Th1/Th2 skewing caused by vaccinations, among other things, creates a situation whereby cells are chronically infected/inflamed. The body then starts to attack those cells, in an effort to remove the infection/inflammation.

A third possibility is the concept of molecular mimicry, which occurs due to the similarity of proteins found in organisms and mammals. Some viruses are made up of proteins that are so similar to proteins contained in our body, that infection (or introduction via vaccination) of one, causes the body to cross-react with similar self-proteins.

This is the case with measles - the viral proteins are so similar to myelin basic protein, that antibodies against measles virus may also cause attack against the myelin sheath.

If auto-antibodies attack the myelin sheath around neurons, nerve impulses cannot conduct properly, which affects coordination, and, depending on the location of the damage, the diagnosis might be multiple sclerosis, autism, ADHD, seizure disorders, Guillaine-Barre Syndrome, Lou Gehrig's disease (ALS), Parkinson's disease, etc.

The location of the cells that are attacked by the immune system will determine the symptoms and eventual diagnosis:

If autoantibodies attack the mucosa of the gastrointestinal tract, the person develops Crohn's disease, colitis or leaky gut syndrome.

If autoantibodies attack the articular surface of the joints, the person develops rheumatoid or juvenile arthritis.

If you develop autoantibodies against your own DNA, you will likely get a diagnosis of lupus.

If autoantibodies attack the insulin-producing cells of the pancreas, the islets of langerhans, you can expect to be diagnosed with juvenile diabetes.

Unfortunately, nobody can say for sure that a vaccine won't produce these unwanted, and serious, side effects before the vaccine is authorized and administered to the public [133].

So far, a number of vaccines have been linked to autoimmune conditions, including:

- The HPV vaccine has been linked to the production of auto-antibodies against the ovaries and thyroid, resulting in primary ovarian failure [134].

- The HPV vaccine has been linked to systemic lupus erythematosus (SLE) autoimmune disorder [135].

- The Hepatitis B vaccine has been linked to chronic fatigue syndrome and fibromyalgia [136].

- The HPV vaccine has been linked to pancreatitis via molecular mimicry [137].

- the HPV vaccine has been linked to rheumatoid arthritis [138].

- The Hepatitis B vaccine has been linked to multiple sclerosis [139].

- The HPV vaccine has been associated with loss of eyesight due to damage to the myelin sheath [140].

- The rubella vaccine is linked to chronic arthritis in adult women [141].

- The MMR vaccine has been linked to autoantibodies against the central nervous system, and the myelin sheath in particular, in children with autism [142].

- The HPV vaccine has been shown to increase antibodies against glutamate receptors in some people [143]. These antibodies have been linked to seizures and epilepsy [144].

Researchers point out that large-scale epidemiological studies have failed, so far, to find a connection between vaccines and autoimmune conditions due to "the limited number of cases, the different classifications of symptoms and the long latency period of the diseases" [145]. The presence of autoantibodies is a predictor of future autoimmune disease, even in patients without symptoms, and may occur years ahead of disease onset [146].

Further, researchers have proposed that there are four groups of people who are at increased risk of autoimmune/inflammatory conditions after vaccination, and this should be considered when weighing up the risks/benefits of vaccination for the individual [147]:

i) Those who have had a previous adverse reaction to vaccines.
ii) Those who have an established autoimmune condition.
iii) Those with a history of allergy.
iv) Those who are prone to developing autoimmunity, which includes those with a family history of autoimmune disorders, those who have tested positive for autoantibodies, smokers, and those with high estrogen and low vitamin D levels - which would likely be those taking birth control or hormone replacement therapy.

SKIN DISORDERS

The skin is the largest organ of the body, and comprises part of the elimination system, along with the liver, kidneys, lungs and intestines. If the other eliminatory organs are not working optimally, the skin will be called upon, to try and remove toxins from the body. Water-soluble wastes may also be removed via sweat.

Given that vaccines contain known toxins, it is hardly surprising that vaccination has been linked to numerous skin disorders.

Psoriasis: is a chronic, inflammatory disease of the skin that causes itchy, scaly patches. It is now recognized as an autoimmune condition, but the antigen/s responsible are unclear [148].

Numerous reports have been published suggesting a link between vaccination and the beginning, or worsening, of psoriasis, namely influenza, tuberculosis and tetanus vaccines [149-153].

A 2015 study published in the Journal of Immunology Research reported on 43 patients suffering from psoriasis triggered by influenza vaccination: "*The short time intervals between vaccination and psoriasis flares in our patients and the lack of other possible triggers suggest that influenza vaccinations may have provocative effects on psoriasis*" [154].

Eczema: causes dry, itchy patches of skin, and affects between 10%-20% of children in the US, and approximately 3% of adults. Even mainstream medicine concedes that eczema is probably "*linked to an overactive response by the body's immune system to an irritant*" [155].

A large birth cohort study of almost 30,000 children found a 9-fold increase in eczema amongst vaccinated children, compared to unvaccinated. Unfortunately, the authors explained away this finding as being due to unvaccinated children visiting the doctor less, and therefore had less chance to be diagnosed [156].

A link between vaccination and eczema was acknowledged back in the 1950's, and researchers even went so far as to recommend that if a person, or a member of their family, was suffering from eczema, they should not be vaccinated [157].

Bullous pemphigoid: is a skin condition that causes large, fluid-filled blisters, usually on areas that often flex, such as lower abdomen, or armpits.

It is thought that bullous pemphigoid occurs as an *immune malfunction,* caused by auto-antibodies against the connective fibers between the skin layers. This results in inflammation, causing itching and blisters [158].

Numerous case studies have been published on the onset of bullous pemphigoid following vaccination - sometimes as early as 24hrs after injection - mostly in older adults, but sometimes in children. The most implicated vaccines were tetanus, influenza, and hepatitis B vaccines [159-162].

Stevens-Johnson Syndrome: is a serious, potentially life-threatening disorder which causes rashes, blistering, and shedding of the skin, usually from a reaction to drugs [163]. There are numerous case studies of Stevens-Johnson Syndrome occurring after vaccination, including varicella, measles, hepatitis B and smallpox vaccines [164-167].

OTHER DISORDERS

Psychiatric Disorders: In early 2017, a study from Yale was published, showing an increased risk of psychiatric disorders in the months following receipt of a vaccine during childhood or adolescence [168].

Although the authors were careful to emphasize that vaccine benefits still outweighed the risks, nevertheless, they noted a possible temporal association with vaccinations in childhood, and diagnoses of anorexia nervosa, obsessive-compulsive disorder (OCD), anxiety, and tic disorders.

Narcolepsy: "*is a sleep disorder that is characterized by excessive sleepiness, sleep attacks, sleep paralysis, hallucinations and, for some, sudden loss of muscle control*" [169].

The incidence of narcolepsy has grown in Finland, Sweden, Ireland, Norway, England, and France after vaccination with AS03-adjuvanted H1N1 (swine flu) vaccine [170-171].

Narcolepsy, with loss of muscle control, is caused by loss of brain cells that secrete hypocretin - a chemical that regulates sleep and wakefulness. The AS03-adjuvanted swine flu vaccine has been shown to induce auto-antibodies against human hyprocretin receptors [172].

Reproductive Disorders/Infertility: In 2012, the British Medical Journal published a case report of a 16-year-old girl who received a cervical cancer vaccine towards the end of 2008. Following that, her menstrual periods became irregular and scant, and by 2011, her menstrual cycle had ceased altogether.

Upon further inspection, it was discovered that all of her remaining eggs were dead - she was totally infertile. She was given a diagnosis of primary ovarian failure, basically premature menopause at 16 years of age [173].

Other cases of premature ovarian failure in young women following vaccination for cervical cancer have since come before the courts [174].

Eye Disorders: Panuveitis and Uveitis have both been reported in association with vaccines [175-176]. Both conditions involve inflammation in the eye, and may lead to vision loss or blindness. Optic neuritis involves inflammation of the optic nerve, which leads to pain and loss of vision - this problem has also been reported following vaccination [177-178].

Hearing Loss: Three days after rubella vaccination, a 27-year-old woman began to experience joint pain, which then led to fever, vomiting, headaches, tinnitus, dizziness, unsteady gait, and eventually, hearing loss in both ears. Audiography at 29 days post-vaccination found complete deafness in both ears, which could not be resolved via steroid treatment [179].

Twenty-five days after receiving MMR vaccine, one young girl broke out in a rash, which then developed into vomiting and malaise, and then poor balance. Soon after, she stopped speaking, and began responding poorly to noise. She was found to be completely deaf in both ears [180].

Other reports of hearing loss following vaccination, have been published in medical journals and mainstream media [181-182].

9.
VACCINES AROUND THE WORLD

Drug companies are not charities, they are 'for-profit' ventures, whose legal responsibility is to their shareholders, to maximise dividend return on investment. How does that mesh with the complex ethical issues of supplying drugs or vaccines to under-developed nations?

The pharmaceutical industry has come under fire for question-able practices in third-world countries. Although the provision of vaccines to third-world countries is hailed as a great human-itarian move, the prioritisation process remains dubious in many instances. Would the billions of dollars spent on vaccine programs to Africa, and other undeveloped parts of the world, be better spent ensuring a nutritious food supply, clean water and sanitation, first?

Take Rwanda, for example. According to UNICEF statistics, Rwanda has 98%-99% vaccination coverage for polio, Hib, diphtheria-tetanus-pertussis...yet 44% of children are stunted due to malnutrition. Eighty-five percent of babies are vac-cinated for tetanus...but only 61% have access to proper sanita-tion [1].

Despite the lack of clean water and sanitation faced by millions of Rwandans, Merck saw fit to donate enough free HPV vaccines to vaccinate 95% of the nation's 11-year-old girls. The freebies ran out after three years, at which time Merck offered the vaccine to the Rwandan government at 'discount prices'. Such donations can have the effect of locking governments into programmes, which they later have to fund themselves, at the expense of more pressing issues, and may be more about 'priming the market' than charity, on the part of the drug company [2].

The GAVI Alliance (The Global Alliance for Vaccines and Immunisation) was created in 2000 "to improve access to new and underused vaccines for children living in the world's poorest countries" [3]. GAVI is an international partnership between public entities, such as the World Health Organization, and private sector, such as pharmaceutical companies. The Bill and Melinda Gates Foundation, a founding partner of GAVI, have donated USD 4.1 billion, to date [4].

Any country with a GNP of less than US$1000 per capita is eligible to apply for GAVI support, which represents roughly half the world's population [5].

Global vaccine initiatives such as these, were credited with slashing the measles death rate in Africa by a whopping 91%. The news of this outstanding success was splashed across media headlines around the world [6], but a further look into the actual data reveals little proof for these sensational claims [7].

The figures are not based on actual reports, but rather, mathematical modelling, which is based upon how many people got vaccinated, how 'effective' the vaccine is (remember that this figure is based apon ability to induce antibodies, which doesn't necessarily equal real-world protection), and based on the as-sumption of what would happen if they hadn't got the vaccine [7].

Even the World Health Organization saw the pitfalls in such an approach, and belatedly attempted to apply some caution [8], saying "*the assessment of a recent change in measles mortality from vaccination is mostly based on statistics predicted from a set of covariates such as the number of live births, vaccine coverage, vaccine effectiveness and case-fatality ratios. It is understandable that estimating causes of death over time is a difficult task. However, that is no reason for us to avoid meas-uring it when we can also measure the quantity of interest di-rectly; otherwise the global health community would continue to monitor progress on a spreadsheet with limited empirical basis. This is simply not acceptable.*"

One wonders how all those measles deaths in the past were even verified? Without access to laboratory testing, how did they ever ascertain whether it was actually measles...or one of nu-merous other infections that manifest similar symptoms?

Indeed, the vast majority of third world countries do not have sufficient data-collection systems in place, to accurately assess information such as cause of death statistics, anyway. In fact, only about one-third of all countries in the world have a func-tional civil registration system in place [9].

Not only do many third-world countries lack a civil registration system, they also lack a pharmacovigilance system. What this means, is that nobody is monitoring for, or reporting on, adverse reactions to vaccines, or any other pharmaceutical drug, in these countries [10].

"The main reasons for this are lack of resources, infrastructure, and expertise. Thus, although access to medicines is increasing in developing countries, there is a danger that their risk benefit profiles in indigenous populations will not be fully monitored and acted upon" [10].

If there is no system to report adverse reactions to vaccines - or any medical treatment - how can we assess what effect the current vaccine programme is really having in undeveloped nations?

In 2011, there were an extra 47,500 cases of Non-Polio Accute Flaccid paralysis (NPAFP) in India, with cases manifesting in direct proportion to doses of oral polio vaccine received [11]. NPAFP is clinically indistinguishable from polio, but twice as deadly. Although these cases were reported on, via the polio surveillance system, *they were not investigated.*

Tens of thousands of vaccine recipients were paralysed...and nobody investigated?

Five deaths following a new pentavalent vaccine in Sri Lanka did get investigated, by the World Health Organization. The investigators felt that three of the deaths may have been linked to the vaccine, however, the World Health Organization revised their classifications soon after, so that deaths seen during post-marketing surveillance can no longer be classified as "consistent with causal association with vaccine" [12].

Vietnam suspended use of the same pentavalent vaccine in 2013, after it was linked to 6 deaths. The WHO used the revised classifications, and concluded that "no fatal adverse event following immunisation (AEFI) has ever been associated with this vaccine" [12].

It seems as though vaccine programs must be implemented at all cost in undeveloped countries. If the citizens are reluctant to comply, other methods are employed.

In a bid to persuade reluctant villagers to have their children vaccinated for polio, the Indian government and UNICEF co-opted religious leaders to promote the vaccine. Islamic leaders gave speeches before Friday prayer services, using quotes from the Koran, to encourage fellow worshippers to accept vaccines. Newspaper columns were prepared and signed off by religious leaders, who also conducted radio question-and-answer sessions [13].

Vaccine hesitancy in remote areas is hardly surprising. As one religious leader put it: "*For decades, the government machinery has not reached out to them; there are no proper roads, no drainage systems, no employment opportunities, no basic facilities – and suddenly a team of health officials arrive there to say we care for your children and therefore we want to vaccinate them*" [13].

Another issue with supplying vaccines to impoverished nations, is ensuring distribution, storage, and administration protocols are followed. This is not always the case, and the consequences can be devastating.

During the writing of this book, it was reported that 15 young children died in South Sudan after a "botched measles vaccination campaign". Authorities said the same syringe was used for four days, and children *as young as 12* were administering vaccines [14].

Fifteen children also died in war-torn Syria after receiving an injection of muscle relaxant, instead of the intended measles vaccine. A doctor at the clinic said many of the children *"had exhibited signs of severe shock about an hour after they had been given the injections, with many suffocating to death as their bodies swelled"* [15].

Parents took legal action when twenty-one babies died following measles-rubella vaccination in Namibia. One doctor, defending the vaccination program was quoted as saying *"in Namibia's case, most children are malnourished and when they get the vaccination there is a likelihood that some might die"* *[16]*.

This brings us to an interesting point, which seems as though it should be self-evident. If a malnourished child is more likely to die from common childhood diseases - and we know they are, in fact, it's estimated that more than half of all deaths in children around the world, are caused by undernutrition [17] - then it seems logical that vaccinating undernourished children would also have a similar effect.

 Dr Archie Kalokerinos, a pioneer doctor in outback Australia, obviously thought the same way: *"They went through Africa, South America and elsewhere, and vaccinated sick and starving children...They thought they were wiping out measles, but*

most of those susceptible to measles died from some other dis-
ease that they developed as a result of being vaccinated. The
vaccination reduced their immune levels and acted like an in-
fection. Many got septicaemia, gastro-enteritis, etcetera, or
made their nutritional status worse and they died from mal-
nutrition. So there were very few susceptible infants left alive
to get measles. It's one way to get good statistics, kill all those
that are susceptible, which is what they literally did" [18].

It has been known for decades that supplementing with Vitamin A substantially reduces mortality rates from infectious diseases in developing countries, and in the case of measles, can
halve the mortality rate [19].

In the early 1990's, control of Vitamin A deficiency in developing nations was declared a major international goal, and lauded
as possibly *the* most cost effective of *all* health interventions
[20-21]. This is because sufficient levels of Vitamin A not only
benefit overall health and immunity, but also prevent blindness. Why is it then, that decades later, a country like Rwanda
has a 98-99% vaccination rate, but only 3% rate of Vitamin A
supplementation [1]?

In his book Science Is God, Professor Horrobin, a doctor from
Nairobi, Kenya, writes "*Medicine, for the underdeveloped*
countries is relatively cheap. It is also emotionally attractive
and draws many dedicated souls and large sums of conscience
money" [22].

Such is not the case, it seems, for simple technological solutions
or agricultural systems that would ensure a locally-produced,
nutritional food supply. Perhaps there is simply not enough

profit motive, or 'wow factor', in such solutions, though they must surely provide far more longer-lasting, and wide ranging economic, health and social benefits, than vaccines for a small handful of specific diseases.

Why not put money and energy towards solving the root cause of the high mortality rate in developing nations - poverty?

Poor countries are forced to strive to reach vaccine targets, in order to ensure the flow of foreign aid money continues. As of March 2019, the USAID website states "The USAID Forward reform initiative ran from 2010-2016. USAID Forward improved the way that the Agency delivers foreign assistance by embracing new partnerships, investing in the catalytic role of innovation, **and demanding a renewed focus on results**" (emphasis added) [23].

At the United Nation's Millennium Summit, in 2000, all 191 member states agreed to an ambitious set of development goals, to be achieved by 2015. These were known as the Millennium Development Goals.

Millennium Goal number 4 was to reduce child mortality, with key measurements being a) under-five mortality rate, b) infant mortality rate, and c) proportion of one-year-old children immunised against measles [24].

Any goal to reduce childhood mortality naturally revolves around the use of vaccines, and in order for developing countries to meet targets and qualify for finance to meet those targets, it behoves them to set up infrastructure, committees and systems, including legislation and national schedules for vaccination [24].

In 2016, the Millennium Development Goals were replaced by the Sustainable Development Goals - 17 goals set by the United Nations General Assembly, to be achieved by 2030. These include even more aggressive goals in relation to vaccines – aiming to have at least 95% of the world's children vaccinated with both measles-containing vaccine, and diphtheria-tetanus-pertussis vaccines. Poor countries are routinely monitored and measured ('named and shamed'), and urged to increase their progress towards these goals [25].

As you can imagine, this constant 'pressure to perform', and potential of international sanctions or withdrawal of aid money, can make governments in poor countries overly zealous to vaccinate their people - just to please foreign agencies and aid donors.

I had a glimpse of this while living in a small pacific island that remains highly dependent on foreign aid money, in order to function. Doctors, being overseas-trained, were given god-like status. Common folk were too ashamed to even ask questions about the treatment that was recommended to them. It would have been a sign of lack of respect. So, when doctors advise vaccinations, people comply without murmur.

My own children were in the local village school one day, just like any other day, and a team of nurses from the local health clinic turned up, and the whole class was lined up, and vaccinated. There were no medical histories, or vaccination history, taken.

The vaccine van (donated by foreign aid money) would go around from house to house, to vaccinate infants and small children. If the child wasn't at home, they would come by every week, until the child was vaccinated. If the parents refused to comply (which was extremely rare, due to aforementioned social customs, and fear of being seen as disrespectful), the parents were pressured by statements, such as "If your child doesn't get vaccinated, she won't be able to attend school" (which was untrue), or "If you don't vaccinate, and some emergency happens, the hospital won't treat your child" (which was also untrue).

One day, after working on a tin roof all day, my husband fainted, and his family members rushed him to hospital. At the out-patients department, while still groggy and 'out of it', nurses injected him with what they explained was 'tetanus' vaccine. He was feeling too faint to realize what was going on, until after it was done.

This is one way that poor countries can meet the ambitious vaccine targets set by powerful outside forces - simply take away the choice to say no.

Being a foreigner, I was not subjected to the same kind of pressure, but I was called into the local health clinic to explain my choice not to vaccinate our son. I went to the appointment armed with papers and facts, and the head nurse was rather taken aback at the information I provided. She noted our son was healthy and growing well and, before ending the appointment, she asked if I could provide her with a copy of the information I had – to which I readily agreed.

I returned a week later with numerous papers and left them with her, for which she thanked me.

She continued to come around the village in the 'vaccine van', vaccinating children, and she always called me by name and said hello...but she never again tried to engage me on the subject of vaccination.

There are numerous reports that people in other developing countries are threatened or fined, if they don't comply with ambitious vaccine targets.

Media reports from Nigeria, revealed that hundreds of parents in one state alone, had been threatened with jail time, for refusing vaccination, during a 4-day polio vaccination drive, targeting 6 million children. Authorities later confirmed that the parents would be prosecuted [26].

In 2016, the Ugandan government announced a new law that would punish non-compliant parents with six months jail time, and anybody making "*public misleading statements about vaccinations could face two years in prison or a fine, under the same law*". A Ugandan baby must have an 'immunization card' in order to have their birth registered, and have a birth certificate. That same immunization card must be shown in order to enter school [27].

One religious group in Uganda, known as Njiri Nkalu, are vehemently opposed to vaccines, believing that God will protect them, rather than man-made vaccines. In 2016, health workers, along with armed police, forcefully entered their homes and vaccinated 200 children. Many of the parents and children tried to flee into nearby sugarcane fields, but were rounded up and vaccinated for polio. One member was heard to say: "*We don't see why you bring all these guns to harass us. Our children are protected by God and we don't need polio vaccines*" [28].

At least ten members of the group were detained by police, but later released without charge [29].

The officers also forcefully entered the homes of Tabliq Muslims who had refused vaccines for their children. The District Commissioner, who accompanied the officers, said "*Although the operation was a success, there are those who were tipped off and disappeared into the bushes with their children. We shall come back to get them*" [30].

In 2015, more than 500 parents were arrested by police in Pakistan, for not allowing their children to have the polio vaccine. They could be released on bail, only if they signed an affidavit that they would allow their children to get the vaccine. A UNICEF team leader in Pakistan explained that "*First the workers (try to) convince them, then their supervisors, then senior members of the community*". If all that coercion and intimidation fails, and the parents still resist, then the police are called to arrest them [31].

It is interesting to note the flurry of legislative activity in UN member states following the new 2030 Sustainable Development Goals, set in 2016.

In 2017 in Romania, the government response to growing parental concerns over vaccines, was to bring in legislation that would see unvaccinated children removed from childcare centres, and schools, and fine the parents up to 2,200 euros. The legislation is to come into effect during 2019 [32].

In France, there is a growing mistrust of pharmaceutical companies in general, and vaccines in particular – a global survey conducted in 2016, found 41% of the French do not agree that vaccines are safe [33]. The government response to this vaccine hesitancy? Legislation to mandate 11 vaccines for all young children, by 2018 [34].

In Germany, new laws effectively turned teachers into 'snitches' by requiring them to report parents to health authorities, if the parents failed to consult their doctor regarding vaccination. Not only could their child be expelled from kindergarten, but the parents face fines of up to 2500 euros. [35].

Measles and diphtheria vaccines for children are compulsory in Singapore, and the government announced in 2016 that parents who fail to comply can be fined $500 for a first offence, and $1000 for second, or subsequent, offences [36].

In January, 2019, hundreds of parents in Jinhu, China, marched on the streets, demanding answers over the expired vaccines given to their children. More than 100 children had suffered fevers, skin rashes, and vomiting – some for months on end – since receiving the vaccines.

"Local authorities eventually found that an entire batch of vaccines was used instead of being destroyed". Many parents claim the same kinds of reactions had been occurring for at least 10 years, and believe expired and faulty vaccines had been used for years.

Riot police from neighbouring counties were called in to quell the protests, and authorities banned regular, and social, media from reporting on 'inflammatory' news about vaccines [37].

During the early part of 2019, in Pakistan, a health worker was murdered, trying to persuade a man to let his children have the oral polio vaccine [38]. This comes amidst reports of an angry mob of parents setting fire to a hospital, after school-children were vaccinated, and 75 students later fell sick. Doctors denied the illness was due to vaccines, and suggested they probably felt sick due to their parent's anxiety over vaccinations [39].

In 2018, a national vaccine drive in Afghanistan saw 70,000 health workers going from door to door, and through the streets, even stopping families at border crossings, to administer polio vaccinations. It was deemed too dangerous to enter some provinces controlled by militants. The Taliban has a deep mistrust of the vaccination agenda, believing it to be a covert agenda to sterilize Muslim children [40].

They are not the only ones deeply suspicious…

In 2003, three states in Northern Nigeria boycotted the oral polio vaccine, due to the alleged discovery of contaminants, including trace amounts of estrogen. The boycott lasted for 15 months [41].

In 2015, Catholic Bishops in Kenya announced that they had tested vials of the tetanus vaccine, then being used to vaccinate women of child-bearing age, and found them laced with beta-HCG, a pregnancy hormone [42]. Suspicions began to arise over the secrecy surrounding the WHO/UNICEF vaccination campaign (vials were delivered to health clinics under police guard), and the unusual policy of 5 doses of tetanus toxoid vaccine, administered every 6 months [43].

Researchers noted that the World Health Organization had been working to engineer an 'anti-fertility' vaccine, conjugated with tetanus toxoid, since at least the 1970's [43].

During the 1990's, numerous reports surfaced that millions of women in Nicaragua, Mexico and Philippines had been targeted by WHO 'anti-fertility' vaccination campaigns, under the guise of 'eliminating neonatal tetanus' [43].

Today, many in Africa remain deeply suspicious about the true motive of aggressive vaccination programs. One group is the infamous Boko Haram (which translates to 'Western education is forbidden'), who came to the world's attention in 2014, when it was reported they had kidnapped 276 school-girls.

It is too dangerous for vaccinators to go into Boko Haram-held territory during national immunization days, but they do manage to get those who are leaving, or fleeing the area..." *At the bus stations, and the state and national border crossings, the lunchbox-toting teams (the polio vaccines are packed into lunchboxes) are there. Peering into cars, lifting the cloaks of women perched on motorbikes to find the babies strapped to their fronts and backs. Squeezing in the little vials of vaccine."*

"If they say no, then we tell them they can go back," said superintendent of immigration, Charles Tashllani, imposing order on Nigeria's border with Niger in Katsina. Here, late in the evening, the Polio Emergency Operations committee reviews

the campaign's first day, which has seen 3,661 teams immunise 28,882 underfives. The detail is such that eight missing marker pens are on the agenda, as is the sacking of two town announcers who did not inform people about the programme" [44].

What many people don't realize is that, in addition to routine childhood vaccines, WHO and other agencies also conduct 'supplemental immunization activities' in poor countries - mass vaccination campaigns that aim to administer *extra* doses of vaccines, to all children.

According to the WHO, there have been *"thousands of these supplementary vaccination campaigns"* with oral polio vaccine since the 1980's. Children are vaccinated regardless of prior vaccine history. The extra doses were not recorded on the child's health cards [45].

Extra doses of measles vaccines are also given. A quick look at the Measles and Rubella Initiative Calendar for 2019 shows they plan on supplementally vaccinating more than 100 million people in sub-Saharan Africa this year – in addition to routine vaccinations [46].

This could potentially result in some children being (over)vaccinated many times (more times than the average Western child), while others (in the most hard-to-reach, or dangerous, places) still receiving no vaccines at all.

In addition to routine vaccinations and supplementary vaccination, poor countries are increasingly used to test experimental vaccines because it's quicker and cheaper, and regulations are less stringent than in western countries *"Development cycles can be reduced thanks to the faster recruitment of subjects from a larger pool of patients. The costs of recruiting patients and paying investigators are lower too"* [47].

M. Nabeel Ghayur, a pharmacologist who worked in drug development in Pakistan says: *"People actually have blind trust in their doctor in South Asia. They have no idea what drug development is, they have no idea what clinical trials are"*.

He said there was little red tape in those countries, and that people would rarely ask about drug side effects and legal issues [48].

Starting in March 2019, an estimated 750,000 babies in Kenya, Ghana and Malawi will be given a new experimental malaria vaccine. The vaccine Mosquirix will be given to children in four doses- at six, seven, nine and 24 months through an injection on the upper arm [49].

The Star newspaper in Kenya reported: *"Mosquirix, also called RTS,S, was first conceived in the 1980s and has undergone all clinical trials, returning less than optimal results"*.

"The vaccine – made by GSK – is only effective in 30 to 50 per cent of patients, says the WHO. Its effectiveness diminishes over time and it disappears fastest in children who are most exposed to malarial mosquito bites. However, because no defence against malaria is perfect, the vaccine is being considered in addition to the existing defences" [50].

GlaxoSmithKline and its backers, including Bill and Melinda Gates Foundation, had already spent $565 million on developing the vaccine, which brought back disappointing results in early testing, and did not even meet the criteria for a malaria vaccine, which requires a *"protective efficacy of more than 50% against severe disease and death, and last longer than one year"* [51].

In 2017, the Global Task Force on Cholera Control launched a very ambitious set of goals, including 90% reduction in cholera deaths by 2030. A year later, the 'largest vaccination drive in history' took place, with over 2 million people vaccinated for cholera in Zambia, Uganda, Malawi, South Sudan and Nigeria [52].

In December 2012, 500 children in Chad received a new experimental meningitis vaccine, and 38 children were later hospitalized, with 7 of the children flown to Tunisia for specialized treatment. The Chadian government declared their "state of health is not worrying", but other sources in Chad claimed the children were paralysed [53-54].

As of January 2019, more than 66,000 people in the Democratic Republic of Congo have been vaccinated with Merck's V920, an experimental Ebola vaccine [55].

A Chinese-made genetically-engineered Ebola vaccine was given to 500 adults in Sierra Leone in 2015, as part of a Phase II trial. The Chinese FDA then approved the vaccine, without any Phase III trials [56].

In 2018, some 20,000 Malawian children were enrolled to receive an experimental typhoid conjugate vaccine [57].

What we can see is that, far from the media impression that children in third-world countries are desperate for vaccines, many are, in fact, over-vaccinated, receiving more vaccines than the typical Western child, yet without adequate systems in place to monitor what affect this might be having.

10.
VACCINE OPPOSITION

It is often assumed that the 'anti-vax' movement began with Andrew Wakefield, and 'that autism study', or former Playboy model Jenny McCarthy's claims that her son's autism was caused by vaccination.

But did these two events really cause thousands of parents to begin questioning vaccines, and getting embroiled in bitter skirmishes on social media?

The truth is, opposition to vaccination is not a new phenomonem – for as long as there have been vaccines, there has been fierce opposition. Originally focused in England, that opposition really gained momentum when the Compulsory Vaccination Act was passed in Victorian England, in 1853.

The main pockets of opposition to compulsory vaccination were among the working class, and the clergy, who believed it was 'un-Christian' to inject people with animal products [1].

Indeed, it was members of the clergy who also fiercely opposed the original practice of inoculation, before vaccination became accepted practice. In 1772, Reverend Edmund Massey, in his sermon entitled "The Dangerous and Sinful Nature of Inoculation" referred to inoculation as 'diabolical operations', [2], while Reverend John Williams in Massachusetts called it the 'devil's work' [3].

It was Reverend William Hume-Rothery, and his wife Mary, who founded the National Anti-Compulsory Vaccination League at Cheltenham, in 1874 [4].

Writing in 1854, John Gibbs, hydrotherapy practitioner and anti-vaccinationist penned [5]: "*Are we to be leeched, bled, blistered, burned, douched, frozen, pilled, potioned, lotioned, salivated...by an act of parliament?*"

The original Vaccination Act, in 1840, had provided free vaccination for the poor, to be administered by the Poor Law guardians. This law, however, was a failure, as the 'lower and uneducated classes' did not take up the offer of free vaccination [6].

The Compulsory Vaccination Act of 1853 went much further - it ordered all babies up to 3 months old be vaccinated (administered by Poor Law Guardians), and in 1867, this was extended up to 14 years of age, and penalties for non-compliance were introduced. Doctors were encouraged to report non-vaccinators to the authorities, by *"financial inducements for compliance and penalties for failure"*.

While the 1853 Act had introduced one-off fines or imprisonment, the 1867 Act strengthened this, to continuous and cumulative penalties, so that parents found guilty of default could be fined continuously, with increasing prison sentences, until their child reached 14 years of age [7].

(As an interesting side-note here, the vaccination laws were not the only incursions of the state during this time, at the expense of personal liberty, and private bodily autonomy. The

Contagious Diseases Acts of 1864, 1866, and 1869, stated that any woman *suspected* of prostitution was required to be medically inspected for venereal disease. If found infected, she was to be confined in hospital for treatment, with or without her consent. The Notification of Infectious Diseases Acts in 1889 and 1899 required that all contagious diseases – except tuberculosis, which is curious, since it was a major killer at the time – be reported to the local medical officer, who could then forcibly remove the patient to hospital, whether they consented or not [6]).

Meanwhile, the vaccination laws were tightened yet further in 1871 (ironically, the same year that a large smallpox epidemic raged across Europe and England – no doubt testament to how 'effective' the compulsory laws had been), making it compulsory for all local authorities to hire Vaccination Officers [7].

In response to these increasingly draconian measures, the Anti-Vaccination League was formed in England, and a number of anti-vaccine journals were started, which "included the *Anti-Vaccinator* (founded 1869), the *National Anti-Compulsory Vaccination Reporter* (1874), and the *Vaccination Inquirer* (1879)".

Numerous other writings and pamphlets were distributed widely – for example, 200,000 copies of an open letter titled 'Current Fallacies About Vaccination', written by Leicester Member of Parliament, P. Taylor, were distributed in 1883 [7].

The vaccination process itself was both painful and inconvenient, for parents and children alike. The vaccinator used a lancet (a surgical knife with sharp, double-edged blade) to cut lines into the flesh, in a scored pattern. This was usually done in several different places on the arm. Vaccine lymph was then smeared into the cuts. Infants then had to be brought back, eight days later, to have the lymph (pus) harvested from their blisters, which was then used on waiting infants [6].

After the stricter 1871 amendments to the law, parents could also be fined 20 shillings for refusing to allow the pus to be collected from their children's blisters, to be used for public vaccination [6].

By this time, severe and sometimes fatal reactions to the vaccine were being reported, and doubts began to grow about how effective the vaccine really was [8].

Even some of those charged with administering the vaccines revolted. In 1875, seven Poor Law Guardians from Keighley, Yorkshire, were imprisoned in York Castle, for refusing to enforce vaccination on all infants.

They became local, and national, heroes for their stand, being dubbed 'The Seven Men of Keighley'. As they were being taken to the train station, bound for prison, their carriage was surrounded by a very large, angry mob of townsfolk, who released the horses, attacked the police officers, and dragged the carriage back into the township.

The seven men were released on the promise that they would voluntarily surrender, once the commotion had subsided. The following day, the seven men surrendered, and were escorted to the train station by a number of well-known local anti-vaccinators, where they departed "amid the cheers of a large crowd of sympathisers" [6].

A number of medical men publicly decried or questioned the practice of vaccination. Edgar M Crookshank, who was the first Professor of Bacteriology at Kings College in London, roundly criticized smallpox vaccination in his large, two-volume study entitled 'Vaccination, Its History and Pathology' [9].

The town of Leicester was a particular hot-bed of anti-vaccine activity, with numerous marches and rallies, demanding for repeal of the law, and advocating other measures of containment, such as isolation of the infected. These rallies attracted up to 100,000 people [10].

The unrest and opposition continued for two decades, and an estimated 6000 prosecutions were carried out, in the town of Leicester alone [11].

The following excerpts from the *Leicester Mercury* bears witness to the deep convictions held by those who refused to submit to the mandatory measures:

"'George Banford had a child born in 1868. It was vaccinated and after the operation the child was covered with sores, and it was some considerable time before it was able to leave the house. Again Mr. Banford complied with the law in 1870. This child was vaccinated by Dr. Sloane in the belief that by going to him they would get pure matter. In that case erysipelas set in, and the child was on a bed of sickness for some time. In the third case the child was born in 1872, and soon after

vaccination erysipelas set in and it took such a bad course that at the expiration of 14 days the child died".

Mr Banford was fined 10 shillings, with the option of seven days imprisonment, for refusing to subject a fourth child to the vaccine [12].

And again...'*By about 7.30 a goodly number of anti-vaccinators were present, and an escort was formed, preceded by a banner, to accompany a young mother and two men, all of whom had resolved to give themselves up to the police and undergo imprisonment in preference to having their children vaccinated. The utmost sympathy was expressed for the poor woman, who bore up bravely, and although seeming to feel her position expressed her determination to go to prison again and again rather than give her child over to the "tender mercies" of a public vaccinator. The three were attended by a numerous crowd and in Gallowtreegate three hearty cheers were given for them, which were renewed with increased vigour as they entered the doors of the police cells [13]"*.

And this: '*A man named Arthur Ward had two children injured through vaccination and refused to submit another one to the operation. A fine was imposed and on 24th November two police officers called for the penalty, or in default to ticket the goods. The husband was out at the market, and the poor woman had no money to pay. The goods downstairs were considered insufficient to cover the amount, and the officers demanded to go upstairs. The woman refused to allow this, and an altercation took place, and harsh language was used by the officers, who threatened to take her husband to prison, terrifying Mrs. Ward. At that time, she was pregnant, and the shock to the system, and the fright, were of such a character that symptoms ensued which ultimately led to a premature confinement, and on 26th December she gave birth to a still-born child. She never recovered and last week she expired. The doctor who had attended Mrs Ward said that although he be-lieved in vaccination he did not think it was the duty of any professional man to carry out the laws in the outrageous and brutal manner in which they were enforced"* [14].

In a letter to the newspaper, one citizen wrote:

'It must strike the reflective observer as rather singular that all the recent smallpox outbreaks have made their appearance among populations where the laws enforcing vaccination have been rigorously and systematically carried out. 96% of births in London are protected by vaccination. May I venture to ask whether medical men who have defended and fostered a system of medical procedure which eighty years' experience has demonstrated a disastrous and humiliating failure ought not to feel honourably bound on public grounds to retrace their steps and confess that vaccination, like other once popular prescriptions of inoculation, bleeding and mercurization, is a serious and mischievous blunder. Every municipality is in possession of evidence establishing the fact that zymotic diseases originate in and are fostered by insanitary conditions, and are preventable by personal and municipal cleanliness" [15].

Eventually, there were so many vaccine refusers in the town of Leicester, that some local magistrates and politicians declared their support for parental rights, and encouraged their peers to do the same [16].

The law was finally relaxed in 1898, when new laws were passed, that allowed for conscientious objection to vaccination [17]. By the end of that same year, more than 200,000 certificates of conscientious objection had been issued, most among the working class, and many were women [18].

By the late 1890's, Leicester had already reported 80% of births were unvaccinated, in Bedfordshire 79%, Northamptonshire 69%, Nottinghamshire 50%, and Derbyshire 48% unvaccinated [18].

Meanwhile in the United States, smallpox outbreaks in the late 1800's led to vaccine campaigns, and subsequent opposition in the formation of The Anti-Vaccination Society of America in 1879, followed by the New England Anti Compulsory Vaccination League in 1882, and the Anti Vaccination League of New York City in 1885 [19].

The homeless and the itinerate were blamed for spreading smallpox, and in 1901, the Boston Board of Health ordered 'virus squads' to vaccinate men staying in cheap boarding rooms. A reporter who accompanied one such squad, described the night-time raid in the Boston Globe [20]:

"Every imaginable threat from civil suits to cold-blooded murder when they got an opportunity to commit it, was made by the writhing, cursing, struggling tramps who were operated upon, and a lot of them had to be held down in their cots, one big policeman sitting on their legs, and another on their heads, while the third held the arms, bared for the doctors".

Following a smallpox outbreak in 1902, the Cambridge Board of Health in Massachusetts mandated vaccination for all city residents. This led to possibly the most important, and controversial, judicial decision regarding public health.

One man, Henning Jacobson, refused to comply with the mandate, on the grounds that it violated his right to care for his own body as he saw fit. The city filed criminal charges against him, which he fought, and lost, in court. He then appealed to the US Supreme Court, which ruled in the State's favour in 1905, giving priority to public health, over individual liberty [21].

The 'anti-vaxxers' have never really gone away in the intervening years, although sometimes they have been more vocal than others, such as in the 1970's, when there was controversy throughout Europe, North America and Britain, about the safety and possible side effects of the diptheria-tetanus-pertussis vaccine [22].

An advocacy group, known as The Association of Parents of Vaccine Damaged Children (APVDC) gained enough public support, that the government was forced to act – passing the Vaccine Damage Payments Act (1979), which provided payment of £10,000 to those who could show that vaccines caused their child's injuries [23].

Vaccination rates for pertussis dropped to less than 50% in many parts of the UK and, much to their surprise, although notification of whooping cough increased, hospital admissions and death rates decreased [24-25]. (This neatly illustrates what has already been discussed in the opening chapters of this book, regarding the immune 'skewing' and 'symptom suppression' caused by vaccinations.)

In 1998, the vaccination argument again came to the forefront, with Andrew Wakefield's case series published in the Lancet. The debacle became so infamous, that it now seems to be the 'go-to' argument used by doctors and paediatricians everywhere, when faced with a so-called 'vaccine-hesitant' parent.

I experienced this first-hand, after the birth of my youngest son. I declined the hepatitis B vaccine for him, and two resident paediatricians found it necessary to come and have a chat with me, about my decision.

They asked me why I had chosen to decline the vaccine.

My answer went something like this: "The hepatitis B vaccine contains aluminium - I do not think it's necessary to inject a newborn baby with a neurotoxin, when his renal and hepatic systems are not even fully functioning yet, nor his blood-brain barrier complete. Not to mention, with myself having tested negative for Hepatitis B, he had virtually nil chance of contracting the *sexually-transmitted* disease any time soon...Given all that, I do not believe the benefits outweigh the risks".

Without even acknowledging what I had just said, the senior of the two paediatricians launched into what was clearly a rehearsed spiel, which was based on two points :-

1. The hepatitis B vaccine is 'harmless', and he had never seen any baby have a reaction to the vaccine. (I could have interrupted him there, to point out that the mother

342

who had roomed in with me the previous night, had a baby who was vaccinated shortly after birth, and mere hours later, had to be resuscitated after he stopped breathing. (Of course, there is no proof that this incident was directly related to the vaccine, however, it would be irresponsible to merely shrug such cases off, as mere co-incidences.)

2. A 'guy' did this study that said vaccines cause autism, but it was later found out to be a fraud, and his study has been completely debunked.

Let's do a little fact-checking…

First, and foremost, the study was authored by 13 different doctors, not just 'a guy' [26].

Secondly, it actually didn't have anything to do with vaccines. The researchers were investigating bowel dysfunction in twelve developmentally-delayed children. They had seen enough similar cases, that they had started to question whether it might be the manifestation of a new syndrome. However, they wrote in the conclusion of their case series:

"We have identified a chronic enterocolitis in children that may be related to neuropsychiatric dysfunction. In most cases, onset of symptoms was after measles, mumps, and rubella immunisation. Further investigations are needed to examine this syndrome and its possible relation to this vaccine" [26].

There was no hypothesis or theory being proven or disproven, merely investigating this disturbing new 'syndrome', and noting that the parents of eight of the children believed the onset of their child's symptoms coincided with MMR vaccination.

Thirdly, Andrew Wakefield has never been charged with, nor convicted of, fraud. The investigation by the General Medical Council, which eventually saw him struck off from the register, was for misconduct, namely, failure to gain approval for the study from the Ethics Committee, and subjecting the children to what they considered unnecessary and invasive testing [27].

Wakefield, and two of his co-authors, were investigated by the General Medical Council. Though they argued that their investigations were simply a by-product of treating the children's severe symptoms, and therefore did not require permission from the Ethics Committee, Andrew Wakefield and Professor Walker-Smith were subsequently found guilty of serious professional misconduct, and their names were ordered to be removed from the register. Another author Dr Simon Murch, was cleared.

Professor Walker-Smith later appealed the decision through the High Court, and won. He was subsequently re-instated to the register, and his name cleared. The conclusion by the High Court judge included this statement: "*the panel's overall conclusion that Professor Walker-Smith was guilty of serious professional misconduct was flawed, in two respects: inadequate and superficial reasoning and, in a number of instances, a wrong conclusion*" [27].

Andrew Wakefield did not pursue his high court appeal, citing financial reasons. His case was complicated by the fact that he had been approached by lawyers, and got involved in a proposed class action against the manufacturers of MMR vaccine. Email correspondence between Wakefield and Walker-Smith during that time reveal that Wakefield felt morally obligated to act as expert witness for the parents of children allegedly harmed by the vaccine, knowing what a David-vs-Goliath battle it would be, and knowing that the vaccine manufacturer would have a slew of expert witnesses to quash their claims [27].

That class action was later dropped on legal advice.

Finally, was the original work published in the Lancet 'thoroughly de-bunked'? Quite the contrary, a slew of subsequent research supported a link between bowel dysfunction and autism [28-31]. Further, that abnormal measles antibodies were implicated in both the bowel dysfunction, and the autism [32-34].

The claims of 'fraud' have appeared to stick, however, and Wakefield's reputation has been thoroughly reduced from respected gastroenterologist, to 'quack', 'charlatan' and 'fraudster' in media circles, despite all evidence showing that his sins are no more severe than what numerous other scientists and researchers engage in regularly, yet go unpunished – as already shown in this book.

Anybody who confesses to have doubts about the safety of efficacy of vaccines, generally receive the same scorn and derision that Andrew Wakefield has received.

Even in the era of smallpox vaccination, the media tended to portray anti-vaxxers in a less-than-flattering light. At the time, the media referred to the debate as a *"conflict between intelligence and ignorance, civilization and barbarism"* [35].

Over the years, anti-vaxxers have been referred to in the media as 'hopeless cranks' who are 'ignorant' and 'deficient in the power to judge' (science), whose 'jabberings' were 'absurdly fallacious' [35].

So, are anti-vaxxers really anti-science?

Not so, says...*science.*

In 2007, Kim, et al, analysed vaccination records of 11,680 children from 19 – 35 months of age, to evaluate maternal characteristics that might influence whether the child was fully vaccinated, or not.

They found that mothers with tertiary degrees and high incomes, were the least likely to fully vaccinate their children, while mothers in poor minority families, without high school diplomas, were most likely to fully vaccinate their children [36].

Similarly, a study in 2008 that investigated the attitudes and beliefs of parents who decided to opt out of childhood vaccine mandates, found that they valued scientific knowledge, were adept at collecting and processing information on vaccines, and had little trust in the medical community [37].

In 2017, the Australian Institute of Health and Welfare released their latest figures on vaccination rates. The national average was 93% of children fully vaccinated, yet in Sydney's upmarket (ie. Populated by highly educated, high income-earning professionals) inner suburbs and northern beaches, as few as 70% of children under 5 were fully vaccinated [38].

The same story was repeated in Melbourne, with the wealthiest - and by association, better educated - suburbs having the lowest vaccination rates. There was an ironic, and rather telling, opening paragraph in The Age, when reporting these figures: "Four of the wealthiest, *healthiest* suburbs of Melbourne have the worst child vaccination rates in the state" [39]

(Were they not vaccinated because they were healthy...or were they healthy because they were not vaccinated?)

And yet again in the state of Queensland..."*Inner-city Brisbane's most well-to-do suburbs are home to some of the worst vaccination rates in the state*" [40].

Statistics gathered from Canada tell a similar story - a higher percentage of anti-vaxxers held a university degree, compared to the national average [41].

It seems that doctors and paediatric specialists are not always in agreement with current vaccine practice either - at least, not when it comes to their own children: "*Ten percent of paediatricians and 21% of paediatric specialists claim they would not follow [CDC] recommendations for future progeny. Despite their education, physicians in this study expressed concern over the safety of vaccines*" [42].

With the vaccine schedule becoming increasingly crowded, and governments moving ever towards compulsory vaccination, the anti-vaccination movement is again gathering momentum.

Increasing numbers of parents are delaying, declining, or opting for alternative vaccine schedules [43-44].

Around the world, scepticism about vaccines is on the rise, and governments are becoming increasingly more forceful in trying to curb the sentiment.

In 2017, the Italian government announced that the number of mandated vaccines for children would increase to 12, with fines of up to 7500 euros for non-compliance. This was met by fierce opposition, as tens of thousands took to the streets to protest, and the law was subsequently amended, by decreasing mandated vaccines from 12 to 10, and reducing the maximum fines from 7500 euros to 3500 euros [45].

This followed a global survey in 2015 by the 'Vaccine Confidence Project' that concluded the European region had the lowest levels of confidence in the safety and effectiveness of vaccines [46].

Countries such as Poland have a growing anti-vax movement, and increasing non-compliance, despite mandatory vaccination policies, and threat of fines for those who fail to vaccinate their children. In 2017, more than 10,000 Poles marched in Warsaw, in protest of mandatory vaccination policies [46-47].

Vaccine confidence has also significantly decreased in the Czech Republic, Finland and Sweden. In Ireland and Denmark, HPV vaccination rates have dropped to less than half, following widespread safety concerns, and coverage of adverse events [46].

Meanwhile, in the West, numerous high-profile people have publicly stated their concerns over the current vaccination situation.

Actor Rob Schneider has long been an outspoken critic against vaccines, and he has lost at least one gig, due to pressure from pro-vaccination groups. In 2014, State Farm dropped Schneider from appearing in their health insurance ads when pro-vaccine activists flooded the company's social media pages with criticism [48].

Darla Shine, wife of White House communications director, hit out at 'measles hysteria' in a series of tweets, in early 2019. Predictably enough, she was widely criticized by mainstream media, despite a large outpouring of support on social media [49]. The Guardian newspaper accused her of 'spreading conspiracy theories' [50].

Australian celebrity chef, Pete Evans, who is well-known for his conversion to the paleo diet, and being critical of water fluoridation, recently endorsed a podcast by Dr Sherri Tenpenny (American osteopathic physician, well-known for her criticisms of vaccines) to his 1.5 million followers on social media, commenting that it was "one of the most important podcasts to listen to".

Amidst the flurry of both well wishes and criticism that followed, president of the Australian Medical Association, Dr Tony Bartone said "*As a highly recognised chef, Pete Evans has a lot of expertise in the kitchen but none whatsoever when it comes to vaccination*," adding that Evans "*should keep out of this discussion all together and leave it to the medical experts*"[51].

Australian indigenous boxer, Anthony Mundine recently took to social media, to warn parents about vaccine dangers, unleashing a flurry of criticism and name-calling, such as 'dangerous clown' [52].

Numerous journal articles have been dedicated to informing doctors how to deal with this issue, including how to 'communicate' with, or counter against, vaccine hesitant parents [53-54].

A growing number of paediatricians have preferred to simply 'fire' unvaccinated children from their practice. As one paediatrician put it: "*In my personal experience (and I have only fired a couple of patients in my entire career), the decision not to vaccinate is one of several differences in opinion, and I am not able to adequately provide care for a patient when their parent clearly does not respect my medical advice*" [55].

One can't help but wonder if insurance incentives play any role in the doctor's decision to cut all ties with unvaccinated patients. A BlueShield (a major insurer in the US healthcare system) incentive scheme document, which has since been removed from their website, revealed that doctors receive a $400 bonus for each two-year old child up-to-date with all recommended vaccines (including two influenza vaccines)...but the entire bonus is lost, if the vaccination rate for the medical practice falls below 63% [56].

At the beginning of 2019, the World Health Organization listed 'Vaccine Hesitancy' ("*the reluctance or refusal to vaccinate despite the availability of vaccines*") as one of the Top 10 Global

Health Threats of 2019, along with non-communicable diseases, antibiotic resistance, air pollution and climate change, and others [57].

This was followed by an opinion piece in The New York Times, titled *How to Inoculate Against Anti-Vaxxers*, which called for tougher vaccine mandates, and removal of conscientious objection clauses (while conceding that anti-vaxxers had waged a successful social media campaign, to cast doubts on vaccine safety) [58].

Social media platforms and search engines have faced backlash – not to mention letters from Democratic Congressman Adam Schiff, about their role in the spread of 'conspiracy theories' and 'vaccine misinformation' [59-60].

Amidst calls for antivaxxers addresses to be made public (TIME magazine, in 2015), fines for being out in public (New York, in 2019, amidst measles outbreak), and parents reported to Child Protective Services for refusing vaccines (various parts of United States, in 2018/2019), this is shaping up to be the defining issue of our generation. History does have a habit of repeating itself – and history has shown that the more totalitarian the government becomes, the more resistant the people become.

Only time will tell how this particular struggle will play out.

11.
FUTURE VACCINES

In 2013, the Pharmaceutical Research and Manufacturers of America (PhRMA) proudly announced that biopharmaceutical companies had 271 new vaccines in development [1].

"The 271 vaccines in development span a wide array of diseases, and employ exciting new scientific strategies and technologies. These potential vaccines – all in human clinical trials or under review by the Food and Drug Administration (FDA) – include 137 for infectious diseases, 99 for cancer, 15 for allergies and 10 for neurological disorders".

A brief example of the vaccines currently being developed, include:

- A vaccine for Alzheimer's disease [2].

- A genetically-engineered nasal vaccine for obesity [3].

- A vaccine for malaria, using genetically-engineered parasites [4].

- A chimeric virus (two viruses genetically engineered/combined into one virus) vaccine for Japanese encephalitis [5].

 - A chimeric virus vaccine for chikungunya fever (a mosquito-borne infection) [6].

- A vaccine for West Nile virus, inactivated with hydrogen peroxide [7].

- A vaccine for Staphylococcus aureus (commonly known as 'Golden Staph') [8].

- A vaccine made from mouse cancer cells, for use in patients with colorectal cancer [9].

- A genetically-engineered vaccine for Pseudomonas aeruginosa - a major cause of hospital-acquired infections [10]. That particular vaccine was tested on ventilated patients in an intensive care unit - as if they didn't already have enough to deal with! In addition, vaccination made no difference to rates of infection...nevertheless, they recommending further testing.

- A vaccine for Vigoo enterovirus 71 – something the vast majority of people have never even heard of. Nevertheless, if it reaches the market, no doubt we'll all be made aware of what a threat the virus poses, and the urgency of being vaccinated against it [11].

- Plant-based oral vaccines for Type-1 diabetes [12].

- A vaccine made from genetically-engineered Listeria, for early-stage pancreatic cancer [13].

- A stem-cell vaccine for metastatic bladder cancer [14].

- Genetically-engineered papaya with an inbuilt vaccine for Taenia solium or T. crassiceps - a type of tapeworm found in pigs and humans [15].

Researchers at University of California are working on a potential vaccine for acne [16].

Other scientists are working towards a vaccine for *stress* [17]. And Associate Professor Martin Moore, at Emory University is in the process of developing a vaccine for the common cold, stressing how inconvenient it is for parents to look after children suffering from a cold, and how dangerous colds can be for those with asthma, or compromised immune systems. There are 160 strains of viruses believed to be responsible for cold symptoms, and the vaccine would include 50 strains [18].

As of April, 2019, scientists at the National Institute of Allergy and Infectious Disease (NIAID) have begun human trials for a universal flu vaccine – *"by focusing the immune system on a portion of the virus that varies relatively little from strain to strain"* [19].

Looking to the future, we are likely to see more DNA vaccines, genetically-engineered vaccines, and potentially...vaccines from China.

DNA VACCINES

In the early 1990's, scientists discovered they could deliver DNA into the skin of mice, by using a gene gun [20]. When they realized that this approach could generate antibody responses, it quickly became the focus of enthusiastic research.

At the annual vaccine meeting, at the Cold Spring Harbor Laboratory in 1992, Merck scientists reported how they forced antibody responses in mice, by injecting them with plasmids, which are typically DNA strands from the cytoplasm of a bacterium or protozoan [21].

Despite high optimism, early clinical trials in humans failed to produce the required antibody response, however, over the following two decades or so, DNA vaccination has been the subject of many research projects, testing different strategies, delivery systems, adjuvants, and formulations [22].

How do DNA vaccines work? Basically, in plain English, the vaccine contains DNA codes for specific antigens. The DNA is injected into the host's cells, which then manufactures the antigen, that is then recognized as foreign by the immune system, and mounts a response [22].

What could possibly go wrong here? If the host's own cells are co-opted into manufacturing the antigen that stimulates the immune response, what is to stop the immune system from attacking host cells or even our very own DNA? It also raises the question, if the DNA plasmid encodes itself into the host DNA, how will the cell know when to stop manufacturing the antigen?

DNA vaccination of mice resulted in a three-fold increase of anti-DNA auto-antibodies, but did not affect the onset or severity of disease in lupus-prone mice. Incredibly, researchers concluded from this, that DNA vaccination is "not associated with induction of unsafe autoimmune sequelae" [23].

However, in 2011, researchers in China found that DNA vaccination caused vitiligo - a disorder where skin loses its colour - and autoimmunity in mice, within 6 weeks of a third injection [24].

One of the major purported benefits of DNA vaccines is that they can be manipulated to bias the required T-helper response [25]. Another 'benefit' is that antibodies may be much longer-lived than conventional vaccines [26], although, what we now know about antibodies, that may not be such a benefit, at all.

Several DNA vaccines have been approved for livestock, but none for humans, as yet, although more than 100 have been, or are currently going, through clinical trials [27]. DNA vaccines can be administered with a needle and syringe, like conventional vaccines, or with a "needle-less device that uses *high-pressure gas to shoot microscopic gold particles coated with DNA directly into cells"* [28].

GENETICALLY-ENGINEERED VACCINES

Several vaccines on the current childhood schedule are manufactured via the use of genetically-engineered viruses or excipients.

The Hepatitis B vaccine, routinely administered to newborns within hours of birth is produced via genetically-engineered yeast [29]. The rotavirus vaccine is also genetically-engineered, using both human and bovine (cow) strains of the virus [30].

Other genetically-engineered vaccines are currently in the development and testing stages [31-32].

There is no way of knowing if, or how, these viruses may react in the host, whether they can cross-react or mutate with other viruses within the host or circulating at the same time, or cross species. Such environmental risk assessments are apparently not necessary before approval for mass use [33-34]

Another ingredient used in vaccine production is recombinant human albumin [35]. Recombinant means 'genetically engineered' or 'genetically modified'. Albumin is a protein made by the liver, found in the clear liquid portion of the blood. This particular product was genetically-engineered to be 'structurally equivalent' to human albumin [36].

A safety study of recombinant human albumin in healthy volunteers had a reaction rate of just under 2% via intramuscular injection [36].

VACCINES MADE IN CHINA

The World Health Organization declared in 2014, that China would enter the global vaccine market, which would result in cheaper vaccines [37]. WHO claimed that vaccine quality for international procurement had already been assured, via their prequalification system.

Unfortunately, China does not have the best track record, when it comes to product safety, as seen in the following examples.

2004: At least 13 babies in China die from malnourishment due to 'fake milk' in their infant formula [38].

2006: Several hundred people die in Panama, after taking cough syrup that was contaminated with diethylene glycol. The product is traced back to China. It is not the first time that toxic cough syrup from China has resulted in mass poisoning - three other prior cases were also traced back to China [39].

2007: Sixty million cans and pouches of pet food is recalled in the US, after thousands of dogs and cats suffer kidney failure. It is later found to contain Aminopterin, a highly toxic cancer drug that has been replaced by less toxic versions. The contaminated ingredient is thought to be wheat gluten imported from China [40].

2008: An estimated 81 human deaths, and thousands of serious adverse reactions, occur in the US after tainted heparin imported from China apparently made its way through several layers of 'testing'.

Heparin is used as a blood thinner, and is made from pig intestine. China supplies about 70% of the global market [41].

2008: Six babies die, and an estimated 300,000 others fall ill, in China, after infant formula is laced with melamine. The manufacturer was aware of the contamination for several months before alerting authorities [42]. It is thought the melamine was added deliberately, to boost protein content.

A spokesman for the World Health Organisation remarked *"The large scale of this event ensures that it was clearly not an isolated accident. It was a large-scale intentional activity to deceive consumers for simple, basic, short-term profits"* [43].

2010: Four babies die in impoverished Shanxi province, after vaccines are left in sweltering heat, and then administered to children. When the China Economic Times newspaper breaks the story, the editor is fired from his job [44].

2014: More than a thousand dog deaths in the United States are linked to pet food imported from China [45].

2016: Approximately 2 million improperly stored, or expired vaccines are sold around China. The main suspect - a hospital pharmacist - had already been convicted of trading illegal vaccines, in 2009. After police discover the illicit trade, almost a year went by, before authorities notified the public, sparking anger and backlash among parents. Ma Guohui, the owner of a shop that sells baby products, says "*The customers worry about fake milk powder, fake medicine, fake vaccines, fake everything*" [46].

2017: Authorities investigate claims of wheat contaminated with heavy metals, grown on polluted land near former battery factories. Some farmers had allegedly sold unknown amounts of the grain to flour mills [47].

2017: Investigations in Tianjin, after reports that a network of 50 underground factories have been using ingredients 'unfit for human consumption' to make products such as soy sauce, for decades. Some of the products were allegedly labelled as well-known brands, such as Nestle [48].

Although the communist nation has made moves towards greater transparency, in an effort to appease consumer concerns, there is still a way to go. For example, the melamine milk scandal in 2008 was allegedly covered up by officials to avoid negative publicity, in the lead-up to the Beijing Olympics, which were due to start the same week [49].

Following the scandal being made public, journalist Zhao Lianhai, whose son fell ill as a result of the contaminated milk, organized protests, and was subsequently imprisoned for 2.5 years.

Angry parents, who claimed their children were injured by substandard vaccines, in 2016, faced intimidation and arbitrary arrest by security officials, when they protested the government's handling of the affair [50]. Yi Wenlong, 47, was placed in detention for 30 days. His crime? Encouraging the public to buy a newspaper, which ran an in-depth story on the vaccine scandal [51].

There also seems to be a lack of transparency in the disciplinary process, regarding safety scandals.

Take Sun Xianze: When the melamine milk scandal broke in 2008, Sun was Food Safety Director at the China Food and Drug Administration. He was stood down for his role in the scandal, and subsequent cover-up, but after a period of 'administrative discipline', he resumed his career at the CFDA, and was put in charge of drug safety, in 2012. Sun Xianze is now deputy commissioner at the CFDA [52].

There are 12,000 drug wholesalers, 5,000 production firms, including 34 vaccine manufacturers, and more than 400,000 drug retailers in China, but according to Li Guoqing, head of the drug supervision at the CFDA, *"there aren't even 500 people with the aptitude to inspect drugs"* [37,50].

According to the China Chamber of Commerce for Import & Export of Medicines & Health Products, China's exports of vaccines for human use was about $26 million in 2010 - with most exports going to developing countries [52].

The first Chinese vaccine to gain WHO pre-qualification was for Japanese encephalitis, in 2013. A second vaccine, for influenza, gained approval in 2015. This stamp of approval from the WHO means that these vaccines are now recommended for bulk purchase by UNICEF, the GAVI Alliance, and other procurement agencies [53].

According to vaccine inserts, there are no vaccines from China currently used in the US vaccine schedule. That's probably a good thing...

In 2012, USA Today revealed serious flaws in the importation system for other pharmaceuticals [54]. According to a General Accountability Office study, the FDA inspects US drug facilities about every 2.5 years, often unannounced.

Contrast that, with inspections about every 14 years to facilities in India and China, and only pre-arranged - no unannounced visits allowed. Up to two-thirds of foreign pharmaceutical sites have never undergone an FDA inspection [54].

Although vaccines currently used in Western countries don't appear to be manufactured in China, there is no guarantee that components in those vaccines are not sourced from China.

As they say, *caveat emptor* – let the buyer beware.

REFERENCES

CHAPTER 1: VACCINE THEORY

[1] Geison GL. The Private Science of Louis Pasteur, Princeton University Press, 1995.

[2] Giese M. Molecular Vaccines: From Prophylaxis to Therapy, Volume 1, Springer.

[3] Wasik B, Murphy M. Rabid: A Cultural History of the World's Most Diabolical Virus, Penguin Books, New York, 2013.

[4] Brock T. Robert Koch: A life in medicine and bacteriology, ASM Press, Washington DC, 1999.

[5] Schultz M. Rudolf Virchow, *Emerg Infect Dis*, 2008, 14(9):1480–1481.

[6] *Berkowsky B*. The Germ Theory: The Traditional Naturopathic Perspective - Part I, *Nat Health Sci, Joseph Ben Hil-Meyer Research, Inc.*

[7] Hume E. Bechamp or Pasteur? A lost chapter in the history of biology, 1923.

[8] Professor Bechamp, *BMJ*, 1908, 1(2471):1150, Available at: https://www.ncbi.nlm.nih.gov/pmc/articles/PMC2436492/?page=1. Accessed May, 2019.

[9] Rosenow E. Transmutations within the Streptococcus-Pneumococcus Group, *J Infect Dis,* 1914, 14(1):1-32.

[10] Cantwell AR Jr. Pleomorphic Bacteria as a Cause of Hodgkin's Disease (Hodgkin's lymphoma): A Review of the Literature, *JOIMR*, 2006;4(1):1.

[11] Pearce R. The viral content of human genomes is more variable than we thought, *BioMed Central*, 25th January, 2019.

[12] Cohen P. Mother's little helper, *New Scientist*, 24th February, 2001.

[13] Grow EJ, Flynn RA, Chavez SL, et al. Intrinsic retroviral reactivations in human preimplantation embryos and pluripotent cells, *Nature*, 2015, 522:221-225].

[14] Medical Research Council, A study of diphtheria in two areas of Great Britain, London, HMSO, 1950.

[15] Brodie M, Park W. Active Immunization Against Poliomyelitis, *Am J Pub Health*, 1936, 26:119–125.

[16] Burnet FM. Measles as an index of immunological function, *The Lancet*, 1968, 292(7568):610-613.

[17] Moseman EA, Iannocone M, Bosurgi L, et al. B cell maintenance of subcapsular sinus macrophages protects against a fatal viral infection independent of adaptive immunity, *Immunity*, 2012, 36(3):415-426.

[18] Aaby P, Knudsen K, Jensen TG, et al. Measles incidence, vaccine efficacy, and mortality in two urban African areas with high vaccination coverage, *J Infect Dis*, 1990, 162(5):1043-1048.

[19] Crone NE, Reder AT. Severe tetanus in immunized patients with high anti-tetanus titers, *Neurology*, 1992, 42(4):761-764.

[20] Maselle SY, Matre R, Mbise R, Hofstad T. Neonatal tetanus despite protective serum antitoxin concentration, *FEMS Microbiol Immunol*, 1991, 3(3):171-175.

[21] Pitisuttithum P, Gilbert P, Gurwith M, et al. Randomized, double-blind, placebo-controlled efficacy trial of a bivalent recombinant glycoprotein 120 HIV-1 vaccine among injection drug users in Bangkok, Thailand, *J Infect Dis*, 2006, 194(12):1661-1761.

[22] ACIP, Pertussis Vaccination: Use of acellular pertussis vaccines among infants and young children recommendations of

the Advisory Committee on Immunization Practices, *MMWR*, 1997, 46(RR-7):1-25.

[23] O'Connor A. Merrill W Chase, 98, Scientist Who Advanced Immunology, *New York Times*, 22nd Jan, 2004.

[24] Moseman EA, Iannocone M, Bosurgi L, et al. B cell maintenance of subcapsular sinus macrophages protects against a fatal viral infection independent of adaptive immunity, *Immunity*, 2012, 36(3):415-426.

[25] Zimmerman RK, Lin CJ, Raviotta JM, Nowalk MP. Do vitamin D levels affect antibody titers produced in response to HPV vaccine? *Hum Vaccin Immunother*, 2015, 11(10):2345-2349.

[26] Røsjø E, Lossius A, Abdelmagid N, et al. Effect of high-dose vitamin D3 supplementation on antibody responses against Epstein–Barr virus in relapsing-remitting multiple sclerosis, *Mult Scler J*, 2017, *23*(3),395–402.

[27] Halstead SB, O'Rourke EJ. Antibody-enhanced dengue virus infection in primate leukocytes, *Nature*, 1977, 265(5596):739-741.

[28] Dejnirattisai W, Jumnainsong A, Onsirisakul N, et al. Cross-reacting antibodies enhance dengue virus infection in humans, *Science*, 2010, 328(5979):745-748

[29] Takada A, Kawaoka Y. Antibody-dependent enhancement of viral infection: molecular mechanisms and in vivo implications, *Rev Med Virol*, 2003, 13(6):387-398.

[30] Sauter P, Hober D. Mechanisms and results of the antibody-dependent enhancement of viral infections and role in the pathogenesis of coxsackievirus B-induced diseases, *Microbes Infect*. 2009, 11:443–51.

[31] Girn J, Kavoosi M, Chantler J. Enhancement of coxsackievirus B3 infection by antibody to a different coxsackievirus strain, *J Gen Virol*, 2002, 83(pt 2):351-358.

[32] Osiowy C, Horne D, Anderson R. Antibody-dependent enhancement of respiratory syncytial virus infection by sera from young infants, *Clin Diagn Lab Immunol*, 1994, 1(6):670-677.

[33] Furuyama W, Marzi A, Carmody AB, et al. Fcγ-receptor Ila-mediated Src signalling pathway is essential for the antibody-dependent enhancement of ebola virus infection, *PLoS Pathogen*, 2016, 12(12):e1006139.

[34] Homsy J, Meyer M, Tateno M, et al. The fc and not CD4 receptor mediates antibody enhancement of HIV infection in human cells, *Science*, 1989, 244(4910):1357-1360.

[35] Wang SF, Tseng SP, Yen CH, et al. Antibody-dependent SARS coronavirus infection is mediated by antibodies against spike proteins, *Biochem Biophys Res Commun*, 2014, 451(2):208-214.

[36] Biryukov S, Angov E, Landmesser ME, et al. Complement and antibody-mediated enhancement of red blood cell invasion and growth of malaria parasites, *EBioMedicine*, 2016, 9:207-216.

[37] Janeway CA Jr, Travers P, Walport M, et al. Immunobiology: The Immune System in Health and Disease, 5th edition, Garland Science, New York, 2001.

[38] Alberts B, Johnson A, Lewis J, et al. Molecular Biology of the Cell, 4th edition, Garland Science, New York, 2002.

[39] Ademokun AA, Dunn-Walters D. Immune Responses: Primary and Secondary, 2010. In: eLS. John Wiley & Sons Ltd, Chichester. https://onlinelibrary.wiley.com/doi/10.1002/9780470015902.a0000947.pub2. Accessed May, 2019.

[40] McMichael AJ, Borrow P, Tomaras GD, et al. The immune response during acute HIV-1 infection: clues for vaccine development, *Nat Rev Immunol*, 2010, 10(1):11-23.

[41] Hatta Y, Hershberger K, Shinya K, et al. Viral Replication Rate Regulates Clinical Outcome and CD8 T Cell Responses during Highly Pathogenic H5N1 Influenza Virus Infection in Mice, *PLoS Pathog*, 2010, 6(10):e1001139..

[42] Microbiology Notes: What Is The Difference Between primary and Secondary Immune Response, http://www.microbiologynotes.com/differences-between-primary-and-secondary-immune-response/, Accessed May, 2019.

[43] Tangye SG, Avery DT, Deenick EK, Hodgkin PD. Intrinsic Differences in the Proliferation of Naive and Memory Human B Cells as a Mechanism for Enhanced Secondary Immune Responses, *J Immunol*, 2003, 170(2):686-694.

[44] Immunity: Oxford Living Dictionaries, https://en.oxforddictionaries.com/definition/immunity. Accessed January, 2019.

[45] Cush J, Kavanaugh A, Stein C. Rheumatology: Diagnosis and Therapeutics, Lippincott Williams & Wilkins, 2005, pp. 78.

[46] ibid. See reference #37.

[47] Eggleton P, Hypersensitivity: Immune Complex Mediated (Type III). In: eLS. John Wiley & Sons Ltd, Chichester, 2013. http://www.els.net/WileyCDA/ElsArticle/refId-a0001138.html. Accessed August, 2017.

[48] Pathway Medicine: Type III Hypersensitivity, http://www.pathwaymedicine.org/type-iii-hypersensitivity, Accessed May, 2019.

[49] Jackson R. Serum Sickness, *J Cutan Med Surg*, 2000, 4(4):223-225.

[50] Francis AH, Martin LG, Haldorson GJ, et al. Adverse reactions suggestive of type III hypersensitivity in six healthy dogs given human albumin, *J Am Vet Med Assoc*, 2007, 230(6):873-879.

[51] Merck: Gardasil Vaccine Insert,

https://www.merck.com/product/usa/pi_circulars/g/gardasil_9/gardasil_9_pi.pdf, Accessed May, 2019

[52] Merck: MMR Vaccine Insert, http://www.merck.com/product/usa/pi_circulars/m/mmr_ii/mmr_ii_pi.pdf, Accessed May, 2019.

[53] FDA: Afluria Quadrivalent Vaccine Insert, https://www.fda.gov/downloads/BiologicsBloodVaccines/Vaccines/ApprovedProducts/UCM518295.pdf, Accessed August, 2017.

[54] Mosmann TR, Coffman RL. TH1 and TH2 cells: different patterns of lymphokine secretion lead to different functional properties, *Annu Rev Immunol*, 1989, 7:145-173.

[55] Mosmann TR, Sad S. The expanding universe of T-cell subsets: Th1, Th2 and more, *Immunology Today*, 1996, 17:138-146.

[56] Singh VK, Mehrotra S, Agarwal SS. The paradigm of Th1 and Th2 cytokines: its relevance to autoimmunity and allergy, *Immunol Res*, 1999, 20:147-161.

[57] Murata Y, Amao M, Hamuro J. Sequential conversion of the redox status of macrophages dictates the pathological progression of autoimmune diabetes, *Eur J Immunol*, 2003, 33:1001-1011.

[58] Wu Z, Turner DR, Oliviera DB. IL-4 gene expression up-regulated by mercury in rat mast cells: a role of oxidant stress in IL-4 transcription, *Int Immunol*, 2001, 13:297-304.

[59] Brummelman J, Raeven RHM, Helm K, et al. Transcriptome signature for dampened Th2 dominance in acellular pertussis vaccine-induced CD4+ T cell responses through TLR4 ligation, *Sci Rep,* 2016, 6:250-64.

[60] Lalor MK, Smith SG, Floyd S, et al. Complex cytokine profiles induced by BCG vaccination in UK infants, *Vaccine*, 2010, 28(6):1635-1641.

[61] Strid J, Callard R, Strobel S. Epicutaneous immunization converts subsequent and established antigen-specific T helper type 1 (Th1) to Th2-type responses, *Immunology*, 2006, 119(1):27-35.

[62] Lienhardt C, Azzurri A, Amedei A, et al. Active tuberculosis in Africa is associated with reduced Th1 and increased Th2 activity in vivo, *Eur J Immunol*, 2002, 32:1605-1613.

[63] Larche M, Robinson DS, Kay AB. The role of T lymphocytes in the pathogenesis of asthma, *J Allergy Clin Immunol*, 2003, 111:450-463.

[64] Roitt I, Brostoff J, Male D. Immunology, 5th Edition, Philadelphia, PA: Mosby, 1998.

[65] Sato M, Goto S, Kaneko R, et al. Impaired production of Th1 cytokines and increased frequency of Th2 subsets in PBMC from advanced cancer patients, *Anticancer Res*, 1998, 18:3951-3955.

[66] Huang M, Wang J, Lee P, et al. Human non-small cell lung cancer cells express a type 2 cytokine pattern, *Cancer Res*, 1995, 55:3847-3853.

[67] Filella X, Alcover J, Zarco MA, et al. Analysis of type T1 and T2 cytokines in patients with prostate cancer, *Prostate*, 2000, 44:271-274.

[68] Gupta S, Aggarwal S, Rashanravan B, Lee T. TH1 and TH2-like cytokines in CD4+ and CD8+ T cells in autism, *J of Neuroimmunol,* 1998, 85:106-109.

[69] Becker Y. The changes in the T-helper 1 (Th1) and T-helper 2 (Th2) cytokine balance during HIV-1 infection are indicative of an allergic response to viral proteins that may be reversed by Th2 cytokine inhibitors and immune response modifiers --a review and hypothesis, *Virus Genes*, 2004, 28(1)5-18.

[70] MacDonell KB, Chmiel JS, Poggensee L, et al. Predicting Progression to AIDS: combined usefulness of CD4 counts and p24 antigenemia, *Am J Med*, 1990, 89(6):706-712.

[71] Matsushita S. Problems in the diagnosis of AIDS, *Rinsho Byori*, 1994, 42(12):1248-1252.

[72] CDC: Notice to Readers: Fever, Jaundice, and Multiple Organ System Failure Associated With 17D-Derived Yellow Fever Vaccination, 1996--2001, *MMWR Weekly*, 50(30):643-645.

[73] Schuil J, van de Putte EM, Zwaan CM, et al. Retinopathy following measles, mumps and rubella vaccination in an immuno-incompetent girl, *Int Opthalmol*, 1998, 22(6):345-7.

[74] Duesberg PH. Inventing the AIDS virus, Regnery Publishing, Washington DC, 1998.

[75] Duesberg P, Koehnlein C, Rasnick D. The Chemical Bases of the Various AIDS Epidemics: Recreational Drugs, Anti-viral Chemotherapy and Malnutrition, *J Biosci*, 2003, 28:383-412.

[76] Mullis K. A hypothetical disease of the immune system that may bear some relation to the acquired immune deficiency syndrome, *Genetica,* 1995, 95:195–197.

[77] Coghlan A. Mystery Over Drug Trial Debacle Deepens, *New Scientist*, 14th August 2006.

[78] Barrios C, Brawand P, Berney M, et al. Neonatal and early life immune responses to various forms of vaccine antigens qualitatively differ from adult responses: Predominance of a Th2-biased pattern which persists after adult boosting, *Eur J Immunol*, 1996, 26(7):1489-1496.

[79] Martinez X, Brandt C, Sadallah F, et al. DNA immunization circumvents deficient induction of T-helper type 1 and cytotoxic T lymphocyte responses in neonates and during early life, *Proc Natl Acad Sci USA*, 1997, 94(16):8726–8731.

[80] Barrios C, Brandt C, Berney M, et al. Partial correction of the Th2/Th1 imbalance in neonatal murine responses to

vaccine antigens through selective adjuvant effects, *Eur J Immunol*, 1996, 26(11):2666-2670.

[81] Bowman LM, Holt PG. Selective Enhancement of Systemic Th1 Immunity in Immunologically Immature Rats with an Orally Administered Bacterial Extract. Clements JD, ed. *Infection and Immunity*, 2001, 69(6):3719-3727.

[82] Baum MK, Miquez-Burbano MJ, Campa A, et al. Selenium and interleukins in persons infected with human immunodeficientcy virus type 1, *J Infect Dis*, 2000, 182:S69-73.

[83] Prasad AS. Effects of zinc deficiency on Th1 and Th2 cytokine shifts, *J Infect Dis*, 2000, 182:S62-68.

[84] Cross ML. Immunoregulation by probiotic lactobacilli: pro-Th1 signals and their relevance to human health, *Clin Appl Immunol Rev*, 2002, 3:115-125.

[85] Breytenbach U, Clark A, Lamprecht J, et al. Flow cytometric analysis of the Th1-Th2 balance in healthy individuals and patients infected with the human immunodeficiency virus HIV) receiving a plant sterol/sterolin mixture, *Cell Biol Int*, 2001, 25:43-49.

[86] Ibid. See reference #37.

[87] Science Daily. New monoclonal antibody develoedp that can target proteins inside cancer cells, https://www.science-daily.com/releases/2013/03/130313160757.htm, Accessed May, 2019.

[88] Coghlan A. Super antibodies break the cell barrier, *New Scientist*, 19th April, 2004.

[89] Kim EJ, Cho D, Kim TS. Efficient induction of T helper type 1-mediated immune responses in antigen-primed mice by anti-CD3 single-chain Fv/interleukin-18 fusion DNA, *Immunology*, 2004, 111(1):27–34.

[90] Abbas AK, Murphy KM, Sher A. Functional diversity of helper T lymphocytes, *Nature*, 1996, 383(6603):787-93.

[91] Nelson KE, Williams C. Infectious Disease Epidemiology: Theory and Practice, Jones and Bartlett Learning, 2007, pp 131.

[92] Hayflick L. Slow Viruses, *Executive Health Report,* Feb. 1981, pp 4.

[93] Talai N. Autoimmunity, in Fudenberg, *Basic Clinical Immunology,* 3rd Ed., Lange, 1980, p. 222.

[94] Dowdle WR, Orenstein WA. Quest for life-long protection by vaccination, *Proc Natl Acad Sci USA,* 1994, 91(7):2464-2468.

[95] World Health Organization, Measles, http://www.who.int/mediacentre/factsheets/fs286/en/. Accessed May, 2019.

[96] National Health Service: MMR Vaccine FAQS, http://www.nhs.uk/Conditions/vaccinations/Pages/mmr-questions-answers.aspx. Accessed May, 2019.

[97] The Immunisation Advisory Centre, Efficacy and Effectiveness, http://www.immune.org.nz/vaccines/efficiency-effectiveness, Accessed May, 2019.

[98] Children's Hospital of Philadelphia, Vaccine History: Development by Year, http://www.chop.edu/centers-programs/vaccine-education-center/vaccine-history/developments-by-year. Accessed May, 2019.

[99] Australian Department of Health, Australian Immunisation Register AIR), http://www.immunise.health.gov.au/internet/immunise/publishing.nsf/Content/ohp-acir.htm. Accessed October, 2017.

[100] Centers for Disease Control and Prevention, Influenza Vaccination Information for Healthcare Workers, https://www.cdc.gov/flu/healthcareworkers.htm. Accessed October, 2017.

[101] Young E. WA mum's fundraiser to avert homelessness highlights vaccine scheme concern, WA Today, 7th January, 2016.

[102] Topley WWC, Wilson GS. The spread of bacterial infection: The problem of herd immunity, *J Hyg*, 1923, 21(3):1923.

[103] Hedrich AW. Monthly estimates of the child population "susceptible" to measles, 1900- 1931, Baltimore, MD, *Am J Hyg*, 1933, 17:613-36.

[104] Godfrey ES. Practical Uses of Diptheria Immunization Records, *Am J Pub Health*, 1933, 23(8):809-812.

[105] Galazka AM, Robertson SE, Oblapenko GP, Resurgence of diptheria, *Euro J Epidemiol*, 1995, 111):95-105.

[106] Spencer DJ, Dull HB, Langmuir AD. Epidemiologic basis for eradication of measles in 1967, *Pub Health Rep*, 1967, 82(3):253-256.

[107] Stuart-Harris C. Prospects for the eradication of infectious disease, *Rev Infect Dis*, 1984, 6(3):405-411.

[108] Katz SL, Hinman AR. Summary and conclusions: measles elimination meeting, 16-17 March 2000, *J Infect Dis,* 2004, 189(S1):S43-S47.

[109] CDC. Frequently Asked Questions About Measles In The US, https://www.cdc.gov/measles/about/faqs.html#measles-elimination, Accessed July, 2017.

[110] Gustafson TL, Lievens AW, Brunell PA, et al. Measles outbreak in a fully immunized secondary school population, *NEJM*, 1987, 316(13):771-774.

[111] De Serres G, Markowski F, Toth E, et al. Largest measles epidemic in North America in a decade--Quebec, Canada, 2011: contribution of susceptibility, serendipity, and superspreading events, *J Infect Dis*, 2013, 207(6):990-8.

[112] Seaver L, Pertussis outbreak at Salinas school, *KSBW8 News*, 19th March, 2015.

[113] Holland M, Zachary CE. Herd immunity and compulsory childhood vaccination: Does the theory justify the law? *Or Law Rev*, 2014, 93(1).

[114] Brelsford D, Knutzen E, Neher JO, Safranek S. Which interventions are effective in managing parental vaccine refusal, *J Fam Pract*, 2017, 66(12):E12-E14.

[115] Goldman B. The Bodyguard: Tapping the Immune System's Secrets, Stanford Medicine, Summer 2011.

[116] Awate S, Babiuk LA, Mutwiri G. Mechanisms of action of adjuvants, *Front Immunol*, 2013, 4:114.

Chapter 2: VACCINE HISTORY

[1] GB Historical GIS / University of Portsmouth, London Gov Of through time | Population Statistics | Total Population, *A Vision of Britain through Time*.

[2] Porter R. The Greatest Benefit to Mankind, Harper Collins, New York, 1997.

[3] Publications of the American Statistical Association, Volume 9, Nos 65-72, 1904-1905, pp 260-261.

[4] Chesney K. The Victorian Underworld, Penguin Books, 1972.

[5] Porter D. Health, Civilization and the State – A History of Public Health From Ancient to Modern Times, Routledge, Oxfordshire, England, 1999.

[6] Mayhew H. A visit to the cholera districts of Bermondsey, *The Morning Chronicle*, 24th September, 1849.

[7] Byrne J. My Chicago, Northwestern University Press, Evanston, Illinois, 1992.

[8] Mann E. Story of Cities #14: London's Great Stink heralds a wonder of the modern world, *The Guardian*, 4th April, 2016.

[9] Radeska T. The 1854 cholera outbreak of Broad Street, Everyone got sick except those who drank beer instead of water, *Vintage News*, 26th September, 2016.

[10] The British and Foreign Medico-Chirurgical Review, Quarterly Journal of Practical Medicine and Surgery, Volume XXXV, John Churchill and Sons, London, Jan-Apr 1865, pp 32-33.

[11] Cole AC. The Irrepressible Conflict 1850-1865: A History of American Life, Volume VII, Macmillan, New York, 1934, p 81.

[12] Formaldehyde and Milk, *JAMA*, 1900; XXXIV(23):1496.

[13] Report of the Council of Hygiene and Public Health of the Citizen's Association of New York, 1865, p 59.

[14] Wertz RW, Wertz DC. Lying In: A History of Childbirth in America, Yale University Press, 1989, p 122.

[15] Loudon I. Maternal mortality in the past and its relevance to developing countries today, Am J Clin Nutr, 2000, 72:241S-246S.

[16] Newman G. Infant Mortality: A Continuing Social Problem, Methueun and Co, London, 1906, p 95.

[17] Horn P. The Victorian Town Child, New York University Press, 1997.

[18] Willoughby WF, de Graffenried C. Child Labor, American Economic Association, Guggenheimer, Weil and Co, Baltimore, 1890, p 16.

[19] Trueman C. Children in the Industrial Revolution, History Learning Site,12th November 2006.

[20] Cheyney EP. An Introduction to the Industrial and Social History of England, Macmillan, New York, 1920, pp 243-244.

[21] Lovejoy OR. Child Labor in the Coal Mines, Child Labor – A Menace to Industry, Education and Good Citizenship, Academy of Political and Social Science, 1906, p 38.

[22] Ibid. See reference #19.

[23] Ibid. See reference #18.

[24] The American Journal of Nursing, 1903, 3(8):664.

[25] Mearns A, Preston WC. The Bitter Cry of Outcast London: An Inquiry Into the Condition of the Abject Poor, James Clarke and Co, London, 1883.

[26] Noble TFX, Straus B, Osheim DJ, et al. Western Civikization: Beyond Boundaries, Volume II, 6th Edition, Wadsworth, Boston, Massachesetts.

[27] Carrington D. The truth about London's air pollution, *The Guardian*, 5th February, 2016.

[28] Vaughan A. Nearly 9500 die every year in London because of air pollution, *The Guardian*, 15th July, 2015.

[29] UK Air, What are the main trends in particulate matter in the UK? Chapter 7, https://www.google.com.au/url?sa=t&rct=j&q=&esrc=s&source=web&cd=1&ved=2ahUKEwiJo6G8r9ffAhXJP3AKHf4dCesQFjAAegQICxAC&url=https%3A%2F%2Fuk-air.de-fra.gov.uk%2Fassets%2Fdocuments%2Freports%2Fa-qeg%2Fch7.pdf&usg=AOvVaw3Qd9bOWTstyEmCOpcmeLA6, Accessed January, 2019.

[30] Stevens EE, Patrick TE, Pickler R. A history of infant feeding, *J Perinat Educ*, 2009, 18(2):32-9.

[31] Hirschman C, Butler M. Trends and differentials in breast feeding: an update, *Demography*, 1981, 18:39-54.

[32] Riordan J, Countryman BA. Basics of breastfeeding. Part I: Infant feeding patterns past and present, *JOGN Nurs, 1980,* 9(4): 207–210.

[33] Oatman-Stanford H. A Filthy History: When New-Yorkers Lived Knee Deep in Trash, Collector's Weekly, https://www.collectorsweekly.com/articles/when-new-york-ers-lived-knee-deep-in-trash/. Accessed Januray, 2019.

[34] Jackson L. Dirty Old London: The Victorian Fight Against Filth, Yale University Press, 2014.

[35] Annual Report of the Metropolitan Board of Health, 1866, Westcott and Co's Printing House, New York, 1987.

[36] Heggie V. Over 200yrs of deadly London air: smogs, fogs and pea soupers, *The Guardian*, 9th December, 2016.

[37] Holick MF. Resurrection of vitamin D deficiency and rickets, *J Clin Invest*, 2006, 116(8):2062-72.

[38] London Catalyst, A reflection on sickness and poverty in London in the late 19th century, https://www.londoncatalyst.org.uk/newsite/wp-content/uploads/2014/11/London-CatalystMofLpovertyessay2013-doc.pdf, Accessed November, 2017.

[39] Lorenz AJ. Scurvy in the Gold Rush, *J Hist Med All Sci*, 1957, 12(4):473–510.

[40] Cormia FE. Tryparsamide in the treatment of Syphilis of the central nervous system, *Bri J Ven Dis*, 1934, 10:99-116.

[41] Swediaur F. Practical observations on the more obstinate and inveterate venereal complaints, J Johnson and C Elliott, London, 1784.

[42] Blumgarten AS. A Text Book of Medicine - For Students in Schools of Nursing, 1937.

[43] Vincent's Semi-Annual United States Register, 1860, p346.

[44] Greene VW. Personal hygiene and life expectancy improvements since 1850: Historic and epidemiologic associations, *Am J Inf Cont*, 2001, 29(4):203-206.

[45] Rosen J. The Effects of Chronic Fear on a Person's Health, Neuroscience Education Institute (NEI), 2017 Conference, https://www.ajmc.com/conferences/nei-2017/the-effects-of-chronic-fear-on-a-persons-health, Accessed January, 2019.

[46] Ibid. See reference #11.

[47] Ibid. See reference #44.

[48] Korsman S, Van Zyl G, Preiser W, et al. Virology: 1st Edition, Elsevier 2012.

[49] The Letters And Works Of Lady Mary Wortley Montagu, New Edition, London, 1887.

[50] Crookshank EM. History and pathology of vaccination: A critical inquiry, HK Lewis, London, 1889.

[51] Act of 4 and 5 Victoria, c. 29, s. 8, July 23, 1840, *English Statues*, 4to., vol. xv, p. 353.

[52] Hammarsten JF, Tattersall W, Hammarsten JE. Who discovered smallpox vaccination? Edward Jenner or Benjamin Jesty? *Trans Am Clin Clim Assoc*, 1979, 90:44-55.

[53] Baron J. The Life of Edward Jenner MD, Vol 2, Cambridge University Press, 1838.

[54] Riedel S. Edward Jenner and the history of smallpox and vaccination, *Proceedings (Baylor University Medical Center)*, 2005, 18(1):21-25.

[55] Pearce CT. Essay on Vaccination, H Bailliere, Regent Street, London, 1868.

[56] Cox JK. Human and bovine tuberculosis, *Vaccination Inquirer*, 1884, Volume 5, p 114.

[57] Hadwen W, *The Case Against Vaccination*, 1896.

[58] The Robinson Library, Edward Jenner: Developer of Vaccination, http://robinsonlibrary.com/medicine/medicine/history/jenner.htm. Accessed March 2019.

[59] Freemasonry Today, Edward Jenner – Freemason and Natural Philosopher, https://www.freemasonrytoday.com/more-news/lodges-chapters-a-individuals/edward-jenner-freemason-and-natural-philosopher, Accessed May, 2019.

[60] Morabia A. Edward Jenner's 1798 report of challenge experiments demonstrating the protective effects of cowpox against smallpox, 2010, JLL Bulletin: Commentaries on the

history of treatment evaluation http://www.jameslindli-brary.org/articles/edward-jenners-1798-report-of-challenge-experiments-demonstrating-the-protective-effects-of-cowpox-against-smallpox/. Accessed March 2019.

[61] Jenner E. An Inquiry Into the Causes and Effects of Variolae Vaccinae, or Cowpox, S Low, London, 1798.

[62] Woodville W. Reports of a series of inoculations for the variolae vaccinae, or cowpox, 1799, James Phillips, London, pp 57-59.

[63] Boylston AW. The origins of vaccination: no inoculation, no vaccination. JLL Bulletin: Commentaries on the history of treatment evaluation, 2012, Available at: http://www.james-lindlibrary.org/articles/the-origins-of-vaccination-no-inocula-tion-no-vaccination/, Accessed March 2019.

[64] The Robinson Library, Edward Jenner: Developer of Vaccination, http://robinsonlibrary.com/medicine/medicine/his-tory/jenner.htm, Accessed March 2019.

[65] Ibid. See reference #53.

[66] Hays JN. The Burdens of Disease: Epidemics and Human Response in Western History, 2009, Rutgers University Press, p. 126.

[67] Ibid. See reference #61.

[68] Seaton EC. A Handbook of Vaccination, Philadelphia, 1868, pp 305-306.

[69] Hodge JW. A Review Of Some Of The False Claims, Erroneous Deductions And Self-Contradictions Of The Upholders Of The Vaccination-Dogma, reprinted from *Medical Century*, September, 1903, p. 5.

[70] First Annual Report of the Commissioner of Health of the Commonwealth of Pennsylvania, 1905-6, by Samuel G. Dixon, M.D., Commissioner of Health, p.48.

[71] Lippincott H. Extracts From A Paper On The Expedition To The Philippine Islands, May 27, 1898, to April 27, 1899, The Philadelphia Medical Journal, April 14, 1900, vol. v, p. 829.

[72] War Department. Annual reports of the Surgeon-General of the United States Army, 1898 - 1902. Accessed from https://catalog.hathitrust.org/Record/005639085.

[73] Ibid. See reference #55.

[74] Address of William Howard Hay, M.D., Pocono, PA., on June 25, 1937, before The Medical Freedom Society.

[75] Vaccination And Smallpox In Japan, *The Vaccination Inquirer*, June 1, 1910, vol. xxxi, p. 48.

[76] Vaccination In Japan, *Health*, July 25, 1908, quoted in *The Vaccination Inquirer*, September 1, 1908, vol. xxx, p.96.

[77] Smallpox In Vaccinated And Re-vaccinated Japan, *The Vaccination Inquirer*, May 1, 1908, vol. xxx, p.28.

[78] Hodge JW. The Failure Of Vaccination To Protect From Smallpox In Re-vaccinated Japan, *Twentieth Century Magazine*, September 1910, 12 2):518-522.

[79] Ibid. See reference #74.

[80] Carque O. Rational Diet: An Advanced Treatise on the Food Question, Health Research Books, 1996.

[81] Syphilis conveyed by the vaccine lymph to 46 children, *The Lancet*, November 16, 1861.

[82] Lee H. Lectures on syphilitic inoculation in 1865, 1866, *The Lancet*, 87(2224):391-394.

[83] Tebb W. Leprosy and Vaccination: The Recrudescence of Leprosy and Its Causation, Swan Sonnenschein and Co, London, 1893.

[84] Melvin AD. The 1908 Outbreak Of Foot-And-Mouth Disease In The United States, *Twenty-fifth Annual report of the Bureau of Animal Industry, for the Year 1908*, USDA, pp. 379-392.

[85] Mohler JR, Rosenau MJ. The Origins Of The Recent Outbreak Of Foot-And-Mouth Disease In The United States, *Bureau of Animal Industry, Circular 147*, USDA, issued June 16, 1909.

[86] McFarland J. Tetanus And Vaccination -- An Analytical Study Of Ninety-five Cases Of This Rare Complication, Journal of Medical Research, 1902, vol. vii, new series, vol. ii, pp. 474-493.

[87] Ibid. See reference #55.

[88] Durbach N. Bodily Matters: The Anti-Vaccination Movement in England, 1853 – 1907, Duke University Press, Durham and London, 2005.

[89] Shelton HM. The Hygienic System, Orthopathy, Vol. VII, 1941.

[90] Hale AR. The Medical Voodoo, Gotham House, Inc., 1935

[91] Dewhurst K. Dr. Thomas Sydenham (1624-1689): His Life and Original Writings, University of California Press, 1966, p.163.

[92] History of Vaccines, Bloodletting, https://www.historyofvaccines.org/content/17th-century-smallpox-treatment. Accessed March 2019.

[93] Blumgarten AS. A Text Book of Medicine - For Students in Schools of Nursing, Macmillan, 1937.

[94] Science Lab. Phenol MSDS, http://www.sciencelab.com/msds.php?msdsId=9926463. Accessed November, 2017.

[95] Toxicology Data Network. Potassium Bromide, https://toxnet.nlm.nih.gov/cgi-bin/sis/search/a?dbs+hsdb:@term+@DOCNO+5044, Accessed November, 2017.

[96] Healthline. Smallpox, https://www.health-line.com/health/smallpox#overview1, Accessed November, 2017.

[97] King V. Arsenic, The History Magazine, 2001, October/November Issue, http://www.history-magazine.com/arsenic.html, Accessed November, 2017.

[98] Vahidnia A, dan der Voet GB, de Wolff FA. Arsenic neurotoxicity – a review, *Hum Exp Toxicol*, 2007, 26:823-832.

[99] Secretary of State of Michigan, First Annual Report Of The Secretary Of State Of The State Of Michigan, Relating To The Registry And Return Of Births, Marriages, and Deaths, For the Year Ending April 5th, 1868 (Lansing, Michigan; John A. Kerr & Co., 1868) 59.

[100] Secretary of State of Michigan, Third Annual Report Of The Secretary Of State Of The State Of Michigan, Relating To The Registry And Return Of Births, Marriages, and Deaths, For The Year 1869 (Lansing, Michigan; W.S. George & Co., 1870) 126.

[101] Secretary of State of Michigan, Fourth Annual Report Of The Secretary Of State Of The State Of Michigan, Relating To The Registry And Return Of Births, Marriages, and Deaths, For The Year 1870 (Lansing, Michigan; W.S. George & Co., 1872) 229.

[102] Secretary of State of Michigan, Seventeenth Annual Report Relating To The Registry And Return Of Births, Marriages, and Deaths In Michigan For The Year 1883 (Lansing, Michigan; W.S. George & Co., 1885) 228.

[103] Secretary of State of Michigan, Nineteeth Annual Report Relating To The Registry And Return Of Births, Marriages, and Deaths In Michigan For The Year 1885 (Lansing, Michigan; Thorp & Godfrey, 1887) 144.

[104] Secretary of State of Michigan, Twenty-Second Annual Report Relating To The Registry And Return Of Births, Marriages, and Deaths In Michigan For The Year 1888 (Lansing, Michigan; Robert Smith & Co., 1890) 211.

[105] Secretary of State of Michigan, Twenty-Fourth Annual Report Relating To The Registry And Return Of Births, Marriages, and Deaths In Michigan For The Year 1890 (Lansing, Michigan; Robert Smith & Co., 1892) 201.

[106] Secretary of State of Michigan, Twenty-Fifth Annual Report Relating To The Registry And Return Of Births, Marriages, and Deaths In Michigan For The Year 1891 With A Review Of The Results Of State Registration For Twenty-Five Years, 1867-1891 (Lansing, Michigan; Robert Smith & Co., 1893) 207.

[107] Secretary of State of Michigan, Twenty-Sixth Annual Report Relating To The Registry And Return Of Births, Marriages, and Deaths In Michigan For The Year 1892 (Lansing, Michigan; Robert Smith & Co., 1894) 206.

[108] Secretary of State of Michigan, Twenty-Eighth Annual Report Relating To The Registry And Return Of Births, Marriages And Deaths in Michigan For The Year 1894 (Lansing, Michigan: Robert Smith Printing Co, 1897) 302.

[109] Secretary of State of Michigan, Twenty-Ninth Annual Report Relating To The Registry And Return Of Births, Marriages And Deaths in Michigan For The Year 1895 (Lansing, Michigan: Robert Smith Printing Co, 1897) 181.

[110] Colmer G. Paralysis in Teething Children, *Am J Med Sci*, 1843, 5:248.

[111] Bradford A. Mercury Poisoning: Causes, Effects & Fish, *LiveScience*, 24th February, 2016, https://www.livescience.com/53837-mercury-poisoning.html. Accessed April 2019.

[112] Schooley T, Weaver MJ, Mullins D, et al. The History of Lead Arsenate Use in Apple Production: Comparison of its Impact in Virginia with Other States, *J Pest Safety Ed*, 2008, 10:21-53.

[113] Cooke J. Treatise of Nervous Diseases, 1824.

[114] Putnam JJ, Taylor EW. Is Acute Poliomyelitis Unusually Prevalent this Season? *Boston Med Surg J*, 1893, 129:509-510.

[115] Science in the Courtroom: The Woburn Toxic Trial, Chemical Industries in Woburn, https://serc.carleton.edu/woburn/issues/chem_industries.html. Accessed April 2019.

[116] Caverley CS. Infantile Paralysis in Vermont, 1894-1922, Published 1924, Available at: https://archive.org/details/infantileparalys00cave/page/16. Accessed May 2019.

[117] CDC, What is Polio, https://www.cdc.gov/polio/about/. Accessed March 2019.

[118] Ibid. See reference #112.

[119] Hough WS, Hurt RH, Ellett WB, et al. Removal of spray residues from apples, *VA Agricultural Exp Station, VPI Bulletin 278*, 1931, Blacksburg VA, p. 16.

[120] Frear DEH, Worthley HN. Study of the removal of spray residues from apples, *J Agric Res*, 1935, 51(1):60-74.

[121] Emerson HC. An Epidemic of Infantile Paralysis in Western Massachusetts in 1908, published in The Occurrence of Infantile Paralysis in Massachusetts in 1908: reported for the Massachusetts State Board of Health, 1909, Available at: https://archive.org/details/b22431779/page/n13. Accessed March 2019.

[122] Scobey PR. The Poison Cause of Poliomyelitis and Obstruction to Its Investigation, Statement prepared for the Select Committee to Investigate the Use of Chemicals in Food Products, United States House of Representatives, Washington, D.C. *From Archive Of Pediatrics*, April, 1952.

[123] Eggers HJ. Milestones in early poliomyelitis research (1840 to 1949), *J Virol*, 1999, 73(6):4533–4535.

[124] The History of Vaccines, Poliovirus Identified, https://www.historyofvaccines.org/content/poliovirus-identified. Accessed April 2019.

[125] Flexner S, Noguchi H. Experiments on the Cultivation of the Microorganism Causing Epidemic Poliomyelitis (From the Laboratories of the Rockefeller Institute for Medical Research, New York), Available at: https://www.ncbi.nlm.nih.gov/pmc/articles/PMC2125080/pdf/461.pdf. Accessed March 2019.

[126] Mansoor F, Hamid S, Mir T, et al. Incidence of traumatic injection neuropathy among children in Pakistan, *La Rev San Medit Orient*, 2005, 11(4): 798-804.

[127] Melnick JL, Ward R. Susceptibility of vervet monkeys to poliomyelitis virus in flies collected at epidemics, *J Infect Dis, 1945,* 77:251.

[128] Zamula E. A new challenge for former polio patients. FDA Consumer, 1991. Food and Drug Administration, Washington, D.C., as quoted in: Melnick JL, Current status of poliovirus infection, *Clin Microbiol Rev*, 1996, 9(3):293-300.

[129] Risse GB. Revolt Against Quarantine: Community Responses to the 1916 Polio Epidemic, Oyster Bay, New York, Available at: https://s3.amazonaws.com/academia.edu.documents/34344634/Oyster_Bay_quarantine001.pdf?AWSAccessKeyId=AKIAIWOWYYGZ2Y53UL3A&Expires=1556177356&Signature=KNhMfi5rCgP3GTPSYKXXnnru2I8%3D&response-content-disposition=inline%3B%20filename%3DRevolt_Against_Quarantine_Community_Resp.pdf. Accessed April 2019.

[130] Merelli A. 100 Years Ago, New York City Declared War Against Polio and Killed 72,000 cats (and 8000 dogs), *Quartz*, 23rd September 2016.

[131] Scobey RR. Is Human Poliomyelitis Caused by an Exogenous Virus? *Arch Ped*, 1954, 71:111.

[132] European Food Safety Authority (EFSA). Scientific opinion of the panel on contaminants in the food chain: arsenic in food, *EFSA J*, 2009, 7(10):1351.

[133] Hood River Glacier, Sprayed Hay Kills Cows and Horses, 22nd April 1920, https://oregonnews.uoregon.edu/lccn/sn97071110/1920-04-22/ed-1/seq-6.pdf. Accessed April 2019.

[134] Berish A. FDR and Polio, Franklin D Roosevelt Presidential Library and Museum, https://fdrlibrary.org/polio. Accessed April 2019.

[135] Goldman AS, Goldman DA. Prisoners of Time: The Misdiagnosis of FDR's 1921 Illness, EHDP Press, 2017.

[136] Ibid. See reference #134.

[137] Encyclopaedia Brittanica Macropaedia, 1986.

[138] Whorton J. Before Silent Spring: Pesticides and public health in pre-DDT America, Princeton University Press, 1974.

[139] Ibid. See reference #122.

[140] Department of Agriculture and Fisheries, Arsenic, https://www.daf.qld.gov.au/animal-industries/animal-health-and-diseases/protect-your-animals/poisonings-of-livestock/arsenic, Accessed November, 2017.

[141] Cormia FE. Tryparsamide in the treatment of syphilis of the central nervous system, *Brit J Ven Dis*, 1934, 10:99-116.

[142] Ibid. See reference #122.

[143] Sleeman J. Cry for Health: Volume 1, The Casualty of Modern Times, Dragon Lair Publishing, 2011.

[144] Houchaus. Ueber Poliomyelitis acuta, *Munch Med Wochenschr* 1909, 56:2353-55.

[145] Lambert SM. A yaws campaign and an epidemic of poliomyelitis in Western Samoa, *J Trop Med Hyg,* 1936, 39:41-46.

[146] Martin JK. Local paralysis in children after injections, *Arch Dis Child,* 1950, 25:1-14.

[147] Lindsay KW, et al. Neurology and Neurosurgery Illustrated. Edinburgh/London/New York: Churchill Livingston, 1986: 100. Figure 15.2. Polio incidence rates obtained from National Morbidity Reports.

[148] Geffen DH. The incidence of paralysis occurring in London children within four weeks after immunization, *Med Officer*, 1950, 83:137-140.

[149] Medical Research Council Committee on Inoculation Procedures and Neurological Lesions. Poliomyelitis and prophylactic inoculation, *The Lancet*, 1956, ii:1223-1231.

[150] Sutter RW, et al. Attributable risk of DTP (Diphtheria and Tetanus Toxoids and Pertussis Vaccine) injection in provoking paralytic poliomyelitis during a large outbreak in Oman, *J Infect Dis,* 1992, 165:444-449.

[151] Strebel PM, et al. Intramuscular injections within 30 days of immunization with oral poliovirus vaccine -- a risk factor for vaccine-associated paralytic poliomyelitis, *NEJM*, 1995, pp. 500+.

[152] Wyatt HV. Provocation poliomyelitis: neglected clinical observations from 1914-1950, *Bull Hist Med,* 1981, 55:543-57.

[153] Townsend-Coles WF, Findlay GM. Poliomyelitis in relation to intramuscular injections of quinine and other drugs, *Trans R Soc Trop Med Hyg,* 1953, 47:77-81.

[154] McCloskey BP. The Relation of Prophylactic Inoculation to the Onset of Poliomyelitis, *The Lancet*, 1950, 255(6606): 659-663.

[155] Mawdsley SE. Polio Provocation: solving a mystery with the help of history, *The Lancet*, 2014, 384(9940):300-301.

[156] Ibid. See reference #126.

[157] Kohler KA, Hlady WG, Banerjee K, Sutter RW. Outbreak of poliomyelitis due to type 3 poliovirus, Northern India, 1999-2000: injections a major contributing factor, *Int J Epidem*, 2003, 32:272-277.

[158] Nathanson N, Kew OM. From Emergence to Eradication: The Epidemiology of Poliomyelitis Deconstructed, *Am J Epidem,* 2010, 172(11):1213–1229.

[159] Authorizing Research on Insecticides, Herbicides, Fungicides, and Other Pesticides by the Secretary of the Interior. 85th Congress, 2nd Session. House of Representatives Report No. 2181. July 16, 1958.

[160] Conis E. DDT Disbelievers: Health and the New Economic Poisons in Georgia after World War II, *Southern Spaces*, 28th October 2016.

[161] Whelan DE. How About DDT: Here's the Lowdown on our War Famed Bug Killer, *Nebraska Farmer*, 6th April 1946.

[162] Apen-Sadler D. Shocking 1940's video shows how US children were sprayed with dangerous pesticide as neighbourhoods were gassed with the 'miracle cure' that could kill mosquitos and end polio, *The Daily Mail*, 6th March 2018.

[163] Oshishky D. Polio: An American Story, Oxford University Press, 2006.

[164] Gray C. Porphyria, *Postgrad Med Journal*, 1956, Available at: https://pmj.bmj.com/content/postgradmedj/32/366/186.full.pdf. Accessed April 2019.

[165] Walker CH, Silby RM, Hopkin SP, Peakall DB, Principles of Ecotoxicology, CRC Press, Boca Raton, FL, 2012.

[166] Deng GD, Zheng BS, Zhai C, et al. Porphyrins as the early biomarkers for arsenic exposure in humans, *Cell Mol Biol*, 2007, 28(5):1147-52.

[167] Nataf R, Skorupka C, Amet L, et al. Porphyrinuria in childhood autistic disorder: implications for environmental toxicity, *Toxicol Appl Pharmacol*, 2006, 214(2):99-108.

[168] Sabin A. *The Epidemiology of Poliomyelitis*, *JAMA*, 1947, 134: 750.

[169] Capps RB. Chapter III: Dengue, US Army Medical Department, Office of Medical History, https://history.amedd.army.mil/booksdocs/wwii/infectiousdisvolii/chapter3.htm. Accessed April 2019.

[170] Ibid. See reference #158.

[171] Halstead LS. A Brief History of Post-Polio Syndrome in America, *Arch Phys Med Rehabil*, 2011, 92:1344-1349.

[172] Sokol B. Fear of Polio in the 1950's, http://www.plosin.com/beatbegins/projects/sokol.html#note04. Accessed March 2019.

[173] Ibid. See reference #163.

[174] Smithsonian National Museum of History, Whatever Happened to Polio: March of Dimes, https://amhistory.si.edu/polio/howpolio/march.htm. Accessed April 2019.

[175] US Department of Health, Education and Welfare, Vital Statistics of the United States 1952, Volume II, Mortality Data, https://www.cdc.gov/nchs/data/vsus/VSUS_1952_2.pdf. Accessed March 2019.

[176] PTA, PTA History: 1950-1959, https://www.pta.org/home/About-National-Parent-Teacher-Association/Mission-Values/National-PTA-History/PTA-History-1950-1959. Accessed March 2019.

[177] Snowden FM. *The Conquest of Malaria: Italy, 1900-1962,* (pp. 200). Frederick W. Hilles Publication Fund of Yale University, 2006..

[178] Francis T, Jr, et al. Evaluation of the 1954 Field Trial of Poliomyelitis Vaccine; Final Report, Ann Arbor, Michigan, Edwards Brothers, Inc., 1957.

[179] Juskewitch JE, Tapia CJ, Windebank AJ. Lessons from the Salk polio vaccine: methods for and risks of rapid translation, *Clin Transl Sci*, 2010, 3(4):182–185.

[180] Thompson D. The Salk Polio Vaccine: 'Greatest Public Health Experiment in History', *CBS News*, 2nd December 2014.

[181] Beddow Bayly M. The Story of the Salk Anti-Poliomyelitis Vaccine, 1956.

[182] Ibid. See reference #179

[183] Plotkin S, Robinson JM, Cunningham G, et al. The complexity and cost of vaccine manufacturing – an overview, *Vaccine*, 2017, 35(33):4064 – 4071.

[184] Michigan Alumnus, Polio Vaccine Announced Effective 60 Years Ago at U-M, http://alumnus.alumni.umich.edu/polio-vaccine-announced-effective-60-years-ago-at-u-m/. Accessed April 2019.

[185] Smith JS. *Patenting the Sun: Polio and the Salk Vaccine*, William Morrow and Co, Inc, New York, 1990.

[186] Ratner H. An Untold Vaccine Story: The Poliomyelitis Surveillance Unit, *Child and Family*, 1993, 21:253- 263.

[187] Offit PA. The Cutter Incident: How America's First Polio Vaccine Led to the Growing Vaccine Crisis, Yale University Press, 2005.

[188] Ratner H. The Untold Vaccine Story, *Child and Family*, 1988, 20:264-269.

[189] Richard Carter. Breakthrough: The Saga of Jonas Salk, Trident Press, New York, 1965.

[190] Ibid. See reference #186.

[191] Shorter E. The Health Century, Doubleday, New York City, 1987.

[192] Times Magazine, *Medicine: Vaccine Snafu, 30th May, 1955*.

[193] McKie R. A Jab for Elvis Helped America Beat Polio. Now Doctors Have Recruited Him Again, *The Guardian*, 24th April 2016.

[194] Noble G. From The Vault: Dr Albert Sabin saved the world from polio, *WCPO Cincinnati*, 21st April 2016.

[195] The History of Vaccines. Developing Oral Polio Vaccine, https://www.historyofvaccines.org/content/koprowski-tests-polio-vaccine-children. Accessed April 2019.

[196] Horstmann DM. The Sabin live poliovirus vaccination trials in the USSR, 1959, *Yale J Biol Med*, 1991, 64(5):499–512.

[197] CDC, Polio Surveillance, Report No. 285, 30th September 1964.

[198] Kinnunen E, Färkkilä M, Hovi T, et al. Incidence of Guillain-Barré syndrome during a nationwide oral poliovirus vaccine campaign, *Neurology*, 1989, 39(8):1034.

[199] Kim SJ, Kim SH, Jee YM, Kim JS. Vaccine-associated paralytic poliomyelitis: a case report of flaccid monoparesis after oral polio vaccine, *J Korean Med Sci*, 2007, 22(2):362–364.

[200] Whittle E, Robertson NRC. Transverse Myelitis after diptheria, tetanus and polio immunisation, *BMJ*, 1977, Available at: https://www.bmj.com/content/bmj/1/6074/1450.full.pdf. Accessed May 2019.

[201] Shibazaki K, Murakami T, Kushida R, et al. Acute disseminated encephalomyelitis associated with oral polio vaccine, *Jap Soc Int Med*, 2006, Available at: https://www.jstage.jst.go.jp/article/internalmedicine/45/20/45_20_1143/_pdf/-char/en. Accessed May 2019.

[202] Hearings Before the Committee on Interstate and Foreign Commerce, House of Representatives, 87th Congress, 2nd Session on HR 10541. May 1962, pp. 94-112.

[203] Ibid. See reference #186.

[204] CDC Prevention Guidelines Database (Archive), https://wonder.cdc.gov/wonder/prevguid/m0046568/m0046568.asp. Accessed April 2019.

[205] Ratner et al. The Present Status of Polio Vaccines, *Ill Med J*, 1960, pp 84-93.

[206] Ibid. See reference #188.

[207] Ibid. See reference #204.

[208] Wringe A, Fine PE, Sutter RW, Kew OM. Estimating the extent of vaccine-derived poliovirus infection, *PLOS One*, 2008, 3(10):e3433.

[209] Dalldorf G, Sickles GM. An Unidentified, Filtrable Agent Isolated From the Feces of Children With Paralysis, *Science,* 1948, 108 (2794):61–62.

[210] Dalldorf G, Sickles GM. A virus recovered from the feces of poliomyelitis patients pathogenic for suckling mice, *J Exp Med*, 1949, 89 (6):567–82.

[211] Racaniello V. Coxsackie NY and the virus named after it, *Virology Blog*, 10 August 2009.

[212] Yui LA, Gledhill RF. Limb paralysis as a manifestation of Coxsackie B virus infection, *Dev Med Child Neurol*, 1991, 33(5):427-38.

[213] Brown GC. Laboratory data on the Detroit poliomyelitis epidemic 1958, *JAMA*, 1960, 172:807-812.

[214] CDC, Outbreak of poliomyelitis, Dominican Republic and Haiti, *MMWR*, 8th December, 2000.

[215] Aycock WL. Tonsillectomy and poliomyelitis, I. Epidemiologic considerations, *Medicine*, 1942, 21:65.

[216] Anderson GW, Rondeau JL. Absence of tonsils as a factor in the development of bulbar poliomyelitis, *Minn Hosp Med Association*, 1954, XXV:319-337.

[217] Grob GN. The Rise and Decline of Tonsillectomy in Twentieth-Century America, *J Hist Med All Sci*, 2007, 62(4):383–421.

[218] Klass P. A Tonsil Remedy is Fitted for a New Century, *The New York Times*, 11th April 2011.

[219] Ibid. See reference #155.

[220] Sandler BP. Diet prevents polio, Lee Foundation for Nutritional Research, Milwaukee, WI, 1951.

[221] Hamel EE, Santisteban GA, Ely JT, Read D.H. Hyperglycemia and reproductive defects in non-diabetic gravidas: a mouse model test of a new theory, *Life Sci*, 1986, 39:1425–8.

[222] Jungeblut CW. Inactivation of poliomyelitis virus by crystalline vitamin C (ascorbic acid), *J Exper Med*, 1935, 62:317-321.

[223] Jungeblut CW, Zwemer RL. Inactivation of diphtheria toxin in vivo and in vitro by crystalline vitamin C (ascorbic acid), *Proc Soc Exper Biol Med*, 1935, 32:1229-1234.

[224] Jungeblut CW. Inactivation of tetanus toxin by crystalline vitamin C (l-ascorbic acid), *J Immunol*, 1937, 33:203-214.

[225] Stone I. The Healing Factor, Chapter 13, Viral Infection, Grosset and Dunlap, 1972.

[226] Klenner FR. The use of vitamin C as an antibiotic, *J App Nutr*, 1953, 6:274-278.

[227] Klenner FR. The treatment of poliomyelitis and other virus diseases with vitamin C. *South Med Surg*, J1949, 111(7):209-214.

[228] Klenner FR. Observations on the dose and administration of ascorbic acid when employed beyond the range of a vitamin in human pathology, *J Appl Nutr*, 1971, 23:61-68.

[229] Chapman W, Shaffer CF. Mercurial diuretics, *Arch lntern Med*, 1947, 79:449-456.

[230] Ibid. See reference #225.

[231] Klenner FR. Massive Doses of Vitamin C and the Virus Diseases, Presented in the Fifty-second Annual Meeting of the Tri-State Medical Association of the Carolinas and Virginia, held at Columbia, February 19th and 20th, 1951. Available at: https://www.seanet.com/~alexs/ascorbate/195x/klenner-fr-southern_med_surg-1951-v103-n4-p101.htm. Accessed April 2019.

[232] NDSU Agriculture Communication, Sheep Susceptible to Polio: Thiamine Deficiencies and Excess Sulfur can cause polio in sheep, 11th March 2013. Available at: https://www.ag.ndsu.edu/news/newsreleases/2013/march-11-2013/sheep-susceptible-to-polio/, Accessed May, 2019.

[233] Berkow R. The Merck Manual of Diagnosis and Therapy 1992, Sixteenth Edition, Merck Research Laboratories, p 969.

[234] Edward JF. Iodine: Its Use in the Treatment and Prevention of Poliomyelitis and Allied Diseases, *The Manitoba Medical Review*, 1954, 34(6): 337-339. Available at: https://6sd6hj41ya-flywheel.netdna-ssl.com/images/pdfs/IO-DINE USE IN THE TREATMENT AND PREVEN-TION OF POLIOMYELITIS - JF ED-WARD RPRNT 76.pdf. Accessed April 2019.

[235] Gould T. A Summer Plague: Polio and its Survivors, Yale University Press, 1997.

[236] Paul JR. A History of poliomyelitis, Yale University Press, New Haven, Connecticut, 1971.

[237] Wyatt HV, Before the Vaccines: Medical Treatments of Acute Paralysis in the 1916 New York Epidemic of Poliomyelitis, *Op Microbiol J,* 2014, 8:144-147.

[238] Solandt DY, et al. The effect of skeletal fixation on skeletal muscle, *J Neurophysiol*, 1943, 6:17-22.

[239] Cohn V. Sister Kenny: The Woman Who Challenged the Doctors, University of Minnesota Press, 1975.

[240] Ibid. See reference #235.

[241] Smithsonian National Museum of American History, Whatever Happened to Polio: The Iron Lung and Other Equipment, https://amhistory.si.edu/polio/howpolio/ironlung.htm. Accessed April 2019.

[242] CDC: Public Health Image Library, https://phil.cdc.gov/details.aspx?pid=6536. Accessed April 2019.

[243] Kenny E. And They Shall Walk, Robert Hale Ltd, 1951.

[244] Vashisht N, Puliyel J. Polio programme: Let us declare victory and move on, *Ind J Med Ethics*, 2012, IX(2):114-117.

[245] Welch A. Symptoms of mysterious polio-like illness parents should watch out for, *CBS News*, 17th October 2018.

[246] Aiello AE, Larson EL. What is the evidence for a causal link between hygiene and infections? *Lancet Infect Dis*, 2002, 2:103-110.

[247] McKeown T. The Origins of Human Disease, Wiley Blackwell Publishers, 1991.

[248] McKinley JB, McKinley SM. The questionable contribution of medical measures to the decline of mortality in the United States in the twentieth century, Health and Society, *The Milbank Memorial Fund Quarterly*, 1977, 55:405-428.

[249] Grove RD, Hetzel AM. Vital Statistic Rates in the United States 1940-1960. https://www.cdc.gov/nchs/data/vsus/vsrates1940_60.pdf Accessed January, 2017.

CHAPTER 3: VACCINE PRODUCTION

[1] Roberts J. The Vaccine Papers, Impact Investigative Media Productions, Wigan UK, 2010.

[2] Sabin AB, Boulger L. History of Sabin attenuated Poliovirus oral live vaccine strains, *I J Biol Stand*, 1973, 115, 115-118.

[3] NPTEL, Lecture 6: Isolation and purification of viruses and components, https://nptel.ac.in/courses/102103039/6, Accessed February, 2019.

[4] MSDS for Trypsin, https://www.lewisu.edu/academics/biology/pdf/trypsin.pdf, Accessed February 2, 2019.

[5] Ibid. See reference #3.

[6] Humane Research Australia, Use of Fetal Calf Serum, http://www.humaneresearch.org.au/campaigns/fetal_calf_serum, Accessed February 2, 2019.

[7] Fletcher MA, Hessel L, Plotkin SA. Human diploid cell strains (HDCS) viral vaccines, *Dev Bio Stand, 1998,* 93:97–107.

[8] Ammerman NC, Beier-Sexton M, Azad AF. Growth and maintenance of Vero cell lines, *Curr Protoc Microbiol*, 2008, Appendix 4:4E.

[9] Omeir RL, Teferedegne B, Foseh GS, et al. Heterogeneity of the tumorigenic phenotype expressed by Madin-Darby canine kidney cells, *Comp Med*, 2011, 61(3):243-250.

[10] VXP Biologics, The Vero Vaccine Production Pipeline, https://www.vxpbiologics.com/the-vero-vaccine-production-pipeline/, Accessed February, 2019.

[11] Sigma Aldrich, Benzonase Nuclease, https://www.sigmaaldrich.com/catalog/product/sigma/e1014?lang=en&region=AU, Accessed February, 2019.

[12] Ibid. See reference #10

[13] Deisher TA, Doan NV, Koyama K, Bwabye S. Epidemiologic and molecular relationship between vaccine manufacture

and Autism Spectrum Disorder prevalence, *Issues Law Med*, 2015, 30(1):47-70.

[14] Oxford Vaccine Group: Vaccine Knowledge Project, Vaccine Ingredients, http://vk.ovg.ox.ac.uk/vaccine-ingredients, Accessed May 2019.

[15] Chuang VT, Otagiri M. Recombinant human serum albumin, *Drugs Today*, 2007, 43(8):547-61.

[16] Precision Vaccinations, 500 million easter eggs could be saved by the FDA, https://www.precisionvaccinations.com/chicken-eggs-produce-90-flu-vaccines, Accessed February 2, 2019.

[17] Singapore Government, Health Science Authority, Understanding Vaccines, Vaccine Development and Production, https://www.hsa.gov.sg/content/hsa/en/Health_Products_Regulation/Consumer_Information/Public_Advisories/Influenza_A_H1N1_information/H1N1_Vaccines/understanding-vaccines--vaccine-development-and-production.html, Accessed January, 2019.

[18] Hayflick L, The limited in vitro lifetime of human diploid cell strains, *Exp Cell Res*, 1965, 37(3):614-636.

[19] Sven G, Plotkin S, McCarthy K. Gamma globulin prophylaxis: Inactivated Rubella virus; Production and biological control of live attenuated rubella virus vaccines, *Am J Dis Child*, 1969, 118(2):372-381.

[20] Coriell Institute for Medical Research. https://catalog.coriell.org/0/Sections/Search/Sample_Detail.aspx?Ref=AG06814-N&PgId=166. Accessed February, 2017.

[21] Coriell Institute for Medical Research. https://catalog.coriell.org/0/Sections/Search/Sample_Detail.aspx?Ref=AG05965-C&PgId=166. Accessed February, 2017.

[22] Wilson PK. Harry Laughlin's eugenic crusade to control the 'socially inadequate' in Progressive Era America, *Patterns of Prejudice*, 2002, 36(1):49–67.

[23] Marsh JH. Eugenics: Keeping Canada Sane, The Canadian Encyclopedia.

[24] Weller TH, Enders JF, Robbins FC, Stoddard MB. Studies on the cultivation of poliomyelitis viruses in tissue culture : I. The propagation of poliomyelitis viruses in suspended cell cultures of various human tissue, *J Immunol*, 1952, 69(6):645-671.

[25] Leiva R. A brief history of human diploid cell strains, *Nat Cath Bioethics Quart*, 2006, 443-451.

[26] E Norrby, email reply to R Leiva in Leiva R. A brief history of human diploid cell strains, *Nat Cath Bioethics Quart*, 2006, 443-451.

[27] FDA. Briefing document: Cell lines derived from human tumors for vaccine manufacture, Vaccines and related biological products advisory committee meeting, 2012. http://www.fda.gov/downloads/AdvisoryCommittees/CommitteesMeetingMaterials/BloodVaccinesandOtherBiologics/VaccinesandRelatedBiologicalProductsAdvisoryCommittee/UCM319573.pdf. Accessed February, 2017.

[28] Ma B, He LF, Zhang YL, et al. Characteristics and viral propagation properties of a new human diploid cell line, Walvax-2, and its suitability as a candidate cell substrate for vaccine production, *Hum Vaccin Immunother*, 2015, 11(4):998-1009.

[29] Binkley C, Johnson CK. Scientists say fetal tissue essential for medical research, *Associated Press*, Aug 11, 2015.

[30] Ibid. See reference #25.

[31] FDA Center for Biologics and Evaluation and Research Advisory Committee Meeting, May 16, 2001. http://www.fda.gov/ohrms/dockets/ac/01/transcripts/3750t1_01.pdf, Accessed February, 2017.

[32] Le Ru A, Jacob D, Transfiguracion J, et al. Scalable production of influenza virus in HEK-293 cells for efficient vaccine manufacturing, *Vaccine*, 2010, 21(7):3661-3671.

[33] Ibid. See reference #31.

[34] Wong A. The Ethics of HEK 293, *Nat Cath Bioethics Quart*, 2006, 6(3):473-495.

[35] Croce P. Vivisection or Science – a choice to make, Fetal Experimentation-Over the top; Part 1, p. 99-108.CIVIS, 1991, Hans Ruesch Foundation.

[36] CDC: Vaccine Excipient & Media Summary, http://www.cdc.gov/vaccines/pubs/pinkbook/downloads/appendices/B/excipient-table-2.pdf. Accessed May, 2019

[37] Ibid. See reference #8.

[38] Osada N, Kohara A, Yamaji T. The genome landscape of the African green monkey kidney-derived Vero cell line, *DNA Research*, 2014, 21:673–83.

[39] FDA: Vaccines and related Biological Products Advisory Committee, November 2005, https://www.fda.gov/ohrms/dockets/ac/05/briefing/5-4188b1_19a.pdf, Accessed September, 2017.

[40] Ibid. See reference #27.

[41] Petricciani JC, Hennessen W. Cells products safety. Background papers from the WHO Study Group on Biologicals, Geneva, 18-19 Nov, 1986, *Dev Biol Stand*, 1987, 68:1-81.

[42] Brown F, Griffiths E, Horaud F, Petricciani JC. Safety of Biological Products Prepared from Mammalian Cell Culture, vol. 93. 1998, Karger, Basel.

[43] Ibid. See reference #13.

[44] Ibid. See reference #27

[45] Ibid. See reference #13.

[46] Testimony of Dr Theresa Deisher to Bioethics and Fetal Tissue Hearing before the Select Investigative Panel of the

Committee on Energy and Commerce of the US House of Representatives, March 2008, https://bioethicsarchive.georgetown.edu/pcbe/transcripts/sept08/deisher_statement.pdf, Accessed February, 2019.

[47] Ibid. See reference #27.

[48] ABC News. How One Woman's Cells Changed Medicine, http://abcnews.go.com/WN/henrietta-lacks-woman-cells-polio-cancer-flu-research-medicine/story?id=9712579, Accessed May 2019.

[49] Watson DM. Cancer Killed Henrietta Lacks - Then Made Her Immortal, *The Virginian Pilot*, 10th May, 2010.

[50] Ibid. See reference #48.

[51] Mittelman D, Wilson JH. The fractured genome of HeLa cells, *Genome Biology*, 2013, 14(4):111.

[52] Masters J R. HeLa cells 50 years on: The good, the bad and the ugly, *Nat Rev Cancer*, 2002, 2(4): 315–319.

[53] Oransky I, Marcus A. Thousands of studies used the wrong cells, and journals are doing nothing, *STAT*, 21st July 2016.

[54] International Cell Line Authentication Committee, The role of ICLAC, https://standards.atcc.org/kwspub/home/the_international_cell_line_authentication_committee-iclac_/, Accessed May 2019.

[55] Ibid. See reference #27.

[56] Choi CW, Park EC, Yun SH, et al. Potential usefulness of *Streptococcus pneumoniae* extracellular membrane vesicles as antibacterial vaccines, *J Immunol Res*, 2017, 2017:7931982.

[57] Mizrachi Nebenzahl Y, Blau K, Kushnir T, et al. Streptococcus pneumoniae cell-wall-localized phosphoenolpyruvate protein phosphotransferase can function as an adhesin: Identification of its host target molecules and evaluation of its potential as a vaccine, *PLoS One*, 2016, 11(3):e0150320.

[58] Di Pasquale A, Preiss S, Tavares Da Silva F, Garçon N. Vaccine Adjuvants: from 1920 to 2015 and Beyond, Harper DM, ed. *Vaccines*, 2015, 3(2):320-343.

[59] CDC: Ingredients of Vaccines - Fact Sheet, https://www.cdc.gov/vaccines/vac-gen/additives.htm, Accessed September 2017.

[60] Vogel F, Hem SL. Vaccines, Saunders Elsevier, Philadelphia, PA, USA: 2004. Immunologic adjuvants, pp. 69–79.

[61] Marrack P, McKee AS, Munks MW. Towards an understanding of the adjuvant action of aluminium, *Nat Rev Immunol*, 2009, 9(4):287-293.

[62] Ibid. See reference #58.

[63] Jeong EJ, Maeng HJ, Lee HJ, et al. Effect of adjuvant on pharmacokinetics, organ distribution and humoral immunity of hepatitis b surface antigen after intramuscular injection to rats, *Arch Pharm Res*, 2012, 35(9):1621-1628.

[64] Exley C, Siesjo P, Eriksson H. The immunobiology of aluminium adjuvants: how do they really work? *Trends Immunol,* 2010, 31(3):103-109.

[65] Petrik MS, Wong MC, Tabata RC, et al. Aluminium adjuvant linked to Gulf War illness induces motor neuron death in mice, *Neuromolecular Med,* 2007, 9(1):83-100.

[66] Shaw CA, Petrik MS. Aluminium hydroxide injections lead to motor deficits and motor neuron degeneration, *J Inorg Biochem*, 2009, *103*(11):1555-1562.

[67] Struys-Ponsar C, Guillard O, van den Bosch de Aguilar P. Effects of aluminum exposure on glutamate metabolism: a possible explanation for its toxicity, *Exp Neurol*, 2000, 163(1):157-164.

[68] Vargas DL, Nascimbene C, Krishnan C, et al. Neuroglial activation and neuroinflammation in the brain of patients with autism, *Ann Neurol*, 2005, 57(1):67-81.

[69] Pardo CA, Vargas DL, Zimmerman AW. Immunity, neuroglia and neuroinflammation in autism, *Int Rev Psychiatry*, 2005, 17(6):485-495.

[70] Exley C, Mamutse G, Korchazhkina O, et al. Elevated urinary excretion of aluminium and iron in multiple sclerosis, *Mult Scler*, 2006, 12(5):533-540.

[71] Lukiw WJ, Bazan NG. Neuroinflammatory signalling upregulation in Alzheimer's disease, *Neurochem Res*, 2000, 25(9-10):1173-1184.

[72] Exley C, House ER. Aluminum in the human brain, *Manatshefte fuer Chemie*, 2011, 142(4):357-363.

[73] Darbre PD. Metalloestrogens: an emerging class of inorganic xenoestrogens with potential to add to the oestrogenic burden of the human breast, *J Appl Toxicol*, 2006, 26(3):191-197.

[74] Mannello F, Tonti GA, Medda V, et al. Analysis of aluminium content and iron homeostasis in nipple aspirate fluids from healthy women and breast cancer-affected patients, *J Appl Toxicol*, 2011, 31(3):262-269.

[75] Darbre PD. Aluminium and the human breast, *Morphologie*, 2016, 100(329):65-74.

[76] Banasik A, Lankoff A, Piskulak A et al. Aluminum-induced micronuclei and apoptosis in human peripheral-blood lymphocytes treated during different phases of the cell cycle, *Environ Toxicol*, 2005, 20(4):401-406.

[77] Darbre PD, Mannello F, Exley C. Aluminium and breast cancer: Sources of exposure, tissue measurements and mechanisms of toxicological actions on breast biology, J Inorg Biochem, 2013, 128:257-261.

[78] Flarend RE, Hem SL, White JL, et al. In vivo absorption of aluminum-containing vaccine adjuvants using 26Al, *Vaccine*, 1997, 15(12-13):1314–1318.

[79] She Y, Want N, et al. Effects of aluminium on immune functions of cultured splenic T and B lymphocytes in rats, *Biol Tr Elem Res*, 2012, 147(1):246-250.

[80] Zhu Y, Li X, Chen C, et al. Effects of aluminum trichloride on the trace elements and cytokines in the spleen of rats, *Food Chem Toxicol*, 2012, 50(8):2911-2915.

[81] Geier DA, King PG, Hooker BS, et al. Thimerosal: clinical, epidemiologic and biochemical studies, *Clin Chim Acta*, 2015, 444:212-220.

[82] Bernard S, Enayati A, Redwood L, et al. Autism: a novel form of mercury poisoning, *Med Hyp*, 2001, 56:462-71

[83] Blaxill MD, Redwood L, Bernard S. Thimerosol and autism? A plausible hypothesis that should not be dismissed, *Med Hyp*, 2004, 62:799-794.

[84] Blaxill MF. What's going on? The question of time trends in autism, *Pub Health Rep*, 2004, 119:536-551.

[85] Federal Register, Volume 47, No. 2, January 5, 1982. https://worldmercuryproject.org/wp-content/uploads/2016/10/1982_Federal_Register_Mercury_in_OTC_products_ANPR.pdf, Accessed January, 2017.

[86] Thimerosal in Vaccines: A Joint Statement of the American Academy of Pediatrics and the Public Health Service, July 09, 2009.

[87] IOM (Institute of Medicine) 2001. Immunization Safety Review: Thimerosal Containing Vaccines and Neurodevelopmental Disorders (Stratton K, Gable A, McCormick M, eds). Washington, DC, National Academy Press.

[88] IOM (Institute of Medicine) 2004. Vaccines and Autism. Immunization Safety Review Committee. Washington, DC, National Academy Press.

[89] Hooker B, Kern J, Geier D, et al. Methodological issues and evidence of malfeasance in research purporting to show thimerosal in vaccines is safe, *Biomed Res Int*, 2014, 2014:247218.

[90] Fagan DG, Pritchard JS, Clarkson TW, Greenwood MR. Organ mercury levels in infants with omphaloceles treated with organic mercurial antiseptic, *Arch Dis Child*, 1977, 52(12):962-4.

[91] Geier DA, Sykes LK, Geier MR. A review of thimerosal (merthiolate) and its ethylmercury breakdown product: specific historical considerations regarding safety and effectiveness, *J Toxicol Env Health*, 2007, 10(8):575-596.

[92] Ibid. See reference #90.

[93] Axton JH. Six cases of poisoning after a parenteral organic mercurial compound (merthiolate). *Postgrad Med J*, 1972, 48(561):417-421.

[94] Heinonen OP, Shapiro S, Monson RR, et al. Immunization during pregnancy against poliomyelitis and influenza in relation to childhood malignancy, *Int J Epidem*, 1973, 2(3):229-235.

[95] Patrizi A, Rizzoli L, Vencenzi C, et al. Sensitization to thimerosal in atopic children, *Contact Dermatitis*, 1999, 40(2):94-97.

[96] Vojdani A, Pangborn JB, Vojdani E, Cooper EL. Infections, toxic chemicals and dietary peptides binding to lymphocyte receptors and tissue enzymes are major instigators of autoimmunity in autism, *Int J Immun Pharm*, 2003, 16(3):189-199.

[97] Mrozek-Budzyn D, Majewska R, Kieltyka A, Augustyniak M. Neonatal exposure to thimerosal from vaccines and child development in the first 3 years of life, *Neurotoxicology and Teratology*, 2012, 34(6):592-597.

[98] Gallagher C, Goodman M. Hepatitis B triple series vaccine and developmental disability in US children aged 1-9 years, *Tox Env Chem*, 2008, 90(5):997-1008.

[99] Geier DA, Geier MA. A meta-analysis epidemiological assessment of neurodevelopmental disorders following vaccines administered from 1994 through 2000 in the United States, *Neuroendocrin Lett*, 2006, 27(4):401-413.

[100] Ibid. See reference #81.

[101] Loison E, Poirier-Beaudouin B, Seffer V, et al. Suppression by thimerosal of ex-vivo CD4+ T cell response to vaccine and apoptosis in primary memory T cells, *PLoS One*, 2014, 9(1):e92705.

[102] Gallagher C, Goodman M. Hepatitis B vaccination of male neonates and autism diagnosis, NHIS 1997-2002, *J Toxicol Env Health*, 2010, 73(24):1665-1677.

[103] Barile JP, Kuperminc GP, Weintraub ES, et al. Thimerosal exposure in early life and neuropsychological outcomes 7-10 years later, *J Ped Psychology*, 2012, 37(1):106-118.

[104] U.S Food and Drug Administration, Vaccines, Blood and Biologics: Thimerosal in Vaccines. http://www.fda.gov/BiologicsBloodVaccines/SafetyAvailability/VaccineSafety/ucm096228.htm#t1, Accessed February 2017.

[105] Vaccine Excipient and Media Summary, Appendix B. http://www.cdc.gov/vaccines/pubs/pinkbook/downloads/appendices/B/excipient-table-2.pdf. Accessed June 2016.

[106] AAP News. Flu vaccine extended to kids 6-23 months, *American Academy of Pediatrics*, August 2002.

[107] Childhood Influenza Vaccination Coverage – United States, 2002 – 2003 Influenza Season, *JAMA*, 2004, 292:2074-2075.

[108] CDC, Prevention and control of influenza: Recommendations of ACIP, *MMWR*, 2005, 54(41):1050-1052.

[109] CDC, Influenza vaccination in pregnancy: practices among obstetrician-gynocologists – US, 2003-2004 influenza season, *MMWR Morb Mortal Wkly Rep*, 2005, 54(41):1050-1052.

[110] Ong CN, Chia SE, Foo SC, et al. Concentrations of heavy metals in maternal and umbilical cord blood, *Biometals*, 2003, 6(1):61-66.

[111] Drasch G, Schupp I, Hofl H, et al. Mercury burden of human fetal and infant tissues, *Eur J Pediatr*, 1994, 153:607-610.

[112] Grandjean P, White R. Neurodevelopmental disorders. In: Tamburlini G, von Ehrenstein OS, Bertollini R, editors. Children's health and environment: a review of evidence. WHO-EEA; Kopenhagen, 2002, 66–78.

[113] Rice D, Barone S. Critical periods of vulnerability for the developing nervous system: evidence from humans and animal models, *Environ Health Perspect*, 2000, 108(3):511–33.

[114] Harada M. Minamata disease: methylmercury poisoning in Japan caused by environmental pollution, *Crit Rev Toxicol*, 1995, 25:1–24.

[115] Kjellstrom T, Kennedy P, Wallis S, Mantell C. Physical and mental development of children with prenatal exposure to mercury from fish. Stage I: Preliminary Tests at Age 4. National Swedish Environmental Protection Board, Solna, Sweden, 1986.

[116] Grandjean P, Weihe P, White RF. Milestone development in infants exposed to methylmercury from human milk, *Neurotoxicology*, 1995, 16(1):27–33.

[117] Grandjean P, Weihe P, White RF, et al. Cognitive deficit in 7-year-old children with prenatal exposure to methylmercury, *Neurotoxicol Teratol*, 1997, 19(6):417–428

[118] Bose-O'Reilly S, McCarty KM, Steckling N, Lettmeier B. Mercury exposure and children's health, *Curr Probl Pediatr Adolesc Health Care*, 2010, 40(8):186-215.

[119] Grandjean P, Murata K, Budtz-Jorgensen E, Weihe P. Cardiac autonomic activity in methylmercury neurotoxicity: 14-year follow-up of a Faroese birth cohort, *J Pediatr*, 2004, 144(2):169–176.

[120] CDC. Preventing pneumococcal disease among infants and young children, *MMWR*, 2000, 49(9):1-38.

[121] CDC. CDC's ACIP expands Hepatitis A vaccination for children, Press Release, Oct 28, 2005.

[122] EPA: Table of drinking regulated drinking water contaminants, https://www.epa.gov/ground-water-and-drinking-water/table-regulated-drinking-water-contaminants, Accessed February, 2017.

[123] Sun W, Xie C, Wang H, Hu Y. Specific role of polysorbate 80 coating on the targeting of nanoparticles to the brain, *Biomaterials*, 2004, 25(15):3065-3071.

[124] Ramge P, Unger RE, Oltrogge JB, et al. Polysorbate 80 coating enhances uptake of polybutylcyanoacrylate nanoparticles by human and bovine primary brain endothelial cells, *Eur J Neuroscience*, 2000, 12(6):1931-1940.

[125] Gulyaev AE, Gelperina SE, Skidan IN, et al. Significant transport of doxorubicin into the brain with polysorbate 80-coated nanoparticles, *Pharm Res*, 1999, 16(10):1564-1569.

[126] ScienceLab: MSDS for polysorbate 80, http://www.sciencelab.com/msds.php?msdsId=9926645, Accessed September, 2017.

[127] Arrowsmith JB, Faich GA, Tomita DK, et al. Morbidity and mortality among low birth weight infants exposed to an intravenous Vitamin E product E-Ferol, *Pediatrics*, 1989, 83(2):244-249.

[128] Alade SL, Brown RE, Paquet A. Polysorbate 80 and E-Ferol Toxicity, *Pediatrics*, 1986, 77(4):593-597.

[129] Bove KE, Kosmetatos M, Wedig KE, et al. Vasculopathic hepatotoxicity associated with E-Ferol syndrome in low-birth-weight infants, *JAMA*, 1985, 254(17):2422-2430.

[130] Gajdova M, Jakubovsky J, Valky J. Delayed effects of neonatal exposure to Tween 80 on female reproductive organs in rats, *Food Chem Toxicol*, 1993, 31(3):183-190.

[131] Ventola CL. The antibiotic resistance crisis: Part 1, *Pharm and Therapeut*, 2015, 40(4):277-283.

[132] Golkar Z, Bagazra O, Pace DG. Bacteriophage therapy: a potential solution for the antibiotic resistance crisis, *J Infect Dev Ctries*, 2014, 8(2):129–136.

[133] Gross M. Antibiotics in crisis, *Curr Biol*, 2013, 23(24):R1063–R1065.

[134] Sengupta S, Chattopadhyay MK, Grossart HP. The multifaceted roles of antibiotics and antibiotic resistance in nature, *Front Microbiol*, 2013, 4:47.

[135] Centers for Disease Control and Prevention, Office of Infectious Disease Antibiotic resistance threats in the United States, 2013. Apr, 2013, https://www.cdc.gov/drugresistance/threat-report-2013/, Accesssed July, 2017.

[136] CDC. Vaccine Excipient and Media Summary, https://www.cdc.gov/vaccines/pubs/pinkbook/downloads/appendices/appdx-full-b.pdf, Accessed May, 2019.

[137] Bloomberg School of Public Health. Vaccine Excipients Per 0.5 mL Dose. John Hopkins University January 2018, http://www.vaccinesafety.edu/components-Excipients.htm, Accessed October, 2018.

[138] Mishra RP, Ovieda-Orta E, Prachi P, et al. Vaccines and antibiotic resistance, *Curr Opin Microbiol*, 2012, 15(5):596-602.

[139] Langdon A, Cook N, Dantas G. <u>The effects of antibiotics on the microbiome throughout development and alternative approaches for therapeutic modulation</u>, *Gen Med,* 2016, 8(39).

[140] Ibid. See reference #136.

[141] Jochems CE, Van der Valk JB, Stafleu FR, Baumans V. The use of fetal bovine serum: ethical or scientific problem? *Altern Lab Animal*, 2002, 30(2):219-227.

[142] WHO: Recombinant protein vaccines produced in insect cells, <u>http://www.who.int/immunization/research/meetings_workshops/Manon_Cox.pdf</u>, Accessed September, 2017.

[143] Victoria JG, Wang C, Jones MS, et al. Viral nucleic acids in live-attenuated vaccines: Detection of minority variants and an adventitious virus, *J Virol,* 2010, 84(12):6033-6040.

[144] Omeir RL, Teferedegne B, Foseh GS, et al. Heterogeneity of the tumorigenic phenotype expressed by Madin–Darby canine kidney cells, *Comp Med,* 2011, 61(3):243-250.

[145] Levenbook IS, Petricciani JC, Elisberg BL. Tumorigenicity of Vero cells, *J Biol Stand*, 1984, 12(4):391-398.

[146] Humane Society International, About Animal Testing, <u>https://www.hsi.org/news-media/about/</u>, Accessed May 2019.

[147] Use of fetal calf serum. <u>http://www.humaneresearch.org.au/campaigns/fetal_calf_serum</u>. Accessed January 2017.

[148] Jochems C, van der Valk J, Stafleu F, Baumans V. The use of fetal bovine serum: ethical or scientific problem? *Alternatives to Laboratory Animals (ATLA)*, 2002, 30:219-227.

[149] Madrigal AC. The Blood Harvest, *The Atlantic*, 26th February, 2014.

[150] Bang, FB. The toxic effect of a marine bacterium on *Limulus* and the formation of blood clots, Biol Bull, 1953, 105:447-448.

[151] Anderson RL, Watson WH, Chabot CC. Sublethal behavioural and physiological effects of the biomedical bleeding process on the American Horseshoe Crab, Limulus Polyphemus, *Biol Bull*, 2013, 225(3):137-151.

[152] Carmichael RH, Botton ML, Shin PK, Cheung SG. Changing Global Perspectives on Horseshoe Crab Biology, Conservation and Management, Springer, 2015.

[153] McCune JM. Development and applications of the SCID-hu mouse model, *Semin Immunol*, 1996, 8(4):187-196.

[154] Koo GC, Hasan A, O'Reilly RJ. Use of humanized severe combined immunodeficient mice for human vaccine development, *Expert Rev Vaccines*, 2009, 8(1):113–120.

[155] National Cancer Institute. Formaldehyde and Cancer Risk, https://www.cancer.gov/about-cancer/causes-prevention/risk/substances/formaldehyde/formaldehyde-fact-sheet. Accessed October, 2017.

[156] US Department of Health and Human Services. What's In Vaccines: Common Ingredients in US Licensed Vaccines, https://www.vaccines.gov/basics/safety/vaccine_ingredients/index.html. Accessed October, 2017.

[157] International Agency for Research on Cancer. IARC Monographs on the Evaluation of Carcinogenic Risks to Humans Volume 88 (2006): Formaldehyde, 2-Butoxyethanol and 1-tert-Butoxypropan-2-ol, http://monographs.iarc.fr/ENG/Monographs/vol88/index.php, Accessed October, 2017.

[158] Ibid. See reference #155.

[159] Songur A, Ozen OA, Sarsilmaz M. The toxic effects of formaldehyde on the nervous system, *Rev Environ Contam Toxicol*, 2010, 203:105-118.

[160] Tong Z, Han C, Luo W, et al. Accumulated hippocampal formaldehyde induces age-dependent memory decline, *Age*, 2013, 35(3):583-596.

[161] <u>Krolovec</u> RD, <u>Morgan</u> WA. Urea-Formaldehyde Fertilizers, Condensation Products of Urea and Formaldehyde as Fertilizer with Controlled Nitrogen Availability, *J Agric Food Chem,* 1954, 2(2):92–95.

[162] University of Hertfordshire, Pesticide Properties Database, <u>https://sitem.herts.ac.uk/aeru/ppdb/en/Reports/359.htm#1</u>, Accessed May 2019.

[163] Science Lab. 2-phenoxyethanol MSDS, <u>http://www.sciencelab.com/msds.php?msdsId=9926486</u>, Accessed October, 2017.

[164] US National Library of Medicine, 2-phenoxyethanol, <u>https://pubchem.ncbi.nlm.nih.gov/compound/2-phenoxyethanol#section=Top</u>, Accessed October, 2017.

[165] Santa Cruz Biotechnology Inc. MSDS: 2- phenoxyethanol, <u>http://datasheets.scbt.com/sc-238193.pdf</u>, Accessed October, 2017.

[166] CDC. Glutaraldehyde, <u>https://www.cdc.gov/niosh/topics/glutaraldehyde/default.html</u>, Accessed October, 2017.

[167] Science Lab. MSDS Glutaraldehyde, <u>http://www.sciencelab.com/msds.php?msdsId=9924161</u>, Accessed October, 2017.

[168] Science Lab. MSDS Cetyltrimethylammonium bromide, <u>http://www.sciencelab.com/msds.php?msdsId=9923367</u>, Accessed October, 2017.

[169] Stanford University. Huntington's Outreach project for Education, About Glutamate Toxicity, <u>https://web.stanford.edu/group/hopes/cgi-bin/hopes_test/about-glutamate-toxicity/</u>, Accessed October, 2017.

[170] Chapman AG. Glutamate and epilepsy, *J Nutr,* 2000, 130(4):10435-10455.

[171] Pitt D, Werner P, Raine CS. Glutamate excitotoxicity in a model of multiple sclerosis, *Nat Med,* 2000, 6(1):67-70.

[172] Blaylock RL, Strunecka A. Immune-glutamatergic dysfunction as a central mechanism of the autism spectrum disorders, *Curr Med Chem*, 2009, 16(2):157-170.

[173] Blaylock RL. A possible central mechanism in autism spectrum disorders, Part 1, *Altern Ther Health Med*, 2008, 14(6):46-53.

[174] Blaylock RL. A possible central mechanism in autism spectrum disorders, Part 2: immunoexcitotoxicity, *Altern Ther Health Med*, 2009, 15(1):60-67.

[175] Merten OW. Virus contaminations of cell cultures – a biotechnological view, *Cytotechnology*, 2002, 39(2):91-116.

[176] Ito M, Melnick JL, Mayor HD. An immunofluorescence assay for studying replication of adeno-satellite virus, *J Gen Virol*, 1967, 1:199-209.

[177] Hoggan MD. Adenovirus associated virus, *Progr Med Virol*, 1970, 12:211–239.

[178] Hughes G. Millions given infected polio vaccine, *Sydney Morning Herald*, 23rd October, 2004.

[179] Rollison DEM, Shah KV. The epidemiology of SV40 infection due to contaminated polio vaccines: relation of the virus to human cancer, 2001, p. 561-584. *In* K. Khalili and G. L. Stoner (ed.), Human polyomaviruses: molecular and clinical perspectives. Wiley-Liss, Inc, New York.

[180] Vilchez RA, Butel JS. Emergent human pathogen Simian Virus 40 and its role in cancer, *Clin Microbiol Rev*, 2004; 17(3):495-508.

[181] Cutrone R, Lednicky J, Dunn G, et al. Some oral poliovirus vaccines were contaminated with infectious SV40 after 1961, *Cancer Res*, 2005, 65(22):10273-10279.

[182] Fitzpatrick M. The Cutter incident: How America's first polio vaccine led to a growing vaccine crisis, *J R Soc Med*, 2006, 99(3):156.

[183] Seeff LB. Yellow Fever vaccine-associated hepatitis epidemic during WWII: Follow-up more than 40 years later, Epidemiology in Military and Veteran Populations: Proceedings of the Second Biennial Conference, 7th March, 1990.

[184] FDA. News Release: Components of Extraneous Virus Detected in Rotarix Vaccine: No Known Safety Risk, FDA Recommends Clinicians Temporarily Suspend Use of Vaccine As Agency Learns More. March 22, 2010. http://www.fda.gov/NewsEvents/Newsroom/PressAnnouncements/ucm205625.htm, Accessed February, 2017.

[185] Ibid. See reference #1.

[186] Ibid. See reference #143.

[187] Ibid. See reference #175.

[188] Taylor DJ, Green NPO, Stout GW. Biological Science. Cambridge University Press, Cambridge, 1998.

[189] Stang A, Petrasch-Parwez E, Brandt S, et al. Unintended spread of a biosafety level 2 recombinant virus, *Retrovirology*, 2009, 6:86.

[190] Heckenlively K, Mikovits J. Plague: One Scientist's Intrepid Search for the Truth about Human Retroviruses and Chronic Fatigue Syndrome (CFS), Autism and Other Diseases, Skyhorse Publishing, 1st edition, 2014.

[191] Johnson AD, Cohn CS. Xenotropic Murine Leukemia Virus-Related Virus (XMRV) and the safety of the blood supply, *Clin Microbiol Rev*, 2016, 29(4):749-757.

[192] Lombardi VC, Ruscetti FW, Das GJ, et al. Detection of an infectious retrovirus, XMRV, in blood cells of patients with chronic fatigue syndrome, *Science*, 2009, 326:585–589.

[193] Mikovits JA, Huang Y, Pfost MA, et al. Distribution of xenotropic murine leukemia virus-related virus (XMRV) infection in chronic fatigue syndrome and prostate cancer, *AIDS Rev*, 2010, 12(3):149-152.

[194] Chernov VM, Chernova VA, Sanchez-Vega JT, et al. Mycoplasma contamination of cell cultures: Vesicular traffic in bacteria and control over infectious agents, *Acta Naturae*, 2014, 6(3):41-51.

[195] Rottem S, Kosower NS, Kornspan, JD. Contamination of Tissue Cultures by Mycoplasmas, Biomedical Tissue Culture, Dr. Luca Ceccherini-Nelli (Ed.), InTech, DOI, 2012.

[196] "Weaponized Mycoplasmas," Dr. Garth L. Nicolson, Lecture presented at the 9th Common Cause Medical Research Foundation Conference, Sudbury, Ontario, Canada on Aug. 29-31, 2008, Published July 29, 2013, Retrieved January, 2017. https://www.youtube.com/watch?v=sT25HhAVhhU

[197] Robinson LB, Wichelhausen RH. Contamination of human cell cultures by pleuropneumonialike organisms, *Science*, 1956, 124(3232):1147-8.

[198] Ibid. See reference #196.

[199] Drexler HG, Uphoff CC. Mycoplasma contamination of cell cultures: Incidence, sources, effects, detection, elimination, prevention, *Cytotechnology*, 2002, 39(2):75-90.

[200] Barile MF, Rottem S. Mycoplasmas in cell cultures, In: Kahane I, Adoni A. Rapid diagnosis of mycoplasmas, Plenum Press, New York, 1993.

[201] Feng SH, Tsai S, Rodriguez J, Lo SC. Mycoplasmal infections prevent apoptosis and induce malignant transformation of interleukin-3-dependent 32D hematopoietic cells, *Mol Cell Biol*, 1999, 19(12):7995-8002.

[202] Zhang S, Wear DJ, Lo S. Mycoplasmal infections alter gene expression in cultured human prostatic and cervical epithelial cells, *FEMS Immunol Med Microbiol*, 2000, 27(1):43-50.

[203] Zhang S, Tsai S, Lo S-C. Alteration of gene expression profiles during mycoplasma-induced malignant cell transformation, *BMC Cancer*, 2006, 6:116.

[204] Lo S-C. Mycoplasmas and AIDS. In: Maniloff J, McElhaney RN, Finch LR, Baseman JB, editors. Mycoplasmas: molecular biology and pathogenesis. Washington (DC): American Society for Microbiology, 1992:525-45.

[205] Nicolson G, Nicolson NL. Diagnosis and treatment of mycoplasmal infections in Gulf War illness-CFIDS patients, *Intl J Occup Med Immunol Toxicol,* 1996, 5:69-78.

[206] Tsai S, Wear DJ, Shih JW-K, Lo SC. Mycoplasmas and oncogenesis: persistent infection and multistage malignant transformation, *Proc Natl Acad Sci USA*, 1995, 92:10197-10201.

[207] Ekbom A, Daszak P, Kraaz W, Wakefield AJ. Crohn's disease after in-utero measles virus exposure, *Lancet*, 1996, 348:516-517.

[208] Taylor-Robinson D. Mycoplasmas in rheumatoid arthritis and other human arthritides, *J Clin Pathol*, 1996, 49:781-782.

[209] Gatti AM, Montanari S. New Quality Control Investigations on vaccines: micro- and nano-contamination, *Int J Vaccines and Vaccination*, 2017, 4(1):00072.

[210] Sharma A, Madhunapantula SV, Robertson GP. Toxicological considerations when creating nanoparticle-based drugs and drug delivery systems? *Exp Op Drug Metab Toxicol*, 2012, 8(1):47-69.

[211] De Jong WH, Borm PJ. Drug delivery and nanoparticles: applications and hazards, *Int J Nanomedicine*, 2008; 3(2):133-49.

[212] Dhawan A, Sharma V. Toxicity assessment of nano-materials: methods and challenges, *Anal Bioanal Chem*, 2010, 398(2):589-605

[213] El-Ansary A, Al-Daihan S. On the toxicity of therapeutically used nanoparticles: an overview, *J Toxicol*, 2009, 2009:754810.

[214] Oberdörster G. Safety assessment for nanotechnology and nanomedicine: concepts of nanotoxicology, *J Intern Med*, 2010, 267(1):89-105.

[215] Gatti AM, Quaglino D, Sighinolfi GL. A morphological approach to monitor the nanoparticle-cell interaction, *Int J Imag Robiotics*, 2009, 2:S09.

[216] Kennedy S. No recall for glass found in vaccines, *The Morning Call*, 10th December, 2016.

[217] AAFP: Possible Glass Particle Contamination Prompts HPV Vaccine Recall, http://www.aafp.org/news/health-of-the-public/20131221hpvvaccrecall.html. Accessed February, 2017.

[218] Expert Briefings: Merck vaccines contaminated with plastic, says FDA, http://www.expertbriefings.com/news/merck-vaccines-contaminated-with-plastic-says-fda/, Accessed September, 2017.

[219] Zhang Y, Sun S, Xing X, et al. Detection and identification of leachables in vaccines from plastic packaging materials using UpLC-QTOF MS with self-built polymer additives library, *Anal Chem*, 2016, 88(13):6749-6757.

[220] Fierce Pharma, Sanofi plant problems result in vaccine shortage, http://www.fiercepharma.com/drug-safety/sanofi-plant-problems-result-vaccine-shortage. Accessed September, 2017.

[221] US Food and Drug Administration, Inspections, Compliance, Enforcement and Criminal Investigations: Warning Letter, Sanofi Pasteur 7/12/12,

https://www.fda.gov/ICECI/EnforcementActions/Warning-Letters/ucm312929.htm. Accessed September, 2017.

[222] Baby Center. Is safety testing for vaccines rigorous enough? https://www.babycenter.com/404_is-safety-testing-for-vaccines-rigorous-enough_11450.bc. Accessed October, 2017.

[223] New York State Department of Health. The Science Behind Vaccine Research and Testing, https://www.health.ny.gov/prevention/immunization/vaccine_safety/science.htm. Accessed October, 2017.

[224] Stang A, Petrasch-Parwez E, Brandt S, et al. Unintended spread of a biosafety level 2 recombinant retrovirus, *Retrovirology*, 2009, 6:86.

[225] Veerasami M, Chitra M, Mohana Subramanian B, et al. Individual and multiplex PCR assays for the detection of adventitious bovine and porcine viral genome contaminants in the commercial vaccines and animal derived raw materials, *J Vet Sci Tech*, 2014, 5:3.

[226] Marcus-Sekura C, Richardson JC, Harston RK, et al. Evaluation of the human host range of bovine and porcine viruses that may contaminate bovine serum and porcine trypsin used in the manufacture of biological products, *J Int Associ Biol Stand*, 2011, 39(6):359-369.

[227] FDA. Guidance for Industry: Content and Format of Chemistry, Manufacturing and Controls Information and Establishment Description Information for a Vaccine or Related product, https://www.fda.gov/BiologicsBloodVaccines/GuidanceComplianceRegulatoryInformation/Guidances/Vaccines/ucm076612.htm#CONTAMINATIONCROSSCONTAMINATIONISSUES. Accessed October, 2017.

CHAPTER 4: THE VACCINE INDUSTRY

[1] Vaccines market worth 48.03 billion by 2021, Markets and Markets. http://www.marketsandmarkets.com/PressReleases/vaccine-technologies.asp, Accessed May, 2019.

[2] Statista, Top 10 pharmaceutical companies based on global vaccine revenues in 2015 and 2022, https://www.statista.com/statistics/314562/leading-global-pharmaceutical-companies-by-vaccine-revenue/, Accessed May 2019.

[3] Tirrell M. The $1.6 billion business of flu, *CNBC*, 19th October, 2015.

[4] Doshi P. Influenza: marketing vaccine by marketing disease, BMJ, 2013; 346.

[5] Ibid. See reference #3.

[6] CDC: Vaccines for children program, https://www.cdc.gov/vaccines/programs/vfc/awardees/vaccine-management/price-list/, Accessed May 2019.

[7] Taylor C. Raising an Autistic Child: Coping with the costs, *Money*, 24th June 2014, http://money.com/money/2918134/cost-raising-autistic-child/, Accessed May, 2019.

[8] Reply to 'Why Fear of Vaccination is Spelling Disaster in the Developing World, Jacob M. Puliyel, Available at: https://jacob.puliyel.com/download.php?id=224. Accessed May 2019.

[9] Fuchs VR. Major trends in the US Health economy since 1950, *NEJM*, 2012, 366:973-977.

[10] Australian Institute of Health and Welfare. 25 Years of Health Expenditure in Australia, https://www.aihw.gov.au/reports/health-welfare-expenditure/25-years-of-health-expenditure-in-australia-1989-90-to-2013-14/contents/table-of-contents, Accessed May 2019.

[11] The Australian Immunisation Handbook. 3.1: Vaccination for Aboriginal nad Torres Strait Islander people. https://beta.health.gov.au/health-topics/immunisation/im-munisation-throughout-life/immunisation-for-aboriginal-and-torres-strait-islander-people, Accessed May 2019.

[12] CDC: Vaccine Management, National Vaccine Advisory Committee Meeting, June 6, 2012, https://www.hhs.gov/sites/default/files/nvpo/nvac/meet-ings/pastmeetings/2012/shuchat_062912.pdf, Accessed May, 2019.

[13] Kluger J. Is drug company money tainting medical education? TIME, 6th March, 2009.

[14] Shnier A, Lexchin J, Mintzes B, et al. Too Few, Too Weak: Conflict of interest policies at Canadian medical schools, *PLoS ONE*, 2013, 8(7):e68633.

[15] Etain B, Guittet L, Weiss N, et al. Attitudes of medical students towards conflict of interest: A national survey in France, *PLoS ONE*, 2014, 9(3):e92858.

[16] Glauser W. Pharma influence widespread at medical schools: study, *Can Med Assoc J,* 2013, 185(13):1121-1122.

[17] Orme M, Reidenberg M. The teaching of clinical-pharmacology in Europe and North-America. *Trends Pharmacol Sci*, 1989, 10(6):224–226.

[18] Adams KM, Kohmeier M, Zeisel SH. Nutrition education in US medical schools: Latest update of a national survey, *Acad Med*, 2010, 85(9):1537-1542.

[19] Kernéis S, Jacquet C, Bannay A, et al. Vaccine education of medical students: A nationwide cross-sectional survey, *Am J Prev Med*, 53(3):e97-e104.

[20] Pelly LP, MacDougall DM, Halperin B, McNeil SA. The Vaxed project: an assessment of immunization education in

Canadian health professional programs, *BMC Med Ed*, 2010, 10:86.

[21] Dr Joseph Mercola, Youtube, 2012, Dr.Mercola interviews Dr.Lawrence Palevsky. Retrieved from https://www.youtube.com/watch?v=Yh4bGWvFcsE. Accessed October, 2017.

[22] Sears RW. The Vaccine Book: Making the Right Decision for Your Child, Little, Brown and Company, 2011.

[23] Ibid. See reference #20.

[24] Berera D, Thompson KM. Medical Student Knowledge, Attitudes, and Practices Regarding Immunization, *J Vaccines Vaccin*, 2015, 6:268.

[25] Maiden S. GPs offered $26m "No Jab No pay" bonus to keep kid's vaccinations up-to-date, *The Daily Telegraph*, 18th April, 2015.

[26] Kolata G, Abelson R, A bonus For health, payable to the doctor, *The New York Times*, 15th April 2005.

[27] Landro L. Health staff get flu shots to avoid penalty, *The Wall Street Journal*, Oct 31, 2013.

[28] NCQA: HEDIS 2017 Measures, Summary Table of Measures, product Lines and Changes, https://www.ncqa.org/wp-content/uploads/2018/07/20170701_HEDIS_2017-Measures.pdf, Accessed May, 2019.

[29] Sifferlin A. Surgeon salary: How much doctors make, *TIME*, 27th April 2012.

[30] Hill M. Ghosts in the medical machine, *Philadelphia Inquirer*, 20th September, 2009.

[31] Petersen M. Madison Ave. Plays Growing Role in Drug Research. *New York Times*, 22nd November, 2002.

[32] Ngai S, Gold JL, Gill SS, Rochon PA. Haunted manu-scripts: Ghost authorship in the medical literature, *Account Res*, 2005, 12:103–114.

[33] Ibid. See reference #30.

[34] McHenry L. Of sophists and spin-doctors: Industry-spon-sored ghostwriting and the crisis of academic medicine, *Mens Sana Monographs*, 2010, 8(1):129-145.

[35] Ibid. See reference #30.

[36] Moynihan R. Doctors' education: the invisible influence of drug company sponsorship, *BMJ*, 2008, 336(7641):416-417.

[37] Katz HP, Goldfinger SE, Fletcher SW. Academia-industry collaboration in continuing medical education: description of two approaches, *J Contin Educ Health Prof*, 2002, 22(1):43-54.

[38] Boseley S. Vaccination campaign funded by drug firm, *The Guardian*, 26th March 2007.

[39] Spurling GK, Mansfield PR, Montgomery BD, et al. Infor-mation from pharmaceutical companies and the quality, quan-tity, and cost of physicians' prescribing: a systematic review, *PLoS Med*, 2010, 7(10):e1000352.

[40] Meier B. In guilty plea, OxyContin maker to pay $600 mil-lion, *New York Times*, 10th May, 2007.

[41] Martin B. On the suppression of vaccine dissent, *Sci Eng Ethics*, 2015, 21(1):143-157.

[42] Neides D. Make 2017 the year to avoid toxins (good luck) and master your domain: Words on Wellness. http://www.cleveland.com/lyndhurst-south-euclid/in-dex.ssf/2017/01/make_2017_the_year_to_avoid_to.html. Accessed May 2019.

[43] Zeltner B. Cleveland clinic doc apologizes for anti-vax col-umn: hospital promises discipline,

http://www.cleveland.com/healthfit/index.ssf/2017/01/cleveland_clinic_doc_apologizes_for_anti_vax_column_hospital_promises_discipline.html. Accessed May 2019.

[44] ABC: Melbourne doctor raided amid claims GP's helping parents avoid vaccinating kids, 10th September, 2017, https://www.abc.net.au/news/2017-09-10/melbourne-doctor-raided-by-health-authorities/8889678. Accessed May 2019.

[45] Cooper A. Banned: Anti-vax GP's career appears to be over, *The Age*, 14th September, 2017.

[46] Paterson A. Residents encouraged to dob in rogue anti-vax doctors, *The Northern Star*, 25th August 2017.

[47] Davey M. Health professionals threatened with disciplinary action if they spread anti-vaxx messages, *The Guardian*, 10th May 2019.

[48] Offit PA, Quarles J, Gerber MA, et al. Addressing parents' concerns: Do multiple vaccines overwhelm or weaken the infant's immune system? *Pediatrics*, 2002, 109(1):124-129.

[49] FACA: Conflicts of interest and vaccine development—Preserving the integrity of the process. Hearing before the Committee On Government Reform, House Of Representatives, 106th Congress, Second Session, JUNE 15, 2000, Serial No. 106–239.

[50] WHO, Global Vaccine Safety: Rotavirus vaccines and intussusception, https://www.who.int/vaccine_safety/committee/topics/rotavirus/rotarix_and_rotateq/Dec_2011/en/, Accessed May 2019.

[51] The Children's Hospital of Philadelphia Administrative policy Manual: Patent and Intellectual property Policy, 2006, pp 16.

[52] Moore J. The Real Health Care Scare, *Huffington Post*, 23rd October, 2009.

[53] BusinessWire: The Merck Company Foundation, The Children's Hospital of Philadelphia and the University of Pennsylvania School of Medicine Announce the Creation of The Maurice R. Hilleman Chair in Vaccinology, 22nd March, 2005, https://www.business-wire.com/news/home/20050322005469/en/Merck-Company-Foundation-Childrens-Hospital-Philadelphia-University, Accessed January, 2019.

[54] Children's Hospital of Philadelphia Research Institute: Paul A. Offit, https://www.research.chop.edu/people/paul-offit, Accessed January, 2019.

[55] Boseley S. Charity and Big pharma make uneasy bedfellows, *The Guardian*, 11th May 2013.

[56] Goodman B. When disease charities partner with drug companies, where does that leave patients? *Association for Healthcare Journalists*, June 4, 2013.

[57] Global Pertussis Initiative. Welcome to the Global Pertussis Initiative GPI website, http://www.globalvaccinesinitiative.org/. Accessed May 2019.

[58] Popescu R. Ethical concerns over whooping cough vaccine, *KPBS*, 15th December, 2010.

[59] Srugo I, Benilevi D, Madeb R, et al. Pertussis infection in fully vaccinated children in day-care centres, Israel, *EID Journal*, 2000, 6(5):526-529.

[60] Paterson JM, Sheppeard V. Nosocomial pertussis infection of infants: still a risk in 2009, *Commun Dis Intell Q Rep*, 2010, 34(4):440-3.

[61] Schnirring L. Researchers find first US evidence of vaccine-resistant pertussis, Center for Infectious Disease Research and Policy, 7th February, 2013. Available at: http://www.cidrap.umn.edu/news-

perspective/2013/02/researchers-find-first-us-evidence-vaccine-resistant-pertussis, Accessed May, 2019.

[62] Sala-Farre MR, Arias-Varela C, Recasens-Recasens A, et al. Pertussis epidemic despite high levels of vaccination coverage with acellular pertussis vaccine, *Enferm Inf Microbiol Clin*, 2015, 33(1):27-31.

[63] Queenan AM, Cassiday PK, Evangelista A. Pertactin-negative variants of Bordetella Pertussis in the United States, *NEJM*, 2013, 368:583-584.

[64] Warfel JM, Zimmerman LI, Merkel TJ. Acellular pertussis vaccines protect against disease but fail to prevent infection and transmission in a non-human primate model, 2013, 111(2):787-792.

[65] Campins-Marti M, Cheng HK, Forsyth K, et al. Recommendations are needed for adolescent and adult pertussis immunisation: rationale and strategies for consideration, *Vaccine*, 2001, 20(5-6):641-646.

[66] Meningitis B vaccine added to UK child immunization scheme, Press Association, 29th March, 2015, https://www.theguardian.com/society/2015/mar/29/uk-first-meningitis-b-vaccine. Accessed January, 2019.

[67] Meningitis Research Foundation: Corporate Support, https://www.meningitis.org/get-involved/corporate-support. Accessed January, 2019.

[68] Meningitis Death: 370,000 sign petition in call for full vaccine cover, Press Association, 18th Feb 2016, https://www.theguardian.com/society/2016/feb/17/meningitis-b-death-290000-sign-petition-vaccine. Accessed January, 2019.

[69] Meningitis Now: Corporate Partners, https://www.meningitisnow.org/support-us/corporate-fundraising/corporate-partners/. Accessed January, 2019.

[70] Mello MM, Abiola S, Colgrove J. Pharmaceutical companies' role in state vaccination policymaking: the case of human papillomavirus vaccination, *Am J Public Health*, 2012, 102(5):893–898.

[71] Picchi A, Drug Ads: $5.2 billion annually - and rising, *CBS News*, 11th March 2016.

[72] Horovitz B, Appleby J, Pharma TV ad spend promoting prescription drugs has increased 62 percent since 2012, *MedCityNews*, 20th March 2017.

[73] Swanson A. Big pharmaceutical companies are spending far more on marketing than research, *The Washington Post*, 11th February, 2015.

[74] Chapman S, Holding SJ, Ellerm J, et al. The content and structure of Australian television reportage on health and medicine, 2005–2009: Parameters to guide health workers, *Med J Aust*, 2009, 191(11):620–624.

[75] Fairness and Accuracy in Reporting: Single-payer and interlocking directorates, The corporate ties between insurers and media companies, http://fair.org/extra/single-payer-and-interlocking-directorates/, Accessed May 2019.

[76] Partnership for New York City: Current Portfolio, https://pfnyc.org/our-investments/current-portfolio/, Accessed May 2019.

[77] Macalister T, James Murdoch quits GlaxoSmithKline board, *The Guardian*, 28th January, 2012.

[78] Deer B, MMR doctor Andrew Wakefield fixed data on autism, *The Sunday Times*, 8th February, 2009.

[79] Murdoch Children's Research Institute: How Murdoch Children's is leading vaccine research, https://www.mcri.edu.au/virgo-video, Accessed May 2019.

[80] Knott M, Ireland J. Media ownership reform call comes as Tony Abbott dines with Rupert Murdoch, *The Sydney Morning Herald*, 12th June, 2014.

[81] Benelli E. The role of media in steering public opinion on healthcare issues, *Health Policy*, 2003, 63: 179–186.

[82] Yoo B-K, Holland ML, Bhattacharya J, et al. Effects of mass media coverage on timing and annual receipt of influenza vaccination among medicare elderly, *Health Services Research*, 2010, 45(5 Pt 1):1287-1309.

[83] Ren J, Peters HP, Allgaier J, Lo Y-Y. Similar challenges but different responses: Media coverage of measles vaccination in the UK and China, *Public Understanding of Science,* 2014, 23(4):366-375.

[84] Wise J. Academics who spoke out on swine flu risks were more likely to have industry links, study finds, *BMJ,* 2013; 347:f6758.

[85] Morrell B, Forsyth R, Lipworth W, et al. Rules of engagement: Journalists' attitudes to industry influence in health news reporting, *Journalism*, 2014, 16(5):596-614.

[86] Tyrawski J, DeAndrea DC. Pharmaceutical companies and their drugs on social media: a content analysis of drug information on popular social media sites, *J Med Internet Res*, 2015, 17(6):e130.

[87] Linkov F, Lovalekar M, LaPorte R. Scientific journals are "faith based": is there science behind peer review? *J Royal Soc Med*, 2006, 99(12):596-598.

[88] King DW, Tenopir C. Scholarly journal and digital database pricing: Threat or opportunity? In: MacKie-Mason M, Lougee W, eds. Bits and Bucks: Economics and Usage of Digital Collections. Boston: MIT Press, 2004.

[89] Gottlieb S. Medical societies accused of being beholden to the drugs industry, *BMJ*, 1999, 319(7221):1321.

[90] Smith R. Medical journals and pharmaceutical companies: uneasy bedfellows, *BMJ*, 2003, 326(7400):1202-1205.

[91] Ibid. See reference #89.

[92] Wilkes MS, Doblin BH, Shapiro MF. Pharmaceutical advertisements in leading medical journals: experts' assessments, *Ann Intern Med*, 1992, 116(11):912-9.

[93] Villanueva P, Peiró S, Librero J, Pereiró I. Accuracy of pharmaceutical advertisements in medical journals, *Lancet*, 2003, 361(9351):27-32.

[94] Guyatt GH, Naylor D, Richardson WS, et al. What is the best evidence for making clinical decisions? *JAMA*, 2000, 284(24):3127-3128.

[95] Smith R. Medical journals are an extension of the marketing arm of pharmaceutical companies, *PLoS Med*, 2005, 2(5):e138.

[96] Wilde MA. At medical journals, writers paid by industry play a big role, *The Wall Street Journal*, 13th December, 2005.

[97] Chaudhry S, Schroter S, Smith R, Morris J. Does declaration of competing interests affect readers' perceptions? A randomised trial, *BMJ*, 2002, 325(7377):1391-1392.

[98] Lundh A, Barbateskovic M, Hrobjartsson A, Gotzche PC. Conflicts of interest at medical journals: The influence of industry-supported randomised trials on journal impact factors and revenue-cohort study, *PLoS One*, 2010, 7(10):e1000354.

[99] Jefferson T, Alderson P, Wager E, Davidoff F. Effects of editorial peer review: a systematic review, *JAMA*, 2002, 287(21):2784-2786.

[100] Godlee F, Gale CR, Martyn CN. Effect on the quality of peer review of blinding reviewers and asking them to sign their reports: a randomized controlled trial, *JAMA*, 1998, 280(3):237-240.

[101] Schroter S, Black N, Evans S, et al. Effects of training on quality of peer review: randomised controlled trial, *BMJ*, 2004, 328(7441):673.

[102] Smith R. The trouble with medical journals, *J Royal Soc Med*, 2006, 99(3):115-119.

[103] Smith R. Lapses at the New England Journal of Medicine, *J Royal Soc Med*, 2006, 99(8):380-382.

[104] Angell M. The truth about drug companies: How they deceive us and what to do about it, Random House, New York, 2005

[105] Kassirer JP. On the take: How medicine's complicity with big business can endanger your health, Oxford University Press, New York, 2004.

[106] Angell M. Drug Companies & Doctors: A Story of Corruption. The New York Review of Books Magazine. http://www.nybooks.com/articles/2009/01/15/drug-companies-doctorsa-story-of-corruption/. Accessed September, 2017.

[107] Singer N. Merck paid for medical journal without disclosure, *New York Times*, 14th May 2009.

[108] Center for Responsive Politics, Pharmaceuticals/Health products, https://www.opensecrets.org/lobby/induscli-ent.php?id=h04&year=2017. Accessed May 2019.

[109] Investopedia, Which industry spends the most on lobbying? http://www.investopedia.com/investing/which-industry-spends-most-lobbying-antm-so/. Accessed May 2019.

[110] Belmonte A. FDA medical adviser: "Congress is owned by pharma", *Yahoo Finance*, 13th March, 2019.

[111] Rosenberg MJ. The agile approach to adaptive research: Optimizing efficiency in clinical development, John Wiley and Sons, New Jersey, 2010.

[112] Ibid. See reference #70.

[113] Editorial: Flogging Gardasil, *Nature Biotech*, 2007, 25:261.

[114] Rosenthal E. Drug makers' push leads to cancer vaccines' fast rise, *New York Times*, 20th August, 2008.

[115] Ferguson A, Johnston E. The other drug war-the politics of big business, *The Sydney Morning Herald*, 27th February 2010.

[116] Stevens M. Howard rescues Gardasil from Abbott poison pill, *The Australian*, 10th November, 2006.

[117] The Sydney Morning Herald, Janette Howard beat cervical cancer, http://www.smh.com.au/news/National/Janette-Howard-beat-cervical-can-cer/2006/10/16/1160850845630.html. Accessed May 2019.

[118] Capital Hill Advisory, Our Company, http://capitalhilladvisory.com.au/company/. Accessed October, 2017.

[119] Willard Public Affairs, David Miles, Principal, http://www.willard.com.au/about-us/, Accessed May, 2019.

[120] The Agenda Group, About: The Right Mix For Your Needs, http://www.theagendagroup.com.au/about/, Accessed May, 2019.

[121] CanTeen, Meet The Board: Kieran Schneemann, https://www.canteen.org.au/about-us/about-canteen/youth-leadership-and-governance/meet-the-board/kieran-schnee-mann/, Accessed May, 2019.

[122] Ferguson A, Johnston E. Making sure pills go down and money flows, *The Sydney Morning Herald*, 27th February, 2010.

[123] Hrabe J. CA Assemblyman resigns to take high-paying job in pharmaceutical industry, *California Political Review*, 27th Dec, 2017.

[124] Lupkin S. Big Pharma Greets Hundreds of ex-Federal Workers at the Revolving Door, *Kaiser Health News*, 25th January, 2018.

[125] Australian Government, Dept of Social Services, 8.1.1. Immunisation Requirement Changes - Part Year Effects and Past Period Claims (FTB) Summary, http://guides.dss.gov.au/family-assistance-guide/8/1/1, Accessed February, 2017.

[126] Australian Technical Advisory Group on Immunisation. The Australian Immunisation Handbook. 10th ed. https://www.immunise.health.gov.au/internet/immunise/publishing.nsf/content/Handbook10-home~handbook10part1~handbook10-1-2, Accessed February, 2017.

[127] California Legislative Information, SB 277 Public Health: Vaccinations, http://leginfo.legislature.ca.gov/faces/billNavClient.xhtml?bill_id=201520160SB277, Accessed May, 2019.

[128] Dunn L, Carroll L. Some doctors helping anti-vaccine parents get medical exemptions, *NBC News*, 28th January, 2019.

[129] Feder Ostrov B. Antivaxxers are paying doctors for "fake" medical exemptions in California, *Vice*, 4th April, 2019.

[130] Gstalter M. California bill would monitor doctors who grant vaccination exemptions, *The Hill*, 27th March, 2019.

[131] Kerridge I, Lowe M, Stewart C. Ethics and law for the health professions, 3rd ed. Sydney: The Federation Press, 2009.

[132] Wolfe S. How independent is the FDA? Frontline, 13th November, 2013. Available at: http://www.pbs.org/wgbh/pages/frontline/shows/prescription/hazard/independent.html. Accessed May, 2019.

[133] House of Commons Health Committee. The Influence of the pharmaceutical industry: Fourth Report of Session 2004-

2005.Published on 5 April 2005 by authority of the House of Commons London: The Stationery Office Limited.

[134] Government of Canada. Funding and Fees, https://www.canada.ca/en/health-canada/services/drugs-health-products/funding-fees.html, Accessed October, 2017.

[135] Productivity Commission. Submission To The Productivity Commission, re: Federal Government Cost Recovery, https://www.pc.gov.au/inquiries/completed/cost-recovery/submissions/medical industry association of australia /sub012.pdf, Accessed October, 2017.

[136] Kennedy S. No recall for glass found in vaccines, The Morning Call, 10th December, 2016.

[137] Office of the Associate Director for Science (OADS). Available Technologies for Licensing, https://www.cdc.gov/od/science/technology/techtransfer/industry/licensing/technologies.htm, Accessed May, 2019.

[138] Office of the Associate Director for Science (OADS). Top Grossing Licensing Agreements for 2014, https://www.cdc.gov/od/science/technology/techtransfer/successstories/licensingagreements.htm, Accessed May, 2019.

[139] FACA: Conflicts of Interest and Vaccine Development: Preserving the Integrity of the Process, Before the Government Reform Committee of the House of Representatives, 106th Congress, June 15, 2000.

[140] Food and Drug Administration (FDA). FDA Science and Mission at Risk, Report of the Subcommittee on Science and Technology, 2007.

[141] Schafly R. Official vaccine policy flawed, *The Medical Sentinel*, 1999, 4(3):106-108.

[142] Ibid. See reference #139.

[143] Brennan Z. Revolving Door Between Industry and FDA Continues to Spin, Regulatory Affairs Professionals Society, 6th September, 2018.

[144] Covington and Burling: Pharma and Biotech, https://www.cov.com/en/practices-and-industries/practices/regulatory-and-public-policy/food-drug-and-device/pharma-and-biotech. Accessed January, 2019.

[145] Bien J, Prasad V. Future jobs of FDA's haematology-oncology reviewers, *BMJ (Online)*, 2016, *354*, [i5055].

[146] Kaplan S. From FDA Expert to Biotech insider: The drug industry thrives on the revolving door, STAT News, https://www.statnews.com/2016/09/27/fda-biopharama-revolving-door-study/. Accessed November, 2018.

[147] The New York Times. He Raised Drug Prices at Eli Lilly. Can He Lower Them for the US? Available at: https://www.nytimes.com/2017/11/26/us/politics/alex-azar-senate-confirmation-hearing-hhs.html, Accessed May 2019.

[148] Bright M, McVeigh T. Meningitis Advisors Funded by Drug Firms, *The Observer*, 3rd Sept, 2000, https://www.theguardian.com/uk/2000/sep/03/tracymcveigh.martinbright, Accessed January, 2019.

[149] US Food and Drug Administration. Clinical Trials: What patients need to know, https://www.fda.gov/forpatients/clinicaltrials/, Accessed October, 2017.

[150] Medicines and Healthcare products Regulatory Agency. Medicines and Medical Devices Regulation: What you need to know, http://www.mhra.gov.uk/home/groups/comms-ic/documents/websiteresources/con2031677.pdf, Accessed October, 2017.

[151] Government of Canada. Clinical trials and drug safety, https://www.canada.ca/en/health-canada/services/healthy-

living/your-health/medical-information/clinical-trials-drug-safety.html. Accessed October, 2017.

[152] Therapeutic Goods Administration. TGA regulatory framework, https://www.tga.gov.au/tga-regulatory-framework. Accessed October, 2017.

[153] Independent. Big pharma and governments are turning a blind eye to corruption, report claims, http://www.independent.co.uk/news/world/politics/big-pharma-and-governments-are-turning-a-blind-eye-to-corruption-report-claims-a7059871.html. Accessed October, 2017.

[154] Roumeliotis G. Blunder at Merck's biggest production site pollutes creek, *InPharma Technologist*, 5th July 2006.

[155] Roumeliotis G. Merck 'delayed or impeded' probe into release from production plant, *InPharma Technologist*, 15th August 2006.

[156] Daily Mail. Drug firms drove swine flu pandemic warning to recoup £billions spent on research, http://www.dailymail.co.uk/news/article-1246370/Drug-firms-drove-swine-flu-pandemic-warning-recoup-billions-spent-research.html, Accessed May, 2019.

[157] Husten L. Merck pleads guilty and pays $950 Million for illegal promotion of Vioxx, *Forbes*, November 22, 2011.

[158] Herper M. David Graham on the Vioxx Verdict, *Forbes*, August 19, 2005.

[159] United States Department of Justice. GlaxoSmithKline to plead guilty and pay $3 billion to resolve fraud allegations and failure to report safety data, https://www.justice.gov/opa/pr/glaxosmithkline-plead-guilty-and-pay-3-billion-resolve-fraud-allegations-and-failure-report. Accessed October, 2017.

[160] Webb J. Why pharma faces so many corruption allegations, *Forbes Business*, 23rd February, 2016.

[161] Bradshaw J. Watchdog fines GSK £37M for paying to keep generic drugs out of UK market, *The Telegraph*, 12th February, 2016.

[162] Hiltzik M. Big Pharma bombshell: Judge finds Merck lied in patent trial, overturns $200 million verdict, *Los Angeles Times*, 9th June, 2016.

[163] Leroux M. EU Threatens GE, Canon, Merck with fines for misleading data, *The Times*, 7th July, 2017.

[164] Davey M. 'Deceitful' big pharma accused of putting lives at risk, *The Age*, 7th April, 2013.

CHAPTER 5: VACCINE SAFETY STUDIES

[1] Evidence Based Medicine Working Group. Evidence based medicine. A new approach to teaching the practice of medicine, *JAMA*, 1992, 268:2420-2425.

[2] Greenhalgh T, Howick J, Maskrey N. Evidence based medicine: a movement in crisis? *BMJ,* 2014, 348:g3725.

[3] Ehrhardt S, Appel LJ, Meinert CL. Trends in National Institutes of Health Funding for Clinical Trials Registered in ClinicalTrials.gov, *JAMA,* 2015, 314(23):2566–2567.

[4] Bodenheimer, T. Uneasy alliance: Clinical investigators and the pharmaceutical industry, *NEJM,* 2000, 342:1539-1544.

[5] PhRMA: Biopharmaceutical industry-sponsored clinical trials: impact on state economies, http://phrma-docs.phrma.org/sites/default/files/pdf/biopharmaceutical-industry-sponsored-clinical-trials-impact-on-state-economies.pdf, Accessed May, 2019.

[6] Wikipedia: Selection bias, https://en.wikipedia.org/wiki/Selection_bias, Accessed May, 2019.

[7] US National Library of Medicine: ClinicalTrials.gov. Hepatitis A vaccine, Inactivated and Measles, Mumps, Rubella and

Varicella Virus Vaccine Live Safety Study, https://www.clini-caltrials.gov/ct2/show/NCT00326183?term=vac-cine&recrs=e&cond=vari-cella&age=0&phase=3&fund=2&rank=4, Accessed May, 2019.

[8] FDA: Infanrix Vaccine Insert, https://www.fda.gov/down-loads/biologicsbloodvaccines/vaccines/approvedprod-ucts/ucm124514.pdf, Accessed May, 2019.

[9] Accord Clinical Research, phase IV trials, https://www.ac-cordclinical.com/clinical-study/types-of-clinical-trials/phase-iv-clinical-trials/, Accessed May, 2019.

[10] Ibid. See reference #7.

[11] Wu T, Hu YM, Li J, et al. Immunogenicity and safety of an E. coli-produced bivalent human papillomavirus (type 16 and 18) vaccine: A randomized controlled phase 2 clinical trial, *Vaccine*, 2015, 33(32):3940-3946.

[12] Treanor JT, Albano FR, Sawlwin DC, et al. Immunogenicity and safety of a quadrivalent inactivated influenza vaccine compared with two trivalent inactivated influenza vaccines containing alternate B strains in adults: A phase 3, randomized noninferiority study, *Vaccine,* 2017, 35(15):1856-1864.

[13] Kang JH, Lee HJ, Kim KH, et al. The immunogenicity and safety of a combined DTaP-IPV//Hib Vaccine compared with individual DTaP-IPV and Hib (PRP~T) vaccines: a randomized clinical trial in South Korean infants, *J Korean Med Sci*, 2016, 31(9):1383-1391.

[14] Nolan TM, Nissen MD, Naz A, et al. Immunogenicity and safety of a CRM-conjugated meningococcal ACWY vaccine administered concomitantly with routine vaccines starting at 2 months of age, *Hum Vaccin Immunother*, 2014, 10(2):280-289.

[15] Ruiz-Aragón J, Márquez Peláez S, Molina-Linde JM, et al. Safety and immunogenicity of 13-valent pneumococcal conjugate vaccine in infants: a meta-analysis, *Vaccine*, 2013, 31(46):5349-5358.

[16] Collins Dictionary: Placebo definition, https://www.collinsdictionary.com/dictionary/english/placebo, Accessed May, 2019.

[17] Castellsagué X, Muñoz N, Pitisuttithum P, et al. End-of-study safety, immunogenicity, and efficacy of quadrivalent HPV (types 6, 11, 16, 18) recombinant vaccine in adult women 24–45 years of age, *Brit J Cancer*, 2011, 105(1):28-37.

[18] Millum J, Grady C. The ethics of placebo-controlled trials: Methodological justifications. *Contemporary clinical trials*, 2013, 36(2):510-516.

[19] Rid A, Saxena A, Baqui AH, et al. Placebo use in vaccine trials: Recommendations of a WHO Expert Panel, *Vaccine*, 2014, 323(7):4708-4712.]

[20] Golomb BA, Erickson LC, Koperski S, et al. What's in Placebos: Who Knows? Analysis of Randomized, Controlled Trials, *Ann Intern Med*, 2010, 153:532–535.

[21] Madan A, Ferguson M, Sheldon E, et al. Immunogenicity and safety of an AS03-adjuvanted H7N1 vaccine in healthy adults: A phase I/II, observer-blind, randomized, controlled trial, 2017, 35(10):1431-1439.

[22] US National Institutes of Health, Immunogenicity and safety study of different formulations of GlaxoSmithKline Biologicals H7N1 Influenza vaccine administered to adults 21 to 64 years of age, https://clinicaltrials.gov/show/NCT01934127, Accessed May, 2019.

[23] Vesikari T, Karvonen A, Borrow R, et al. Results from a Randomized Clinical Trial of Coadministration of RotaTeq, a Pentavalent Rotavirus Vaccine, and NeisVac-C, a

Meningococcal Serogroup C Conjugate Vaccine, *Clin Vacc Immunol,* 2011, 18(5):878-884.

[24] Munoz FM, Bond NH, Maccato M, et al. Safety and Immunogenicity of Tetanus Diphtheria and Acellular Pertussis (Tdap) Immunization During Pregnancy in Mothers and Infants: A Randomized Clinical Trial, *JAMA,* 2014, 311(17):1760-1769.

[25] De Vito C, Manzoli L, Marzuillo C, et al. A systematic review evaluating the potential for bias and the methodological quality of meta-analyses in vaccinology, *Vaccine,* 2007, 25(52):8794-806.

[26] Lievre M, Menard J, Bruckert E. et al. Premature discontinuation of clinical trial for reasons not related to efficacy, safety, or feasibility, *BMJ,* 2001, 322:603-605.

[27] Psaty BM, Rennie D. Stopping medical research to save money. A broken pact with researchers and patients, *JAMA,* 2003, 289:2128-2131.

[28] Canadian Association of University Teachers: The Olivieri Report, https://www.caut.ca/docs/af-reports-indepedent-committees-of-inquiry/the-olivieri-report.pdf?sfvrsn=0, Accessed May, 2019.

[29] Rennie D. Thyroid Storm, *JAMA,* 1997, 277(15):1238–1243.

[30] GlaxoSmithKline, Package Insert, Infanrix, https://www.gsksource.com/pharma/content/dam/GlaxoSmithKline/US/en/Prescribing_Information/Infanrix/pdf/INFANRIX.PDF, Accessed May, 2019.

[31] FDA. Vaccine Insert, Menactra©, https://www.fda.gov/downloads/BiologicsBloodVaccines/Vaccines/ApprovedProducts/UCM131170.pdf, Accessed May, 2019.

[32] World Health Organization. Clinical Evaluation of Vaccines, http://www.who.int/biologicals/vaccines/clinical_evaluation/en/, Accessed May, 2019.

[33] U.S FDA, Workshop on Non-clinical Safety Evaluation of Preventative Vaccines: Recent Advances and Regulatory Considerations, 2002. http://www.fda.gov/downloads/BiologicsBloodVaccines/GuidanceComplianceRegulatoryInformation/Guidances/Vaccines/UCM092170.pdf, Accessed May, 2019.

[34] World Health Organization (WHO). Weekly and epidemiological record, 7th Jan, 2005, http://www.who.int/wer/2005/wer8001.pdf, Accessed May, 2019.

[35] Zinka B, Penning R. Unexplained cases of sudden infant death shortly after hexavalent vaccination. Letter to Editor. Response to the comment by H.J. Schmitt et al, *Vaccine*, 2006, 24: 5785-5786.

[36] Ottaviani G, Lavezzi AM, Maturri L. Sudden infant death syndrome (SIDS) shortly after hexavalent vaccination another pathology in suspected SIDS? *Virchows Arch*, 2006, 448:100-104.

[37] European Medicines Agency: Committee for Human Medicinal Products, Note for Guidance on the Clinical Evaluation of Vaccines, Available at: http://www.ema.europa.eu/docs/en_GB/document_library/Scientific_guideline/2009/09/WC500003875.pdf. Accessed May 2019.

[38] Chalmers I. Underreporting research is scientific misconduct, *JAMA,* 1990, 263:1405-1408.

[39] Ross JS, Tse T, Zarin DA, et al. Publication of NIH funded trials registered in ClinicalTrials.gov: cross sectional analysis, *BMJ,* 2012, 344:d7292.

[40] Vogel G. Long-suppressed study finally sees light of day, *Science,* 1997, 276:525-526.

[41] Abbasi K. The missing data that cost $20bn, *BMJ,* 2014, 348:g2695.

[42] Jefferson T, Jones M, Doshi P, et al. Oseltamivir for influenza in adults and children: systematic review of clinical study reports and summary of regulatory comments, *BMJ,* 2014, 348:g2545.

[43] Ibid. See reference #7.

[44] Smith R. Medical journals and pharmaceutical companies: uneasy bedfellows, *BMJ,* 2003, 326(7400):1202-1205.

[45] Als-Nielsen B, Chen W, Gluud C, Kjaergard LL. Association of funding and conclusions in randomized drug trials: A reflection of treatment effect or adverse events? *JAMA,* 2003, 290(7):921–928.

[46] Chopra SS. Industry funding of clinical trials: Benefit or bias? *JAMA,* 2003, 290(1):113–114.

[47] GlaxoSmithKline: Infanrix insert, https://www.gsksource.com/pharma/content/dam/GlaxoSmithKline/US/en/Prescribing_Information/Infanrix/pdf/INFANRIX.PDF. Accessed May, 2019.

[48] Merck, MMR insert, http://www.merck.com/product/usa/pi_circulars/m/mmr_ii/mmr_ii_pi.pdf, Accessed May, 2019.

[49] Cancer Australia: Children's Cancer Statistics, https://childrenscancer.canceraustralia.gov.au/about-childrens-cancer/statistics. Accessed September, 2017.

[50] Poplack DG. Acute lymphoblastic leukemia in childhood. In: Altman AJ (ed) The Pediatric clinics of North America. Saunders Philadelphia, 1985, pp 669–697.

[51] O'Byrne KJ, Dalgleish AG. Chronic immune activation and inflammation as the cause of malignancy, *Brit J Cancer*, 2001, 85(4):473-83.

[52] Dalgleish AG, O'Byrne KJ. Chronic immune activation and inflammation in the pathogenesis of AIDS and cancer, *Adv Cancer Res*, 2002, 84:231-76.

[53] Letter, Daily Mail, 25th Jan, 2001.

[54] Innis MD, Letter to the Editor: Immunization and Childhood Leukaemia, The Lancet, 13th March 1965, i605.

[55] Buckley JD, Buckley CM, Ruccione K, et al. Epidemiological characteristics of childhood acute lymphocytic leukemia: Analysis by immunophenotype, The Children's Cancer Group, *Leukemia*, 1994, 8(5):856-864.

[56] Ivanovski P, Ivanovski I. Childhood acute lymphoblastic leukemia is triggered by the introduction of immunization against diphtheria, *Med Hyp*, 2007, 68(2):324-327.

[57] Akinmoladun VI, Arinola OG, Elumelu-Kupoluyi T, Eriba LO. Evaluation of humoral immunity in oral cancer patients from a Nigerian referral centre, *J Maxillofac Oral Surg*, 2013, 12(4):410-3.

[58] Flexner S, Jobling JW. On the promoting influence of heated tumor emulsions on tumor growth, *Proc Soc Exp Biol Med*, 1907, 4:156-169.

[59] Clerici M, Clerici E. The tumor enhancement phenomenon: Reinterpretation from a Th1/Th2 perspective, *J Nat Can Inst*, 1996, 88(7):461.

[60] Kaliss N. Immunological enhancement of tumor homografts in mice: a review, *Cancer Res*, 1958, 992-1003.

[61] Lalor MK, Smith SG, Floyd S, et al. Complex cytokine profiles induced by BCG vaccination in UK infants, *Vaccine*, 2010, 28(6):1635-1641.

[62] Wei LH, Kuo ML, Chen CA, et al. Interleukin 6 promotes cervical tumor growth by VEGF-dependent angiogenesis via a STAT3 pathway, *Oncogene*, 2003, 22:1517–1527.

[63] Culig Z, Puhr M. Interleukin-6: A multifunctional targetable cytokine in human prostate cancer, *Mol Cell Endocrin*, 2012, 360(1-2):52-58.

[64] Becker C, Fantini MC, Wirtz S, et al. IL-6 signaling promotes tumor growth in colorectal cancer, *Cell Cycle*, 2005, 4(2):220-223.

[65] Little DT, Ward HR. Premature ovarian failure 3 years after menarche in a 16-year-old girl following human papillomavirus vaccination, *BMJ Case Reports*, 2012, doi:10.1136/bcr-2012-006879.

[66] Wetzstein C. HPV Vaccine Cited in Infertility Case, The Washington Times, November 11, 2013.

[67] DeLong G. A lowered probability of pregnancy in females in the USA aged 25–29 who received a human papillomavirus vaccine injection, *J Toxicol Enviro Health*, 2018, 81(14):661-674.

[68] Donahue JG, Kieke BA, King JP et al. Association of spontaneous abortion with receipt of inactivated vaccine containing H1N1pdm09 in 2010-11 and 2011-12, *Vaccine*, 2017, 35(40):5314-5322.

[69] Tietze C, Lewit S. Abortion, *Scientific American*, 1969, 220:21.

[70] Cheadle C. Dropping Fertility Rates are a Threat to the Global Economy, Business Insider, 28th November, 2016.

[71] Levine H, Jørgensen N, Martino-Andrade A, et al. Temporal trends in sperm count: a systematic review and meta-regression analysis, *Hum Reprod Update*, 2017, 23(6): 646–659.

[72] Stein R, Sperm counts plummet in western men, study finds, *NPR*, 31st July 2017.

[73] Andersson AM, Jensen TK, Juul A et al. Secular decline in male testosterone and sex hormone binding globulin serum levels in Danish population surveys, *J Clin Endocrin Metab*, 2007, 92(12): 4696–4705.

[74] Travison TG, Araujo AB, Amy B, et al. A population-level decline in serum testosterone levels in American men, *J Clin Endocrinol Metab*, 2007, 92(1): 196–202.

[75] Perheentupa A, Mäkinen J, Laatikainen T, et al. A cohort effect on serum testosterone levels in Finnish men, *Euro J Endocrinol*, 2013, *168*(2):227-233.

[76] Boaz NT. Essentials of biological anthropology, 1999, Prentice Hall, New Jersey.

[77] Thacker HL. Does early menstruation mean earlier menopause? https://speakingofwomenshealth.com/column/does-early-menstruation-mean-early-menopause, Accessed May, 2019.

[78] ABC News, Vaccine Boycott Grows in Northern Nigeria, 24th February, 2004.

[79] Kenya Conference of Catholic Bishops: Press Statement by the Kenya Conference of Catholic Bishops, http://www.kccb.or.ke/home/news-2/press-statement-by-the-kenya-conference-of-catholic-bishops/, Accessed March, 2019.

[80] Kenya Conference of Catholic Bishops: Catholic Health Commission of Kenya, http://www.kccb.or.ke/home/commission/12-catholic-health-commission-of-kenya/, Accessed March 2019.

[81] Oller JW, Shaw CA, Tomljenovic L, et al. HCG found in WHO tetanus vaccine in Kenya raises concern in the developing world, *Op Acc Lib J*, 2017, 4:e3937.

[82] Obara V, License of industrial lab Agriq-Quest suspended, *Business Daily*, 12th January, 2017.

[83] Corvelva, Study on the chemical composition of Hexyon, Available at: https://drive.google.com/file/d/12e3OocT1hSM-GULzvFg3DcoM_XyGZMRur/view, Accessed May, 2019.

[84] Hayes TB, Collins A, Lee M, et al. Hermaphroditic, demasculinized frogs after exposure to the herbicide atrazine at low ecologically relevant doses, *Proc Nat Acad Sci*, 2002, 99(8):5476-5480.

[85] US EPA memorandum, "Sulfluramid – Amount of A.I. in Raid Max Roach Bait." To Mike Mendelsohn, PM Team Reviewer, Registration Division (7505C). From Linda L. Talor, Ph.D., Toxicology Branch II, Health Effects Division (7509C) and Marcia van Gemert, Ph.D., Chief, Toxicology Branch II/HED (7509C), August 10, 1994.

[86] Centers for Disease Control, Parent's Guide to Childhood Immunizations, https://www.cdc.gov/vaccines/parents/tools/parents-guide/parents-guide-part4.html, Accessed May, 2019.

[87] European Medicines Agency: Note for Guidance on the Clinical Evaluation of Vaccines, http://www.ema.europa.eu/docs/en_GB/document_library/Scientific_guideline/2009/09/WC500003875.pdf. Accessed September, 2017.

[88] Tomljenovic L, Shaw C. Aluminum vaccine adjuvants: Are they safe? *Curr Med Chem*, 2011, 18(17):2630-7.

[89] Liu HF, Li W, Lu MB, Yu LJ. Pharmacokinetics and risk evaluation of DNA vaccine against Schistosoma japonicum, *Parasitol Res*, 2013, 112(1):59-67.

[90] Mitkus RJ, King DB, Walderhaug MO, Forshee RA. A comparative pharmacokinetic estimate of mercury in U.S. infants following yearly exposures to inactivated influenza vaccines containing thimerosal, *Risk Analysis*, 2014, 34:735–750.

[91] Hughes RG, Blegen MA. Chapter 37: Medication Administration Safety in Patient Safety and Quality: An Evidence-

Based Handbook for Nurses, Agency for Healthcare Research and Quality, 2008.

[92] Institute of Medicine Committee on the Assessment of Studies of Health Outcomes Related to the Recommended Childhood Immunization Schedule. The Childhood Immunization Schedule and Safety: Stakeholder Concerns, Scientific Evidence and Future Studies. Washington, DC: *The National Academies Press,* 2013.

[93] Institute of Medicine, The childhood immunization schedule and safety: stakeholder concerns, scientific evidence and future studies (2013), https://www.nap.edu/read/13563/chapter/2#4, Accessed May, 2019.

[94] US National Library of Medicine: Genetics Home Reference, MTHFR gene, https://ghr.nlm.nih.gov/gene/MTHFR, Accessed May, 2019.

[95] Nazki FH, Sameer AS, Ganaie BA. Folate: metabolism, genes, polymorphisms and the associated diseases, *Gene*, 2014, 533(1):11-20.

[96] Dean L. Methylenetetrahydrofolate Reductase Deficiency. *Medical Genetics Summaries.* NCBI; Available at: https://www.ncbi.nlm.nih.gov/books/NBK66131/, Accessed May, 2019.

[97] MTHFR.Net: MTHFR Basics From Dr Erlich, http://mthfr.net/mthfr-basics-from-dr-erlich/2012/03/01/, Accessed May, 2019.

[98] Friso S, Choi S-W, Girelli D, et al. A common mutation in the 5,10-methylenetetrahydrofolate reductase gene affects genomic DNA methylation through an interaction with folate status, *Proc Natl Acad Sci USA*, 2002, 99(8):5606-5611.

[99] Fisher MC, Cronstein BN. Meta-analysis of methylenetetrahydrofolate reductase (MTHFR) polymorphisms affecting methotrexate toxicity, *J Rheumatol,* 2009, 36(3):539-545.

[100] Pu D, Shen Y, Wu J. Association between MTHFR gene polymorphisms and the risk of autism spectrum disorders: a meta-analysis, *Autism Res*, 2013, 6(5):384-92.

[101] Ulrich CM, Yasui Y, Storb R, et al. Pharmacogenetics of methotrexate: toxicity among marrow transplantation patients varies with the methylenetetrahydrofolate reductase C677T polymorphism, *Blood*, 2001, 98:231-234.

[102] Aaby P, Mogensen SW, Rodrigues A, Benn CS. Evidence of increase in mortality after the introduction of Diphtheria–Tetanus–Pertussis vaccine to children aged 6–35 Months in Guinea-Bissau: A time for reflection? *Front PubHealth*, 2018, 6:79.

[103] Aaby P, Jensen H, Simondon F, Whittle H. High-titer measles vaccination before 9 months of age and increased female mortality: do we have an explanation? *Semin Paediatr Infect Dis*, 2003, 14(3):220-232.

[104] Danish DOX, Most of you think we know what our vaccines are doing – we don't, Peter Aaby, https://www.youtube.com/watch?v=NPNHYAevTwg. Accessed May 2019.

[105] Misra S. Randomized double blind placebo control studies, the "Gold Standard" in intervention-based studies, *Ind J Sex Trans Dis,* 2012, 33(2):131-134.

[106] Institute of Medicine. 2013. *The Childhood Immunization Schedule and Safety: Stakeholder Concerns, Scientific Evidence, and Future Studies*. Washington, DC: The National Academies Press.

[107] WavesNZ. The 1992 IAS Survey of Vaccinated and Unvaccinated Children, http://wavesnz.org.nz/wp-content/uploads/2015/02/The-1992-IAS-NZ-Survey-of-Vaccinated-vs.-Unvaccinated-Children.pdf, Accessed May, 2019.

[108] Scribd. Roosendaal study of vaccinated vs unvaccinated children in the Netherlands, https://www.scribd.com/doc/60166949/Roosendaal-study-of-vaccinated-vs-unvaccinated-children-in-the-Netherlands-Results-Survey#scribd, Accessed May, 2019.

[109] Schmitz R, Poethko-Muller C, Reiter S, Schlaud M. Vaccination status and health in children and adolescents, *Dtsch Artebl*, 2011, 108(7):99-104.

[110] VaccineInjury.info. State of health in unvaccinated children, http://web.archive.org/web/20130122020332/http://www.vaccineinjury.info/vaccinations-in-general/health-unvaccinated-children/survey-results-illnesses.html, Accessed May, 2019.

[111] Mawson AR, Ray BD, Bhuiyan AR, Jacob B. Pilot comparative study on the health of vaccinated and unvaccinated 6- to 12-year-old US children, *J Transl Sci*, 2017, 3(3):1-12.

[112] Michels KB, Rothman KJ. Update on unethical use of placebos in randomised trials, *Bioethics*, 2003, 17(2):188-204.

[113] Martinson BC, Anderson MS, deVries R. Scientists behaving badly, *Nature*, 2005, 435:737-738.

[114] Smith R. Medical journals are an extension of the marketing arm of pharmaceutical companies, *PloS Med*, 2005, 2(5):e138.

[115] Horton R. Offline: What is medicine's 5 sigma? Comment, The Lancet, 2015, 385:1380.

[116] Freedman DH. Lies, Damned Lies, And Medical Science, *The Atlantic*, November, 2010.

CHAPTER 6: PREGNANCY, INFANTS & THE ELDERLY

[1] Harper SA, Fukuda K, Uyeki TM, et al. Prevention and control of influenza: recommendations of the advisory committee on immunization practices (ACIP*), MMWR Recomm Rep,* 2004, 53(6):1-40.

[2] Herberts C, Melgert B, van der Laan JW, et al. New adjuvanted vaccines in pregnancy: what is known about their safety? *Exp Rev Vaccines*, 2010, 9(12):1411-1422.

[3] Goldman GS. Comparison of VAERS fetal-loss reports during three consecutive influenza seasons: was there a synergistic fetal toxicity associated with the two-vaccine 2009/2010 season, *Hum Exp Toxicol*, 2013. 32(5):464-475.

[4] CDC. Updated recommendations for use of tetanus toxoid, reduced diptheria toxoid and acellular pertussis vaccine in pregnant women and persons who have or anticipate having close contact with an infant aged <12 months---advisory committee on immunization practices (ACIP), 2011, *MMWR*, 60(41):1424-1426.

[5] Lam C, Octavia S, Ricafort L, et al. Rapid increase in pertactin-deficient Bordetella pertussis isolates, Australia, *J Emerg Infect Dis*, 2014, 20(4):626-633.

[6] Martin SW, Pawloski L, Williams M, et al. Pertactin-negative bordetella pertussis strains: evidence for a possible selective advantage, *Clin Infect Dis*, 2015, 60(2):223-227.

[7] Althouse BM, Scarpino SV. Asymptomatic transmission and the resurgence of bordetella pertussis, *BMC Med*, 2015, 13:146.

[8] Meyer U, Engier A, Weber L, et al. Preliminary evidence for a modulation of fetal dopaminergic development by maternal immune activation during pregnancy, *Neuroscience*, 2008, 154(2):701-709.

[9] Malkova NV, Yu CZ, Hsiao EY, et al. Maternal immune activation yields offspring displaying mouse versions of the three core symptoms of autism, *Brain Behav Immun*, 2012, 26(4):607-616.

[10] Bauman MD, Iosif AM, Smith SEP, et al. Activation of the maternal immune response during pregnancy alters behavioural development of rhesus monkey offspring, *Biol Psych*, 2014, 75(4):332-341.

[11] Shi L, Smith SEP, Malkova N, et al. Activation of the maternal immune system alters cerebellar development in the offspring, *Brain Behav Immun*, 2009, 23(1): 116-123.

[12] Pendyala G, Chou S, Jung Y, et al. Maternal immune activation causes behavioural impairments and altered cerebellar cytokine and synaptic protein expression, *Neuro Psych*, 2017, 42(7):1435-1447.

[13] Garay PA, Hsiao EY, Patterson PH, McAllister AK. Maternal immune activation causes age- and region-specific changes in brain cytokines in offspring throughout development, *Brain Behav Immunol*, 2013, 31:54-68.

[14] Smith SE, Li J, Garbett K, Mirnics K, Patterson PH. Maternal immune activation alters fetal brain development through interleukin-6, *J Neurosci*, 2007, 27(40):10695-10702.

[15] Nyffeler M, Meyer U, Yee BK, et al. Maternal immune activation during pregnancy increases limbic GABAa receptor immunoreactivity in the adult offspring; implications for schizophrenia, *Neuroscience*, 2006, 143(1):51-62.

[16] Zuckerman L, Weiner I. Maternal immune activation leads to behavioural and pharmacological changes in the adult offspring, *J Psych Res*, 2005, 39(3):311-323.

[17] Zuckerman L, Rehari M, Nachman R, Weiner I. Immune activation during pregnancy in rats leads to a postpubertal emergence of disrupted latent inhibition, dopaminergic

hyperfunction, and altered limbic morphology in the offspring: a novel neurodevelopmental model of schizophrenia, *Neuro Psych*, 2003, 28(10):1778-1789.

[18] Knuesel I, Chicha L, Britschgi M, et al. Maternal immune activation and abnormal brain development across CNS disorders, *Nat Rev Neurol*, 2014, 10:643-660.

[19] Munoz FM, Greisinger AJ, Wehmanen AO, et al. Safety of influenza vaccination during pregnancy, *Am J Ob Gyn*, 2005, 192(4):1098-1106.

[20] De Gregorio E, Caproni E, Ulmer JB. Vaccine adjuvants: mode of action, *Front Immunol*, 2013, 4:214.

[21] Zerbo O, Qian Y, Yoshida C, et al. Association Between Influenza Infection and Vaccination During Pregnancy and Risk of Autism Spectrum Disorder, *JAMA Pediatr,* 2017, 171(1):e163609.

[22] Heinonen OP, Shapiro S, Monson RR, et al. Immunization During Pregnancy Against Poliomyelitis and Influenza in Relation to Childhood Malignancy, *Int J Epidemiol*, 1973, 2(3):229–236

[23] Black SB, Shinefield HR, France EK, et al. Effectiveness of influenza vaccine during pregnancy in preventing hospitalizations and outpatient visits for respiratory illness in pregnant women and their infants, *Am J Perinatol*, 2004, 21(6):333-339.

[24] France EK, Smith-Ray R, McClure D, et al. Impact of maternal influenza vaccination during pregnancy on the incidence of acute respiratory illness visits among infants, *Arch Pediatr Adolesc Med*, 2006, 160(12):1277-1283.

[25] Oxford Vaccine Group, Respiratory Syncytial Virus, https://www.ovg.ox.ac.uk/research/respiratory-syncytial-virus-rsv, Accessed May, 2019.

[26] Haelle T, Group B Strep Vaccine for Pregnant Women Found Safe, Effective in Phase 2 trial, *Forbes*, 12th January 2016.

[27] CDC, Respiratory Syncytial Virus Infection (RSV), https://www.cdc.gov/rsv/high-risk/infants-young-children.html. Accessed March 2019.

[28] Dudas RA, Karron RA. Respiratory syncytial virus vaccines, *Clin Microbiol Rev*, 1998, 11(3):430-439.

[29] Delgado MF, Coviello S, Monsalvo AC, et al. Lack of antibody affinity maturation due to poor Toll-like receptor stimulation leads to enhanced respiratory syncytial virus disease, *Nat Med*, 2008, 15(1):34-41.

[30] FierceBiotech, Novavax craters after phase III RSV F vaccine failure; seeks path forward, https://www.fiercebiotech.com/biotech/novavax-craters-after-phase-iii-rsv-f-vaccine-failure-seeks-path-forward. Accessed March 2019.

[31] CNBC, Novavax is down 80%. Here's why its been really hard to develop an RSV vaccine, https://www.cnbc.com/2016/09/16/heres-why-its-been-really-hard-to-develop-a-vaccine-for-rsv.html. Accessed March, 2019.

[32] Novavax, Press Release: Novavax announces topline results from Phase 3 PrepareTM Trial of Resvax TM for prevention of RSV disease in infants via maternal immunization, http://ir.novavax.com/news-releases/news-release-details/novavax-announces-topline-results-phase-3-preparetm-trial. Accessed March 2019.

[33] Novavax, Bill & Melinda Gates Foundation, https://novavax.com/page/19/bill-and-melinda-gates-foundation. Accessed March 2019.

[34] Bill and Melinda Gates Foundation, How We Work, Grant: Novavax, Inc,

https://www.gatesfoundation.org/How-We-Work/Quick-Links/Grants-Database/Grants/2015/09/OPP1127647. Accessed March 2019.

[35] Downham MA, Scott R, Sims DG, Webb JK, Gardner PS. Breast-feeding protects against respiratory syncytial virus infections, *Br Med J*, 1976, 2(6030):274-276.

[36] UNICEF Progress for Children, Nutrition Indicators: Exclusive Breastfeeding, https://www.unicef.org/progress-forchildren/2006n4/index_breastfeeding.html. Accessed March 2019].

[37] Oxford Vaccine Group: Vaccine Knowledge Project, Respiratory Syncytial Virus, http://vk.ovg.ox.ac.uk/rsv. Accessed April 2019.

[38] Justia Patents, Vaccine, https://patents.justia.com/patent/20130089571, Accessed April 2019.

[39] Justia Patents, Compositions comprising OPA Protein Epitopes, https://patents.justia.com/patent/20100183676. Accessed April 2019.

[40] Oxford Vaccine Group, Matthew Snape, https://www.ovg.ox.ac.uk/team/matthew-snape. Accessed April 2019.

[41] Anti-RSV Immunogens and methods of Immunization, https://patents.google.com/patent/US8846056?oq=vaccine+inassignee:centers+inassignee:for+inassignee:disease+inassignee:control. Accessed April 2019.

[42] WHO/GlaxoSmithKline, Maternal GBS Vaccine, Immaculada Margarit PD-VAC Meeting, Geneve, 7th September, 2015, https://www.who.int/immunization/research/meetings_workshops/12_Group_B_Strep.pdf?ua=1. Accessed March 2019.

[43] Ibid. See reference #26.

[44] Ibid. See reference #42.

[45] Waly M, Oteanu H, et al. Activation of methionine synthase by insulin-like growth factor-1 and dopamine: a target for neurodevelopment toxins and thimerosal, *Mol Psychiatry*, 2004, 9(4):358-370.

[46] Blaylock RL. Excitotoxicity: a possible central mechanism in fluoride neurotoxicity, *Fluoride*, 2004, 37(4):264-277.

[47] Epstein HT. Growth spurts during brain development: Implications for educational policy and practice, 1978. In J. S. Chall, & A. F. Mirsky (Eds.), Education and the brain). Chicago: University of Chicago Press, pp. 343–370.

[48] Kolb B, Fantie BD. Development of the Child's Brain and Behaviour. In C.R. Reynolds, E. Fletcher-Janzen (eds.), Handbook of Clinical Child Neuropsychology, Springer Publishing, 2009.

[49] EPA: Neurodevelopmental Disorders, https://www.epa.gov/sites/production/files/2015-10/documents/ace3_neurodevelopmental.pdf, Accessed May, 2019.

[50] Holt PG, Upham JW, Sly PD. Contemporaneous maturation of immunologic and respiratory functions during early childhood: implications for development of asthma prevention strategies, *J Allergy Clin Immunol*, 2005, 116(1):16-24.

[51] Chelvarajan RL, Collins SM, Doubinskaia IE, et al. Defective macrophage function in neonates and its impact on unresponsiveness of neonates to polysaccharide antigens, *J Leukoc Biol*, 2004, 75(6):982-994.

[52] Chelvarajan L, Popa D, Liu Y, et al. Molecular mechanisms underlying anti-inflammatory phenotype of neonatal splenic macrophages, *J Leukoc Biol*, 2007, 82(2):403-416.

[53] Romagnani S. Biology of human TH1 and TH2 cells, *J Clin Immunol*, 1995, 15(3):121-129.

Kate William

[54] Cryan JF, Dinan TG. More than a gut feeling: the microbiota regulates neurodevelopment and behavior, *Neuropsych Rev*, 2015, 40:241-242.

[55] Maloney RD, Desbonnet L, Clarke G et al. The microbiome: stress, health and disease, *Mamm Genome,* 2014, 25:49-74.

[56] Jamieson AM. Influence of the microbiome on response to vaccination, *Human Vaccin Immunother*, 2015, 11(9):2329-2331.

[57] Plenge-Bönig A, Soto-Ramírez N, Karmaus W, et al. Breastfeeding protects against acute gastroenteritis due to rotavirus in infants, *Eur J Pediatr*, 2010, 169:1471.

[58] Moon SS, Wang Y, Shane AL, et al, Inhibitory effect of breast milk on infectivity of live oral rotavirus vaccines, *Pediatr Infect Dis J*, 2010, 29(10):919-923.

[59] Alzheimer's Association. 2017 Alzheimer's Disease Facts and Figures, https://www.alz.org/facts/. Accessed October, 2017.

[60] Speech by Hugh Fudenburg, 1st Annual Public Conference on Vaccination, National Vaccine Information Center, Arlington.

[61] Verreault R, Laurin D, Lindsay J, Serres GD. Past exposure to vaccines and subsequent risk of Alzheimer's disease, *CMAJ*, 2001, 165(11):1495-1498.

[62] Tomljenovic L. Aluminum and Alzheimer's disease: after a century of controversy, is there a plausible link? *J Alzheimer's Dis*, 2011, 23(4):567-598.

[63] Exley C. Aluminium and Alzheimer's disease: The science that describes the link, 1st Edition; Elsevier Science: Amsterdam, 2001.

[64] Mutter J, Naumann J, Schneider R, Walach H. Mercury and alzheimer's disease, *Fortschr Neurol Psyciatr*, 2007, 75(9):528-38.

452

[65] Mutter J, Curth A, Naumann J, et al. Does inorganic mercury play a role in Alzheimer's disease: A systematic review and an integrated molecular mechanism, *J Alzheimers Dis*, 2010, 22(2):357-74.

[66] Osterholm MT, Kelley NS, Sommer A, Belongia EA. Efficacy and effectiveness of influenza vaccines: a systematic review and meta-analysis, *Lancet Infect Dis*, 2012, 12(1):36-44.

[67] Simonsen L, Reichert TA, Viboud C, et al. Impact of influenza vaccination on seasonal mortality in the US elderly population, *Arch Intern Med*, 2005, 165(3):265-272.

[68] US Dept Health and Human Services, Senior Schedule, https://www.vaccines.gov/who_and_when/seniors/index.html, Accessed May, 2019.

[69] Boraschi D, Italian P. Immunosenescence and vaccine failure in the elderly: strategies for improving response, *Immunol Lett*, 2014, 162:346-353.

[70] National Centre for Immunisation Research and Surveillance. Zoster vaccine for Australian adults, http://ncirs.org.au/ncirs-fact-sheets-faqs/zoster-vaccine-australian-adults, Accessed May, 2019.

[71] CDC. Fluzone High Dose Seasonal Influenza Vaccine, https://www.cdc.gov/flu/prevent/qa_fluzone.htm?CDC_AA_refVal=https%3A%2F%2Fwww.cdc.gov%2Fflu%2Fprotect%2Fvaccine%2Fqa_fluzone.htm, Accessed May, 2019.

[72] WebMD. Seniors need 2 pneumonia vaccines, CDC panel says, https://www.webmd.com/healthy-aging/news/20150203/seniors-need-2-pneumonia-vaccines-cdc-advisory-panel-says#1, Accessed May, 2019.

[73] Ala. Code § 22-21-10(d).

[74] N.C. Gen. Stat. Ann. § 131E-113(a).

[75] Del. Admin. Code § 3201-6.3.1.

[76] Aird H. Influenza epidemic: Six deaths confirmed at Tasmania's Strathdevon aged care home, ABC News, 2nd September, 2017.

[77] Le Messurier D. The biggest mistakes Australians are making in the influenza outbreak, *News.com.au*, 5th September 2017.

CHAPTER 7: OTHER VACCINATION ISSUES

[1] Nakayama T, Maehara N, Sadaki K, Makino S. Long-term regulation of interferon production by lymphocytes from children inoculated with live measles virus vaccine, *J Infect Dis*, 1988, 158(6): 1386-1390.

[2] Goldstein D, Laszlo J. The roles of interferon in cancer therapy: a current perspective, *Canc J Clin*, 1988, 38(5): 258-277.

[3] Hussey GD, Goddard EA, Hughes J, et al. The effect of Edmonston-Zagreb and Schwarz measles vaccines on immune response in infants, *J Infect Dis*, 1996, 173(6):1320-1326.

[4] Imai K, Matsuyama S, Miyake S, et al. Natural cytotoxic activity of peripheral-blood lymphocytes and cancer incidence: an 11-year follow-up study of a general population, *Lancet*, 2000, 356(9244):1795-1799.

[5] Eibl MM, Mannhealter JW, Zlabinger G. Abnormal T-lymphocyte subpopulations in healthy subjects after tetanus booster immunization, *NEJM*, 1984, 310(3):198-199.

[6] Toraldo R, Tolone C, Catalanotti P, et al. Effects of measles-mumps-rubella vaccination on polymorphonuclear neutrophil functions in children, *Acta Pediatr*, 1992, 81(11):887-890.

[7] Ehrengut W. Susceptibility to infection after vaccination, *Br Med J*, 1972, 1(5801):683.

[8] Martinez X, Brandt C, Saddallah F, et al. DNA immunization circumvents deficient induction of T helper type 1 and cytotoxic T lymphocyte responses in neonates and during early life, *Proc Natl Acad Sci*, 1997, 94(16):8726-8731.

[9] Cowling BJ, Fang VJ, Nishiura H, et al. Increased risk of non-influenza respiratory virus infections associated with receipt of inactivated influenza vaccine, *Clin Infect Dis*, 2012, 54(12):1778-1783.

[10] Bodewes R, Kreijtz JH, Baas C, et al. Vaccination against human influenza A/H3N2 virus prevents the induction of heterosubtypic immunity against lethal infection with avian influenza A/H5N1 virus, *PloS One*, 2009, 4(5):e5538.

[11] Miller E, Goldacre M, Pugh S, et al. Risk of aseptic meningitis after measles, mumps, and rubella vaccine in UK children, *Lancet*, 1993, 341(8851):979-982.

[12] Sugiura A, Yamada A. Aseptic meningitis as a complication of mumps vaccination, *Pediatr Infect Dis J*, 1991, 10(3):209-213.

[13] Dourado I, Cunha S, Teixara MG, et al. Outbreak of aseptic meningitis associated with mass vaccination with a Urabe-containing measles-mumps-rubella vaccine, *Am J Epidemiol*, 2000, 151(5): 524-530.

[14] Brisson M, Gay NJ, Edmunds WJ, Andrews NJ. Exposure to varicella boosts immunity to herpes zoster: implications for mass vaccination against chickenpox, *Vaccine*, 2002, 20(19-20):2500-2507.

[15] Goldman GS, King PG. Vaccination to prevent varicella: Goldman and King's response to Myers' interpretation of Varicella Active Surveillance Project Data, *Hum Exp Toxicol*, 2014, 33(8):886-893.

[16] Brisson M, Edmunds WJ. Varicella vaccination in England and Wales: cost-utility analysis, *Arch Dis Child*, 2003, 88(10):862-869.

[17] Damm O, Ultsch B, Horn J, et al. Systematic review of models assessing the economic value of routine varicella and herpes zoster vaccination in high-income countries, *BMC Public Health*, 2015, 15:533.

[18] van Lier A, Lugner A, Opstelten W, et al. Distribution of health effects and cost effectiveness of varicella vaccination are shaped by the impact on herpes zoster, Ebio Med, 2015, 2(10):1494-1499.

[19] Gershon AA. The history and mystery of VZV in saliva, *J Infect Dis,* 2011, 204(6):815-816.

[20] Alain S, Dommergues MA, Jacquard AC. State of the art: Could nursing mothers be vaccinated with attenuated live virus vaccine? *Vaccine,* 2012, 30(33):4921-4926.

[21] Eckerle I, Keller-Stanislawski B, Eis-Hubinger AM. Non-febrile seizures after Mumps, Measles, Rubella and Varicella-zoster virus combination vaccination with detection of measles virus RNA in serum, throat and urine, *Clin Vaccine Immunol,* 2013, 29(7):1094-1096.

[22] Laassr M, Lottenback K, Beishe R, et al. Effect of different vaccination schedules on excretion of Oral Poliovirus vaccine strains, *J Infect Dis,* 2005, 192(12):2092-2098.

[23] La Russa P, Steinberg S, Meurice F, Gershon A. Transmission of vaccine strain varicella zoster virus from a healthy adult with vaccine-associated rash to susceptible household contacts, *J Infect Dis,* 1997, 176:1072-1075.

[24] Dunn G, Klapsa D, Wilton T, et al. Twenty eight years of poliovirus replication in an immunodeficient individual: impact on the global polio eradication initiative, *PloS Pathogens*, 2015, 11(8):e1005114.

[25] Burns CC, Diop OM, Sutter RW, Kew OM. Vaccine-derived polioviruses, *J Infect Dis*, 2014, 210(S1):S283–293.

[26] Hovi T, Shulman L, van der Avoort H, et al. Role of environmental poliovirus surveillance in global polio eradication and beyond, *Epidemiol Inf*, 2012, 1:1–13.

[27] Rivera L, Pena LM, Stainier I, et al. Horizontal transmission of a human rotavirus vaccine strain—a randomized, placebo- controlled study in twins, *Vaccine,* 2011, 29:9508–9513.

[28] Barclay VC, Sim D, Chan BHK, et al. The evolutionary consequences of blood-stage vaccination on the rodent malaria plasmodium chabaudi, *PloS Biol*, 2012, 10(7):e1001368.

[29] Read AF, Baigent SJ, Powers C, et al. Imperfect vaccination can enhance the transmission of highly virulent pathogens, *PloS Biol*, 2015, 13(7):e1002198.

[30] Franzo G, Tucciarone CM, Cechinato M, Drigo M. Porcine circovirus Type 2 (PCV2) evolution before and after the vaccine introduction, *Sci Rep*, 2016, 6:39458.

[31] Miller JJ, Saito TM, Silverberg RJ. Parapertussis: clinical and serologic observations, *J Pediatr,* 1941, 19:229-240.

[32] Eldering G, Kendrick PL. Incidence of parapertussis in the Grand Rapids area as indicated by 16 years' experience with diagnostic cultures, *Am J Public Health,* 1952, 42:27-31.

[33] Trembath B. Whooping cough "breaking through" vaccines, *ABC News Online*, 21st March, 2012.

[34] He Q, Viljanen MK, Arvilommi H, et al. Whooping cough caused by Bordetella pertussis and Bordetella parapertussis in an immunized population, *JAMA*, 1998, 280(7):635-637.

[35] Long GH, Karanikas AT, Harvill ET, et al. Acellular pertussis vaccination facilitates *Bordetella parapertussis* infection in a rodent model of bordetellosis**,** *Proc Biol Sci*, 2010, 277(1690):2017-2025.

[36] CDC. Meeting of the Board of Scientific Counselors, Office of Infectious Diseases Centers for Disease Control and Prevention Tom Harkins Global Communication Center Atlanta, Georgia, Dec 11, 2013. http://www.cdc.gov/maso/facm/pdfs/bscoid/2013121112_bscoid_minutes.pdf (page 6). Accessed February, 2017.

[37] Martin SW, Pawloski L, Williams M, et al. Pertactin-negative Bordetella pertussis strains: evidence for a possible selective advantage, *Clin Infect Dis*, 2015, 60(2):223-227.

[38] Kaplan SL, Barson WJ, Lin PL, et al. Serotype 19A Is the most common serotype causing invasive pneumococcal infections in children, *Pediatrics*, 2010, 125(3):429-436.

[39] Dagan R. Impact of pneumococcal conjugate vaccine on infections caused by antibiotic-resistant streptococcus pneumoniae, *Clin Microbiol Infect*, 2009, 3:16-20.

[40] Hsu KK, Shea KM, Stevenson AE, et al. Changing serotypes causing childhood invasive pneumococcal disease: Massachusetts, 2001-2007, *Paediatr Infect Dis J*, 2010, 29(4):289-293.

[41] Hendrickson DJ, Blumberg DA, Joad JP, et al. Five-fold increase in pediatric parapneumonic empyema since introduction of pneumococcal conjugate vaccine, *Pediatr Infect Dis J*, 2008, 27(11): 1030-1032.

[42] Ribeiro GS, Reis JN, Cordeiro SM, et al. Prevention of haemophilus influenzae type b (Hib) meningitis and emergence of serotype replacement with Type A strains after introduction of Hib immunization in Brazil, *J Infect Dis*, 2003, 187:109-116.

[43] Perdue DG, Bulkow LR, Gellin BG, et al. Invasive haemophilus influenza type b disease in Alaskan residents aged 10 years or older before and after infant vaccination programs, *JAMA*, 2000, 283(23): 3089-3094.

[44] Bender JM, Cox CM, Mottice S, et al. Invasive haemophilus influenzae disease in Utah children: an 11 year population-based study in the era of conjugate vaccine, *Clin Infect Dis*, 2010, 50(7):e41-46.

[45] Giufre M, Cardines R, Caporali MG, et al. Ten years of Hib vaccination in Italy: prevalence of non-encapsulated Haemophilus influenzae among invasive isolates and the possible impact on antibiotic resistance, *Vaccine*, 2011, 29(22):3857-3862.

[46] McConnell A, Tan B, Scheifele D, et al. Invasive infections caused by haemophilus influenzae serotypes in twelve canadian IMPACT centers, 1996-2001, *Paediatr Infect Dis J*, 2007, 26(11):1025-1031.

[47] Ulanova M, Tsang RS. Haemophilus influenzae serotype a as a cause of serious invasive infections, *Lancet Infect Dis*, 2014, 14(1):70-82.

[48] Lahra MM, Enriquez RP, National Neisseria Network. Australian meningococcal surveillance program annual report, 2015, *Commun Dis Intell Q Rep*, 2016, 40(4):e503-511.

[49] Baccarini C, Ternouth A, Wieffer H, Vyse A. The changing epidemiology of meningococcal disease in North America, 1945-2010, *Hum Vaccin Immunother*, 2013, 9(1):162-171.

[50] Patel MS. Australia's century of meningococcal disease: development and the changing ecology of an accidental pathogen, *Med J Aust*, 2007, 186(3):136-141.

[51] Aubusson K. All high school seniors offered free meningococcal vaccine to combat rising W strain, *Sydney Morning Herald*, Feb 6, 2017.

[52] Henry S. A Pox on My Child: Cool! *The Washington Post*, September 2005.

[53] Romagnani S. Biology of human TH1 and TH2 cells, *J Clin Immunol*, 1995, 15:121-129.

[54] Silverberg JI, Norowitz KB, Kleiman E, et al. Varicella zoster virus (wild type) infection, but not varicella vaccine, in late childhood is associated with delayed asthma onset, milder symptoms and decreased atopy, *Pediatr Asthma Allergy Immunol*, 2009, 22:15-20.

[55] Illi S, von Mutius E, Lau S, et al. Early childhood infectious diseases and the development of asthma up to school age: a birth cohort study, *BMJ*, 2001, 322:390-395.

[56] Sasco AJ, Paffenbarger RS, Jr. Measles infection and Parkinson's disease, *Am J Epidemiol*, 1985, 122:1017-1031.

[57] Cramer DW, Vitoris AF, Pinheiro SP, et al. Mumps and ovarian cancer: modern interpretation of an historic association, *Cancer Causes Control*, 2010, 21(8):1193-1201.

[58] West RO. Epidemiological studies of malignancies of the ovaries, *Cancer*, 1966, 19(7):1001-1007.

[59] Wrensch M, Weinber A, Wiencke J, et al. History of chickenpox and shingles and prevalence of antibodies to varicella-zoster virus and three other herpesviruses among adults with glioma and controls, *Am J Epidemiol*, 2005, 161:929-938.

[60] Wolpert S. Childhood infections provide lifelong protection against flu viruses that come from animals, *UCLA Newsroom*, 10th November, 2016.

[61] Mota C. Infantile Hodgkins' disease: remission after measles, *BMJ*, 1973, 2(5863):421.

[62] Aref S, Bailey K, Fielding A. Measles to the Rescue: A Review Of Oncolytic Measles Virus, *Viruses,* 2016, 8(10):294.

[63] Msaouel P, Dispenzieri A, Galanis E. Clinical testing of engineered oncolytic measles virus strains in the treatment of cancer: An overview, *Curr Opin Mol Ther*, 2009, 11(1):43-53.

[64] Lederberg J. Letter-to-the-editor, *Science*, Oct 20, 1967:313.

[65] Choi SW, Friso S. Epigenetics: A New Bridge Between Nutrition and Health, *Adv Nutri*, 2010, 1:8-16.

[66] Hou L, Zhang X, Wang D, Baccarelli A. Environmental chemical exposures and human epigenetics, *Int J Epidemiol*, 2012, 41(1):79-105.

[67] Paschos K, Allday MJ. Epigenetic reprogramming of host genes in viral and microbial pathogenesis, *Trends in Microbiol*, 2010, 18(10):439-447.

[68] Carlquist JF, Anderson JL. Pharmacogenetic mechanisms underlying unanticipated drug reactions, *Discov Med*, 2011, 11(60):469-478.

[69] Adhya D, Basu A. Epigenetic modulation of host: new insights into immune evasion by viruses, *J Biosci*, 2010, 35:647-663.

[70] Stanford Medicine: Viral Proteins May Regulate Human Embryonic Development, http://med.stanford.edu/news/all-news/2015/04/viral-proteins-may-regulate-human-embry-onic-development.html. Accessed May 2019.

[71] Intramural Research Program, Germ-Free Mice, https://irp.nih.gov/catalyst/v19i4/germ-free-mice. Accessed April, 2019.

[72] Zimmermann P, Curtis N. The influence of the intestinal microbiome on vaccine responses, *Vaccine*, 2018, 36(30):4433-4439.

[73] Biesbroek G, Wang X, Keijser B, et al. Seven-valent pneumococcal conjugate vaccine and nasopharyngeal microbiota in healthy children, *Emerg Infect Dis*, 2014, 20(2):201-210.

[74] van Gils EJM, Hak E, Veenhoven RH, et al. Effect of seven-valent pneumococcal conjugate vaccine on *Staphylococcus aureus* colonisation in a randomised controlled trial, *PloS ONE*, 2011, 6:e20229.

[75] Camilli R, Vescio MF, Giufre M, et al. Carriage of hae-mophilis influenzae is associated with pneumococcal vaccina-tion in Italian children, *Vaccine*, 2015, 33(36):4559-4564.

[76] Sanicas M. Can we find a vaccine for Staph Aureus? *World Economic Forum*, 19th February 2016.

[77] Spijkerman J, Prevaes SM, van Gils EJ, et al. Long-term effects of pneumococcal conjugate vaccine on nasopharyngeal carriage of S. pneumoniae, S. aureus, H. influenzae and M. ca-tarrhalis, *PloS One*, 2012, 7(6):e39730.

[78] Luczynski P, McVey Neufeld KA, Oriach CS, et al. Growing up in a bubble: Using germ-free animals to assess the influence of the gut microbiota on brain and behaviour, *Int J Neuropsy-chopharmacol*, 2016, 19(8):pyw020.

[79] NZ Ministry of Health. Tips following immunisation, https://www.health.govt.nz/your-health/healthy-living/im-munisation/tips-following-immunisation, Accessed May, 2019.

[80] Schlune A, Mayatepek E. Glutathione synthetase defi-ciency – An inborn error of the gamma-glutamyl cycle, *J Pedi-atr Sci,* 2011, 3(70):2505–2509.

[81] Lu SC. Regulation of glutathione synthesis, *Mol Aspects Med*, 2009, 30:42–59.

[82] Griffith OW. Biologic and pharmacologic regulation of mammalian glutathione synthesis, *Free Radic Biol Med*, 1999, 27:922–935.

[83] Mitchell JR, Jollow DJ, Potter WZ, et al. Acetaminophen-induced hepatic necrosis. IV. Protective role of glutathione, *J Pharmacol Exp Ther*, 1973, 187:211–217.

[84] Davis DC, Potter WZ, Jollow DJ, Mitchell JR. Species dif-ferences in hepatic glutathione depletion, covalent binding and hepatic necrosis after acetaminophen, *Life Sci*, 1974, 14:2099–2109.

[85] Adams JB, Baral M, Geis E, et al. The severity of autism is associated with toxic metal body burden and red blood cell glutathione levels, *J Toxicol,* 2009, 2009:532640.

[86] Torres AR. Is fever suppression involved in the etiology of autism and neurodevelopmental disorders? *BMC Pediatr,* 2003, 2:3–9.

[87] Schultz ST, Klonoff-Cohen HS, Wingard DL, et al. Acetaminophen (paracetamol) use, measles-mumps rubella vaccination, and autistic disorder: The results of a parent survey, *Autism,* 2008, 12(3):293–307.

[88] Schultz ST. Can autism be triggered by acetaminophen activation of the endocannabinoid system? *Acta Neurobiol Exp,* 2010, 70(2):227–231.

[89] Becker KG, Schultz ST. Similarities in features of autism and asthma and a possible link to acetaminophen use, *Med Hypotheses,* 2010, 74(1):7–11.

[90] Kristensen DM, Lesné L, Le Fol V, et al. Paracetamol (acetaminophen), aspirin (acetylsalicylic acid) and indomethacin are anti-androgenic in the rat foetal testis, *Int J Androl,* 2012, 35(3):377-384.

[91] Albert O, Desdoits-Lethimonier C, Lesné L, et al. Paracetamol, aspirin and indomethacin display endocrine disrupting properties in the adult human testis in vitro, *Hum Reprod,* 2013, 28(7):1890-1898.

[92] Frye CA, Bo E, Calamandrei G, et al. Endocrine disrupters: a review of some sources, effects, and mechanisms of actions on behaviour and neuroendocrine systems, *J Neuroendocrinol,* 2012, 24(1):144-159.

[93] Colborn T. Neurodevelopment and endocrine disruption, *Environ Health Perspect,* 2004, 112(9):944-949.

[94] Liew Z, Ritz B, Rebordosa C, et al. Acetaminophen use during pregnancy, behavioral problems, and hyperkinetic disorders, *JAMA Pediatr,* 2014, 168(4):313–320.

[95] Avella-Garcia CB, Julvez J, Fortuny J, et al. Acetaminophen use in pregnancy and neurodevelopment: attention function and autism spectrum symptoms, *Int J Epidem*, 2016, 45(6):1987–1996,

[96] DrugWatch. Tylenol, https://www.drugwatch.com/tylenol/, Accessed May, 2019.

[97] Machado GC, Maher CG, Ferreira PH, et al. Efficacy and safety of paracetamol for spinal pain and osteoarthritis: systematic review and meta-analysis of randomised placebo-controlled trials, *BMJ,* 2015, 350:h1225

[98] Ibid. See reference #87.

[99] Squires RH, Jr, Shneider BL, Bucuvalas J, et al. Acute liver failure in children: the first 348 patients in the pediatric acute liver failure study group, *J Pediatr*, 2006, 148:652–658.

[100] Mischkowski D, Crocker J, Way BM. From painkiller to empathy killer: acetaminophen (paracetamol) reduces empathy for pain, *Soc Cog Affect Neuro,* 2016, 11(9):1345–1353.

[101] Congressional Record: Research and Scientific Integrity, House of Representatives, July 29, 2015, https://www.congress.gov/congressional-record/2015/7/29/house-section/article/H5602-1, Accessed May, 2019.

[102] PR Newswire, CDC blocks testimony of CDC whistleblower, says World Mercury project, http://www.prnewswire.com/news-releases/cdc-blocks-testimony-of-vaccine-whistleblower-says-world-mercury-project-300347376.html, Accessed May, 2019.

[103] Alliance for Human Research Protection, Principal research investigator for CDC Utah autism data filed whistleblower lawsuit, http://ahrp.org/lawsuit-by-principal-

investigator-for-cdc-utah-autism-data-filed-whistleblower-lawsuit/, Accessed May, 2019.

[104] Solomon L, Merck has some explaining to do over its MMR vaccine claims, Huffington Post, 27th November, 2014.

[105] Alliance for Human Research protection, Former Merck scientists sue Merck alleging MMR vaccine efficacy fraud, http://ahrp.org/former-merck-scientists-sue-merck-alleging-mmr-vaccine-efficacy-fraud/, Accessed May, 2019.

[106] Corrigan S, Former science chief: MMR fears coming true, *Daily Mail*, 22nd May, 2016.

[107] Health Resources Services Administration (HRSA), National Vaccine Program, https://www.hrsa.gov/vaccinecompensation/about/titlexxiphsvaccines1517.pdf, Accessed May, 2019.

[108] Vaccine Supply and Innovation, National Research Council (US) Division of Health Promotion and Disease Prevention, Washington (DC): National Academies Press (US), 1985.

[109] US Department of Health and Human Services, The National Vaccine Injury Compensation program https://www.hrsa.gov/vaccine-compensation/index.html, Accessed May, 2019.

[110] Holland MS, Krakow RJ. Brief of Amici Curiae National Vaccine Information Center, Its Co-Founders and 24 other organizations in support of petitioners. In: *Bruesewitz v. Wyeth* filed with Supreme Court of the United States June 1, 2010.

[111] Vernick JS, Mair JS, Tenet SP, Sapsin JW. Role of litigation in preventing product-related injuries *Epidemiol Rev,* 2003, 25(1):90-98.

[112] Supreme Court of the United States. *Bruesewitz v. Wyeth* No. 09-152. Justice Scalia delivering opinion Feb. 22, 2011, https://www.supremecourt.gov/opinions/10pdf/09-152.pdf, Accessed May, 2019.

[113] National Vaccine Information Centre: Gao Review, https://www.nvic.org/cmstemplates/nvic/pdf/vicp/nvic-gao-response-on-vicp-07112014.pdf, Accessed May, 2019.

[114] US Department of Health and Human Services, Vaccine Compensation Data, https://www.hrsa.gov/sites/default/files/hrsa/vaccine-compensation/data/monthly-stats-may-2019.pdf, Accessed May, 2019.

[115] US Department of Health and Human Services, Vaccine Injury Table, https://www.hrsa.gov/sites/default/files/vaccinecompensation/vaccineinjurytable.pdf, Accessed May, 2019.

[116] DHHS. Final Rule: National Vaccine Injury Compensation Program Revision of the Vaccine Injury Table. *Federal Register* Feb. 8, 1995, 60(26):7678-7695.

[117] The National Vaccine Injury Compensation Program: Awareness, Perception, and Communication Considerations. Presented Oct. 2010 by Banyan Communications and Altarum Institute to the Advisory Commission on Childhood Vaccines in June 2010. Provided by NVIC to GAO staff July 2014.

[118] Rubin R. Court rules autism not connected to vaccines, *USA Today, 13th* Feb, 2009.

[119] U.S. Court of Federal Claims, Omnibus Autism Proceeding: Guidance to Petitioners on How to Exit the Vaccine Program. Oct. 10, 2012.

[120] Health Resources Services Administration (HRSA). Advisory Commission on Childhood Vaccines (ACCV) Transcript: Comments of Vince Matanoski, Deputy Director, Torts Branch, Dept. of Justice (pp. 25-26) Sept. 5, 2013.

[121] Williams WW, Peng JL, O'Halloran A, et al. Surveillance of vaccine coverage among adult populations - 2014, *MMWR*, 2016, 65(1):1-36

[122] Centers for Disease Control (CDC). Recommended schedule for active immunization of normal infants and children, *DHHS,* 1983.

[123] American Medical Association Council on Ethical and Judicial Affairs, "Reporting Adverse Drug and Medical Device Events" Code of medical ethics: reports of the Council on Ethical and Judicial Affairs of the American Medical Association, 1993, 4:183-189.

[124] Wood AJ. Thrombotic thrombocytopenic purpura and clopidogrel: a need for new approaches to drug safety, *N Engl J Med*, 2000, 342(24):1824-1826.

[125] Institute of Medicine, Preventing Medication Errors: Quality Chasm Series, Washington DC: National Academy Press, 2006.

[126] Congressional Record: Mercury in Medicine Report, Available at: https://www.gpo.gov/fdsys/pkg/CREC-2003-05-21/pdf/CREC-2003-05-21-pt1-PgE1011-3.pdf, Accessed May, 2019.

[127] Juretic M. Exanthema subitum, a review of 243 cases, *Helv Paed Acta*, 1963, 18:80-95.

[128] Centers for Disease Control and Prevention, Manual for the Surveillance of Vaccine-preventable Diseases: Diptheria, https://www.cdc.gov/vaccines/pubs/surv-manual/chpt01-dip.html, Accessed May, 2019.

[129] Centers for Disease Control and Prevention, Manual for Surveillance of Vaccine-preventable Diseases: Measles, https://www.cdc.gov/vaccines/pubs/surv-manual/chpt07-measles.html, Accessed May, 2019.

[130] Francombe H. Measles diagnosis unreliable, *Australian Doctor*, Feb 18, 2000.

[131] Society to Improve Diagnosis in Medicine. Reducing Harm From Diagnostic Error, http://www.improvediagnosis.org/, Accessed October, 2017.

CHAPTER 8: VACCINE SIDE EFFECTS

[1] Nobel Lecture: Charles Richet, The Nobel Prize in Medicine or Physiology, 1913. https://www.nobelprize.org/nobel_prizes/medicine/laureates/1913/richet-lecture.html. Accessed January, 2017.
[2] Wells HG. Studies on the chemistry of anaphylaxis, *J Inf Dis*, 1908, 5:449-483.
[3] Ratner B, Untracht S, Hertzmark F. Allergy to viral and Rickettsial vaccines – influence of repeated inoculations on the acquisition of egg allergy, *N Engl J Med*, 1952, 246:533-536.
[4] Yamane N, Uemura H. Serological examination of IgE- and IgG-specific antibodies to egg protein during influenza virus immunization, *Epidem Infect*, 1988, 100:291-299.
[5] Nakayama T, Aizawa C, Kuno-Sakai H. A clinical analysis of gelatin allergy and determination of its causal relationship to the previous administration of gelatin-containing acellular pertussis vaccine combined with diptheria and tetanus toxoids. *J Allergy Clin Immunol*, 1999, 103:321-325.
[6] Jones SW. Peanut oil used in new vaccine; product patented for Merck said to extend immunity, *New York Times*, 19th September, 1964.
[7] Gecher P (Editor). Encyclopedia of Emulsion Technology: Applications, Marcel Dekker, 1985, p191.
[8] Hotchkiss M. Princeton researcher digs into the contested peanut allergy epidemic. https://www.princeton.edu/main/news/archive/S37/46/79G28/index.xml?section=topstories. Accessed May, 2019.

[9] Horino A, Taneichi M, Naito S, Ami Y, Suzaki Y. Cytokine production by spleen cells from mice with ovalbumin-specific, IgE-selective unresponsiveness induced by ovalbumin-liposome conjugate. *Allergology Int*, 1997, 46(4):249-253.

[10] Birmingham N, Thanesvorakul S, Gangur V. Relative immunogenicity of commonly allergenic food versus rarely allergenic and non-allergenic foods in mice, *J Food Prot*, 2002, 65(12):1988-1991.

[11] IOM (Institute of Medicine). Adverse effects of vaccines: evidence and causality, Washington DC: The National Academies Press, 2012.

[12] Wakefield AJ, Murch SH, Anthony A, et al. Ileal-lymphoid hyperplasia, non-specific colitis, and pervasive developmental disorder in children, *The Lancet*, 1998, 351(9103):637-641.

[13] Science summary: CDC Studies on Thimerosal in Vaccines. https://www.cdc.gov/vaccinesafety/pdf/cdcstudiesonvaccinesandautism.pdf. Accessed 29th January, 2017.

[14] US Department of Health and Human Services: Office of Inspector General, Fugitive Profiles, https://oig.hhs.gov/fraud/fugitives/profiles.asp. Accessed May 2019.

[15] Verstraeten T, Davis RL, Gu D, DeStefano F. Increased risk of developmental neurologic impairment after high exposure to thimerosal-containing vaccine in first month of life, *Proceedings of the Epidemic Intelligence Service Annual Conference*, April, 2000.

[16] Verstraeten T, Davis RL, DeStefano F, et al. Safety of thimerosal-containing vaccines: a two-phased study of computerized health maintenance organization databases, *Pediatrics*, 2003, 112(5): 1039-1048.

[17] Hooker B, Kern J, Geier D, et al. Methodological issues and evidence of malfeasance in research purporting to show thimerosal in vaccines is safe, *Biomed Res Int*, 2014, 2014:247218.

[18] Blaylock RI. The danger of excessive vaccination during brain development, *Medical Veritas*, 2008, 5(1):1727-1741.

[19] Blaylock RI. Chronic microglial activation and excitotoxicity secondary to excessive immune stimulation: possible factors in Gulf War Syndrome and autism. *J Amer Phys Surg*, 2004, 9(2):46-52.

[20] Vargas DL, Nascimbene C, Zimmerman AW, Pardo CA. Brain inflammation found in autism. *Annals of Neurology*, 2005, 57:67-81.

[21] Delong G. A positive association found between autism prevalence and childhood vaccination uptake across the U.S population, *J Toxicol Enviro Health*, 2011, 74(14): 903-916.

[22] Tomljenovic L, Shaw CA. Do aluminium vaccine adjuvants contribute to the rising prevalence of autism? *J Inorg Biochem*, 2011, 105(11): 1489-1499.

[23] Deisher TA, Doan NV, Omaiye A, et al. Impact of environmental factors on the prevalence of autistic disorder after 1979, *J Public Health Epidem*, 2014, 6(9):271-284.

[24] Aran A, Eylon M, Harel M, et al. Lower circulating endocannabinoid levels in children with autism spectrum disorder, *Mol Autism*, 2019, 10:2.

[25] Acharya N, Penukonda S, Shcheglova T, et al. Endocannabinoids regulate immunity in the gut, *Proc Nat Acad Sci*, 2017, 114(19):5005-5010.

[26] Dotsey E, Ushach I, Pone E, et al. Transient cannabinoid receptor 2 blockade during immunization heightens intensity and breadth of antigen-specific antibody responses in young and aged mice, *Sci Rep*, 2017, 7:42584.

[27] Schultz ST, Gould GG. Acetaminophen Use for Fever in Children Associated with Autism Spectrum Disorder, *Autism Open Access*, 2016, 6(2):170.

[28] Cherrin P, Gherardi RK. Emergence of a new entity, macrophagic myofascitis, *Rev Rhum Engl Ed*, 1998, 65:541-542.

[29] Authier FJ, Cherin P, Creange A, et al. Central nervous system disease in patients with macrophagic myofascitis, *Brain*, 2001, 124:974-983.

[30] Papo T. Macrophagic myofascitis: focal or systemic? *Joint Bone Spine*, 2003, 70:242-245.

[31] Gherardi RK, Coquet M, Cherin P, et al. Macrophagic myofascitis lesions assess long-term persistence of vaccine-derived aluminium hydroxide in muscle, *Brain*, 2001, 124(9):1821-1831.

[32] Israeli E, Agmon-Levin N, Blank M, Shoenfeld Y. Macrophagic myofascitis a vaccine (alum) autoimmune-related disease, *Clin Rev Allergy Immunol*, 2011, 41(2):163-168.

[33] Gherardi R, Eidi H, Crepeaux G, et al. Biopersistence and brain translocation of aluminium adjuvants of vaccines, *Front Neurol, 2015*. https://doi.org/10.3389/fneur.2015.00004, Accessed May, 2019.

[34] Mount HR, Boyle SD, Aseptic and bacterial meningitis: Evaluation, treatment and prevention, *Am Fam Physician*, 2017, 96(5):314-322.

[35] Miller E, Farrington P, Goldacre M, et al, Risk of aseptic meningitis after measles, mumps, and rubella vaccine in UK children, *The Lancet*, 1993, 341(8851):979-982.

[36] Miller E, Andrews N, Stowe J, et al. Risks of Convulsion and Aseptic Meningitis following Measles-Mumps-Rubella Vaccination in the United Kingdom, *Am J Epidem*, 2007, 165(6):704–709.

[37] Autret E, Jonville-Bera AP, Galy-Eyraud C, Hessel L. Aseptic meningitis after mumps vaccination, *Therapie*, 1996, 51(6):681-3.

[38] Fujinaga T, Motegi Y, Tamura H, Kuruome T. A prefecture-wide survey of mumps meningitis associated with measles, mumps and rubella vaccine, *Pediatr Infect Dis J*, 1991, 10(3):204-209.

[39] Dourado I, Cunha S, Teixeira MG, et al. Outbreak of aseptic meningitis associated with mass vaccination with a Urabe-containing measles-mumps-rubella vaccine: implications for immunization programs, *Am J Epidemiol*, 2000, 151(5):524-30.

[40] Khalfan S, Aymard M, Lina B, et al. Epidemics of aseptic meningitis due to enteroviruses following national immunization days in Bahrain, *Ann Trop Paed*, 1998, 18(2):101-109.

[41] CDC, Acute Flaccid Myelitis, https://www.cdc.gov/acute-flaccid-myelitis/index.html. Accessed May 2019.

[42] Goldschmidt D. AFM: CDC identifies 31 states with 116 confirmed cases of polio-like illness, CNN, 28th November 2018.

[43] Snoderly J. Polio-like illness reaches WV, official confirms, West Virginia News, 11th April 2019.

[44] Cunningham AS. Outbreaks of acute flaccid myelitis in the US, BMJ, 2018, 363:k5246.

[45] National Institute of Neurological Disorders and Stroke, Transverse Myelitis Fact Sheet, https://www.ninds.nih.gov/Disorders/Patient-Caregiver-Education/Fact-Sheets/Transverse-Myelitis-Fact-Sheet, Accessed May 2019.

[46] Karussis D, Petrou P. The spectrum of post-vaccination inflammatory CNS demyelinating syndromes, *Autoimmunity Reviews*, 2014, 13(3):215-224.

[47] Nakamura N, Nokura K, Zettsu T, et al. Neurologic complications associated with influenza vaccination: two adult cases, *Intern Med*, 2003, 42(2):191-194.

[48] Anne Dachel. Coleman 1, Youtube, https://www.youtube.com/watch?v=XucLg8iTkH8. Accessed May 2019.

[49] Chang H, Lee HL, Yeo M, et al. Recurrent optic neuritis and neuromyelitis optica IgG following first and second human papillomavirus vaccinations, *Clin Neurol Neurosurg*, 2016, 144:126-128.

[50] Cho JH, Park Y, Woo N. A case of neuromyelitis optica spectrum disorder following seasonal influenza vaccination, *Mult Scler Rel Dis*, 2019, 30:110-113.

[51] MCT Law, Neuromyelitis Optica or Devic's Disease, https://www.mctlaw.com/vaccine-injury/neuromyelitis-optica-or-optic-neuritis/. Accessed May 2019.

[52] Huynh W, Cordato DJ, Kehdi E, et al. Post-vaccination encephalomyelitis: literature review and illustrative case, *J Clin Neurosci*, 2008, 15(12):1315-22.

[53] Sekiguchi K, Yasui N, Kowa H, et al. Two Cases of Acute Disseminated Encephalomyelitis Following Vaccination Against Human Papilloma Virus, *Intern Med*, 2016, 55(21):3181–3184.

[54] O'Neill J. Did Flu Shot Cause 9-Year Old To Go Blind, Become Paralyzed? Yahoo, 5th November 2015.

[55] Mehta P, Kaye W, Raymond J, et al. Prevalence of Amyotrophic Lateral Sclerosis – United States, 2014, *MMWR Weekly*, 2018, 67(7);216–218.

[56] Su F, Goutman SA, Chernyak S, et al. Association of Environmental Toxins With Amyotrophic Lateral Sclerosis. *JAMA Neurol*. 2016;73(7):803–811.

[57] Ibid.

[58] Mayo Clinic, Amyotrophic Lateral Sclerosis (ALS), https://www.mayoclinic.org/diseases-conditions/amyo-trophic-lateral-sclerosis/symptoms-causes/syc-20354022. Accessed May 2019.

[59] Grady D. A Second Drug is Approved to Treat A.L.S, The New York Times, 5th May, 2017.

[60] ALS Association, ALS Ice Bucket Challenge Commitments, http://www.alsa.org/fight-als/ice-bucket-challenge-spend-ing.html#clin-pilot-2016. Accessed May 2019.

[61] Military Health System, Vaccine Recommendations by AOR, https://www.health.mil/MHSHome/Mili-tary%20Health%20Topics/Health%20Readiness/Immuniza-tion%20Healthcare/Vaccine%20Recommendations/Vac-cine%20Recommendations%20by%20AOR#NORTHCOM. Accessed May 2019.

[62] Hikiami R, Yamakado H, Tatsumi S, et al. Amyotrophic Lateral Sclerosis after Receiving the Human Papilloma Virus Vaccine: A Case Report of a 15-year-old Girl, *Intern Med*, 2018;57(13):1917–1919.

[63] Roos, PM, Vesterberg O, Syversen T et al. Metal Concentrations in Cerebrospinal Fluid and Blood Plasma from Patients with Amyotrophic Lateral Sclerosis, *Biol Trace Elem Res*, 2013, 151: 159.

[64] Senerviratne U. Guillain Barre Syndrome, *Postgrad Med J*, 2000, 76:774-782.

[65] Hardy A. 'Straight Back to Barbarism' : Antityphoid inoculation and the Great War, 1914, *Bull Hist Med*, 2000, 74: 265-290.

[66] Ibid. See reference #64.

[67] Garloch K. Former Mooresville child compensated by federal "vaccine court", *Charlotte Observer*, 28th February, 2015.

[68] CDC, Data and Statistics for Cerebral Palsy, https://www.cdc.gov/ncbddd/cp/data.html. Accessed May 2019.

[69] Nabi S, Methylmercury and Minamata Disease: *Toxic Effects of Mercury*, Springer, New Delhi, 2014, pp. 187–199.

[70] US Food & Drug Administration, Mercury in Plasma-Derived Products, https://www.fda.gov/vaccines-blood-biologics/safety-availability-biologics/mercury-plasma-derived-products. Accessed May 2019.

[71] Foster K. Doctors believe they have discovered the cause of multiple sclerosis, *The Daily Telegraph*, 24th July 2018.

[72] <u>Kaplanski G, Retornaz F, Durand J, Soubeyrand J.</u> Central nervous system demyelination after vaccination against hepatitis B and HLA haplotype, *J Neurol Neurosurg Psychiatry*, 1995, 58(6):758-759.

[73] Herroelen L, de Keyser J, Ebinger G. Central-nervous-system demyelination after immunisation with recombinant hepatitis B vaccine, *The Lancet*, 1991, 338(8776):1174-1175.

[74] Mikaeloff Y, Caridade G, Suissa S, Tardieu M. Hepatitis B vaccine and the risk of CNS inflammatory demyelination in childhood, *Neurology*, 2009; 72(10):873-880.

[75] Le Houézec D. Evolution of multiple sclerosis in France since the beginning of hepatitis B vaccination, *Immunol Res*, 2014, 60(2-3):219–225.

[76] Porter R. The longest goodbye: A father's agonizing account of why baby Christopher's body has been in a mortuary for 21 years, *Daily Mail*, 2nd August 2008.

[77] WHO. International Statistical Classification of Diseases and Related Health problems, 10th Revision, Geneva Switzerland: World Health Organization, 1992.

[78] CDC. Table 31. Number of infant deaths and infant mortality rates for 130 selected causes, by race, United States, 2006, *Natl Vital Stat Rep*, 2009, 57:110-112.

[79] Bergman AB, Beckwith JB, Ray CG. Sudden Infant Death Syndrome. Proceedings of the Second International Conference on Causes of Sudden Death in Infants, Seattle and London, University of Washington press, 1970:18.

[80] Bergman AB. The "discovery" of Sudden Infant Death Syndrome, New York, USA, Praeger Publishers, 1989.

[81] Howson CP, Howe CJ, Fineberg HV. Adverse Effects of Pertussis and Rubella Vaccines: A Report of the Committee to Review the Adverse Consequences of Pertussis and Rubella Vaccines. Washington (DC), *National Academies Press*, 1991.

[82] Werne J, Garrow I. Fatal anaphylactic shock: occurrence in identical twins following second injection of diphtheria toxoid and pertussis antigen, *JAMA*, 1946, 131:730-735.

[83] Roberts SC. Vaccination and cot deaths in perspective, *Archives of Disease in Childhood*, 1987, 62(7):754-759.

[84] Baker JP. The pertussis vaccine controversy in Great Britain, 1974-1986, *Vaccine*, 2003, 21:4003-4010.

[85] Norman P, Gregory I, Dorling D, Baker A. Geographical Trends in Infant Mortality 1970-2006, *Health Stat Q*, 2008, 40:18-29.

[86] Cherry JD, Brunell PA, Golden GS, Karzon DT. Report of the Task Force on Pertussis and Pertussis Immunization—1988, *Pediatrics*, 1988, 81(6):933-984.

[87] National Institute of Child Health and Human Development, Key Moments in Safe to Sleep History: 1994-2003, https://safetosleep.nichd.nih.gov/activities/SIDS/progress, Accessed May, 2019.

[88] Malloy MH, MacDorman M. Changes in the classification of sudden unexpected infant deaths: United States, 1992-2001, *Pediatrics*, 2005, 115:1247-1253.

[89] Ibid.

[90] Ridgway D. Disputed Claims for Pertussis Vaccine Injuries Under the National Vaccine Injury Compensation Program, *J Investig Med*, 1998, 46:168–74.

[91] Ottaviani G, Lavezzi AM, Matturri L. Sudden Infant Death Syndrome (SIDS) shortly after hexavalent vaccination: another pathology in suspected SIDS? *Virchows Arch*, 2006, 448:100-104.

[92] Zinka B, Rauch E, Buettner A, et al. Unexplained cases of sudden infant death shortly after hexavalent vaccination, *Vaccine*, 2006, 24:5779-5780.

[93] Zinka B, Penning R. Unexplained cases of sudden infant death shortly after hexavalent vaccination. Letter to Editor. Response to the comment by HJ Schmitt et al. *Vaccine*, 2006, 24:5785-5786.

[94] CDC. Sudden Infant Death Syndrome (SIDS), https://www.cdc.gov/vaccinesafety/Concerns/sids.html, Accessed May 2019.

[95] Miller NZ, Goldman GS. Infant mortality rates regressed against number of vaccine doses routinely given: is there a biochemical or synergistic toxicity? *Hum Exp Toxicol*, 2011, 30(9):1420-1428.

[96] Kuhnert R, Hecker H, Poethko-Muller C, et al. A modified self-controlled case series method to examine association between multidose vaccines and death, *Stat Med*, 2011, 30(6):666-77.

[97] Traversa G, Spila-Alegiani S, Bianchi C, et al. Sudden Unexpected Deaths and Vaccinations during the First Two Years

of Life in Italy: A Case Series Study, *PLoS ONE*, 2011, 6(1):e16363.

[98] The Justice Gap. Shaken Baby Syndrome and the fight for justice, http://thejusticegap.com/2012/08/shaken-baby-syndrome-and-the-fight-for-justice/, Accessed October, 2017.

[99] Reid S. The Shaken Baby Martyr: Top brain doctor who was struck off for controversial claims speaks out on how jailed parents could be innocent, *The Daily Mail*, December 10, 2016.

[100] Dyer O. Brain haemorrhage in babies may not indicate violent abuse, *BMJ*, 2003, 326(7390):616.

[101] Ibid. See reference #99.

[102] Ibid.

[103] Innocent.org. The Tragedy of Sally Clark 1965-2007, https://innocent.org.uk/2016/04/30/the-tragedy-of-sally-clark-1965-2007/, Accessed May, 2019.

[104] Author Unknown. Was Sally Clark's child killed by a vaccine? *The Spectator Archive*, 19 May, 2007, pp 20.

[105] Ibid. See reference #103.

[106] Ibid.

[107] Ibid. See reference #101.

[108] New York State Department of Health, Shaken Baby Syndrome – Facts and Figures, https://www.health.ny.gov/prevention/injury_prevention/shaken_baby_syndrome/sbs_fact_sheet.htm, Accessed January, 2019.

[109] Joyce T, Huecker MR. Pediatric Abusive Head Trauma (Shaken Baby Syndrome). In: StatPearls [Internet]. Treasure Island, Florida, StatPearls Publishing, 2018.

[110] Green MA. A practical approach to suspicious death in infancy--a personal view, *J Clin Pathol*, 1998, 51(8):561-3.

[111] Lynøe N, Elinder G, Hallberg B, et al. Insufficient evidence for 'shaken baby syndrome' - a systematic review, 2017, 106(7):1021-1027.

[112] Kalokerinos A. SBS: An Abusive Diagnosis, 2008, available at https://pdfs.semanticscholar.org/bb7e/8347403638ac98691c58f32f40ea3f4ba678.pdf. Accessed January, 2019.

[113] Ibid.

[114] Schectman G, Byrd JC, Gruchow HW. The influence of smoking on vitamin C status in adults, *Am J Pub Health*, 1989, 79(2):158-162.

[115] Preston AM, Rodriguez C, Rivera CE, Sahai H. Influence of environmental tobacco smoke on Vitamin C status in children, *Am J Clin Nutrition*, 2003, 77(1):167-172.

[116] Yousef MI, El-Morsy AMA, Hassan MS. Aluminium-induced deterioration in reproductive performance and seminal plasma biochemistry of male rabbits: protective role of ascorbic acid, *Toxicology*, 2005, 215(1-2):97-107.

[117] Clemetson CAB. Vaccinations, innoculations and ascorbic acid, *J Orthomol Med*, 1999, Vol 14, 3rd Quarter.

[118] Parrot JL, Richet G. Accroissement de la sensabilité a histamine chez le cobaye soumís a un Régime scorbutogène, *CR Soc Biol*, 1945, 139:1072-1075.

[119] O'Leary ST, Glanz JM, McClure DL, et al. The risk of immune thrombocytopenic purpura after vaccination in children and adolescents, *Pediatrics*, 2012, 129(2):248-55.

[120] Woo EJ, Wise RP, Menschik D, et al. Thrombocytopenia after vaccination: case reports to the US Vaccine Adverse Event Reporting System, 1990-2008, *Vaccine*, 2011, 29(6):1319-1323.

[121] Mayo Clinic, Neutropenia (low neutrophil count), https://www.mayoclinic.org/symptoms/neutropenia/basics/definition/sym-20050854, Accessed May, 2019.

[122] Durbin AP, Whitehead SS, Shaffer D, et al. A Single Dose of the DENV-1 Candidate Vaccine rDEN1Δ30 Is Strongly Immunogenic and Induces Resistance to a Second Dose in a

Randomized Trial. Halstead SB, ed, *PLoS Neglected Tropical Diseases*, 2011, 5(8):e1267.

[123] Hanissian AS, et al. Vasculitis and myositis secondary to rubella vaccination, *Arch Neurol*, 1973, 28:202-204.

[124] Fox BC, Peterson A. Leukocytoclastic vasculitis after pneumococcal vaccination, *Am J Infect Control*, 1998, 26(3):365-6.

[125] Ozaki T, et al. Henoch-Schonlein Purpura after measles immunization, *Acta Paed Jap*, 1989, 31:484-486.

[126] Shimada S, Watanabe T, Sato S. A patient with Kawasaki disease following influenza vaccinations, *Paed Infect Dis J*, 2015, 34(8):913.

[127] de Carvalho JF, Pereira RM, Shoenfeld Y. Systemic poly-arteritis nodosa following hepatitis B vaccination, *Eur J Intern Med*, 2008, 19(8):575-578.

[128] CDC. About Kawasaki Disease, https://www.cdc.gov/kawasaki/about.html, Accessed November, 2017.

[129] Chang RK. Hospitalizations for Kawasaki Disease Among Children in the United States, 1988-1997, *Pediatrics*, 2002, 109(6):e87.

[130] Tseng HF, Sy LS, Liu IL, et al. Postlicensure surveillance for pre-specified adverse events following the 13-valent pneumococcal conjugate vaccine in children, *Vaccine*, 2013, 31(22):2578-83.

[131] Merck. Vaccine Insert for Rotateq, http://www.who.int/immunization_standards/vaccine_quality/RotaTeq_Product_Insert.pdf, Accessed November, 2017.

[132] Shoenfeld Y, Agmon-Levin N. ASIA - autoimmune/inflammatory syndrome induced by adjuvants, *J Autoimmun*, 2011, 36(1):4-8.

[133] European Medicines Agency, Note for Guidance on the Clinical Evaluation of Vaccines,

http://www.ema.europa.eu/docs/en_GB/document_library/Scientific_guideline/2009/09/WC500003875.pdf. Accessed October, 2017.

[134] Colafrancesco S, Perricone C, Tomljenovic L, Shoenfeld Y. Human papillomavirus vaccine and primary ovarian failure: another facet of the autoimmun/inflammatory syndrome induced by adjuvants, *Am J Reprod Immunol*, 2013, 70(4):309-316.

[135] Gatto M, Agmon-Levin N, Soriano A, et al. Human papillomavirus vaccine and systemic lupus erythematosus, *Clin Rheumatol*, 2013, 32(9):1301-1307.

[136] Agmon-Levin N, Zafrir Y, Kivity S, et al. Chronic fatigue syndrome and fibromyalgia following immunization with the hepatitis B vaccine: another angle of the autoimmune/inflammatory syndrome induce by adjuvants, *Immunol Res*, 2014, 60(2-3):376-383.

[137] Bizjak M, Bruck O, Praprtonik S, et al. Pancreatitis after human papillomavirus vaccination: a matter of molecular mimicry, *Immunol Res*, 2016, Epub ahead of print.

[138] Anaya JM, Reyes B, Perdomo-Arciniegas AM, et al. Autoimmune/auto-inflammatory syndrome induced by adjuvants (ASIA) after quadrivalent human papillomavirus vaccination in Colombians: a call for personalised medicine, *Clin Exp Rheumatol*, 2015, 33(4):545-548.

[139] Hernan MA, Jick SS, Olek MJ, Jick H. Recombinant hepatitis B vaccine and the risk of multiple sclerosis: a prospective study, *Neurology*, 2004, 63(5):838-842.

[140] DiMario FJ Jr, Hajjar M, Ciesielski T. A 16-year-old girl with bilateral visual loss and left hemiparesis following an immunization against human papilloma virus, *J Child Neurol*, 2010, 25(3):321-327.

[141] Howson CP, Katz M, Johnston RB Jr, Fineberg HV. Chronic arthritis after rubella vaccination, *Clin Infect Dis*, 1992, 15(2):307-312.

[142] Singh VK, Lin SX, Newell E, Nelson C. Abnormal measles-mumps-rubella antibodies and CNS autoimmunity in children with autism, *J Biomed Sci*, 2002, 9(4):359-364.

[143] Takahashi Y, Matsudaira T, Nakano H, et al. Immunological studies of cerebrospinal fluid from patients with CNS symptoms after human papillomavirus vaccination, *J Neuroimmunol*, 2016, 298:71-78.

[144] Matsuura R, Hamano S, Ikemoto S, et al. Epilepsy with myoclonic atonic seizures and chronic cerebellar symptoms associated with antibodies against glutamate receptors N2B and D2 in serum and cerebrospinal fluid, *Edu J Int League Against Epilepsy*, 2017, 19(1):94-98.

[145] Guimaraes LE, Baker B, Perricone C, Shoenfeld Y. Vaccines, adjuvants and autoimmunity, *Pharmacol Res*, 2015, 100:190-209.

[146] Harel M, Shoenfeld Y. Predicting and preventing autoimmunity, myth or reality? *Ann N Y Acad Sci*, 2006, 1069:322-345.

[147] Soriano A, Nesher G, Shoenfeld Y. Predicting post-vaccination autoimmunity: who might be at risk? *Pharmacol Res*, 2015, 92:18-22.

[148] Valdimarsson H, Thorleifsdottir RH, Sigurdardottir SL, et al. Psoriasis—as an autoimmune disease caused by molecular mimicry, *Trends Immunol*, 2009, 30(10):494–501.

[149] Raaschou-Nielsen W. Psoriasis vaccinalis; report of two cases, one following B.C.G. vaccination and one following vaccination against influenza, *Acta Dermato-Venereologica*, 1955, 35(1):37–42.

[150] Koca R, Altinyazar HC, Numanoğlu G, Ünalacak M. Guttate psoriasis-like lesions following BCG vaccination, *J Trop Ped*, 2004, 50(3):178–179.

[151] Macias VC, Cunha D. Psoriasis triggered by tetanus-diphtheria vaccination, *Cut Ocul Toxicol*, 2013, 32(2):164–165.

[152] Shin MS, Kim SJ, Kim SH, et al. New onset guttate psoriasis following pandemic H1N1 influenza vaccination, *Ann Dermatol*, 2013, 25(4):489–492.

[153] Sbidian E, Eftekahri P, Viguier M, et al. National survey of psoriasis flares after 2009 monovalent H1N1/seasonal vaccines, *Dermatology*, 2014, 229(2):130-135.

[154] Tahsin Gunes A, Fetil E, Akarsu S, et al. Possible triggering effect of influenza vaccination on psoriasis, *J Immunol Res*, 2015, 2015:258430.

[155] WebMD. Skin conditions and eczema, https://www.webmd.com/skin-problems-and-treatments/guide/atopic-dermatitis-eczema#1, Accessed May, 2019.

[156] McKeever TM, Lewis SA, Smith C, Hubbard R. Vaccination and allergic disease: A birth cohort study, *Am J Pub Health*, 2004, 94(6):985-989.

[157] Reynolds AH, Joos HA. Eczema vaccinatum, *Pediatrics*, 1958, 22(2):259-267.

[158] Mayo Clinic, Bullous pemphigoid, https://www.mayoclinic.org/diseases-conditions/bullous-pemphigoid/symptoms-causes/syc-20350414, Accessed May, 2019.

[159] Erbagci Z. Childhood bullous pemphigoid following Hepatitis B immunization, *J Dermatol*, 2002, 29(12):781-785.

[160] Baykal C, Okan G, Sarica R. Childhood bullous pemphigoid developed after the first vaccination, *J Am Acad Dermatol*, 2001, 44(2 Suppl):348-50.

[161] de la Fuente S, Hernandez-Martin A, de Lucas R, et al. Postvaccination bullous pemphigoid in infancy: report of three new cases and literature review, *Pediatr Dermatol*, 2013, 30(6):741-744.

[162] Baroero C, Coppo P, Bertolino L, et al. Three case reports of post immunization and post viral Bullous Pemphigoid: looking for the right trigger, *BMC Pediatrics*, 2017, 17(1):60.

[163] Mayo Clinic. Stevens-Johnson Syndrome, https://www.mayoclinic.org/diseases-conditions/stevens-johnson-syndrome/symptoms-causes/syc-20355936, Accessed May, 2019.

[164] Chopra A, Drage LA, Hansom EM, Touchet NL. Stevens-Johnson syndrome after immunization with smallpox, anthrax, and tetanus vaccines, *Mayo Clin Proc*, 2004, 79(9):1193-1196.

[165] Christou EM, Wargon O. Stevens-Johnson syndrome after varicella vaccination, *Med J Aust*, 2012, 196(4):240-241.

[166] Hazir T, Abbas KA. Stevens-Johnson Syndrome following measles vaccination, *J Pak Med Assoc*, 1997, 47(10):264-5.

[167] Ball R, Ball LK, Wise RP, et al. Stevens-Johnson syndrome and toxic epidermal necrolysis after vaccination: reports to the vaccine adverse event reporting system, *Pediatr Infect Dis J*, 2001, 20(2):219-23.

[168] Leslie DL, Kobre RA, Richmand BJ, et al. Temporal association of certain neuropsychiatric disorders following vaccination of children and adolescents: A pilot case–control study, *Front Psych*, 2017, 8:3.

[169] Sleep Foundation. Narcolepsy, https://sleepfoundation.org/narcolepsy/content/what-narcolepsy, Accessed May, 2019.

[170] Heier MS, Gautvik KM, Wannag E, et al. Incidence of narcolepsy in Norwegian children and adolescents after

vaccination against H1N1 influenza A, *Sleep Med*, 2013, 14(9):867–871.

[171] Partinen M, Kornum BR, Plazzi G, et al. Narcolepsy as an autoimmune disease: the role of H1N1 infection and vaccination, *Lancet Neurol*, 2014, 13(6):600–613.

[172] Ahmed SS, Volkmuth W, Duca J, et al. Antibodies to influenza nucleoprotein cross-react with human hypocretin receptor 2, *Sci Transl Med*, 2015, 7(294):294ra105.

[173] Little DT, Ward HR. Premature ovarian failure 3 years after menarche in a 16-year-old girl following human papillomavirus vaccination, *BMJ Case Reports*, 2012, bcr-2012-006879.

[174] Wetzstein C. HPV Vaccine Cited in Infertility Case, *The Washington Times*, 11th November, 2013.

[175] Esmaei B, Winkelman JZ. Uveitis associated with varicella virus vaccine, *Am J Opthalmol*, 1999, 127:733-734.

[176] Wells MB, Garg S. Bilateral panuveitis after influenza vaccination, *Retin Cases Brief Rep*, 2009, 3(4):386-387.

[177] Moradian S, Ahmadieh H. Early onset optic neuritis following Measles-Rubella Vaccination, *J Ophthal Vis Res,* 2008, 3(2):118-122.

[178] De Giacinto C, Guaglione E, Leon PE, et al. Unilateral Optic Neuritis: A rare complication after Measles-Mumps-Rubella vaccination in a 30-year-old woman, *Case Reports Ophthal Med*, 2016, 2016:8740264.

[179] Hulbert TV, Larsen RA, Davis CL, et al. Bilateral hearing loss after measles and rubella vaccination in an adult, *N Engl J Med*, 1991, 325:134.

[180] Stewart BJA, P Rabhu BU. Reports of sensorineural deafness after measles, mumps and rubella immunisation, *Arch Dis Child*, 1993, 69:153-154.

[181] Güçlü O, Dereköy FS. Sudden Hearing Loss after Rabies Vaccination. *Balk Med J,* 2013, 30(3):327-328.

[182] The Telegraph. Rogue strain of MMR vaccine 'caused deafness', 5th September, 2012, https://www.telegraph.co.uk/news/health/news/9521728/Rogue-strain-of-MMR-vaccine-caused-deafness.html, Accessed May, 2019.

CHAPTER 9: VACCINES AROUND THE WORLD

[1] UNICEF, Statistics: Rwanda, https://www.unicef.org/infobycountry/rwanda_statistics.html#114. Accessed September, 2017.

[2] Green AR. Drug donations are great, but should Big pharma be setting the agenda? *The Guardian*, 29th March, 2013.

[3] GAVI. GAVI's mission, http://www.gavi.org/about/mission/, Accessed May, 2019.

[4] GAVI: The Vaccine Alliance, The Bill and Melinda Gates Foundation, http://www.gavi.org/funding/donor-profiles/bmgf/. Accessed September, 2017.

[5] World Health Organization, Global Alliance for Vaccines and Immunization, http://www.who.int/mediacentre/factsheets/fs169/en/. Accessed September, 2017.

[6] Nullis C. Measles deaths down 91% in Africa, *The Washington Post*, 29th November, 2007.

[7] Wolfson LJ, Strebel PM, Gacic-Dobo M, et al. Has the 2005 measles mortality reduction goal been achieved? A natural history modelling study, *The Lancet*, 2007, 369(9557):191-200.

[8] Bulletin of the World Health Organization, Decide monitoring strategies before setting targets, http://www.who.int/bulletin/volumes/85/6/07-042887/en/, Accessed May, 2019.

[9] Rao C, Bradshaw D, Mathers CD. Improving death registration and statistics in developing countries: a lesson from sub-saharan Africa, *SA J Dem*, 2004, 9(2):81-99.

[10] Pirmohamed M, Atuah KN, Dodoo ANO, Winstanley P. Pharmacovigilance in developing countries, *BMJ,* 2007, 335(7618):462.

[11] Vashisht N, Puliyel J. Polio programme: Let us declare victory and move on, *Indian J Med Ethics*, 2012, 9(2):11-117.

[12] Puliyel J, Phadke A. Letter: Deaths following pentavalent vaccine and the revised AEFI classification, *Indian J Med Ethics*, July 4, 2017. http://ijme.in/wp-content/uploads/2017/07/20170704_deaths_following_pentavalent.pdf, Accessed May, 2019.

[13] Pisharoty S. Interview: Muslim clerics to address misconceptions on ongoing measles-rubella vaccine drive, *The Wire*, 24th April, 2017.

[14] Forster K. South Sudan: 15 children die due to botched measles vaccinations, *The Independent*, 2nd June, 2017.

[15] BBC, Syrian children's deaths "caused by vaccine mix-up", http://www.bbc.com/news/world-middle-east-29251329, Accessed May, 2019.

[16] Haidula T. Parents sue over vaccine deaths, *The Namibian*, 5th August, 2016.

[17] Caulfield LE, de Onis M, Blossner M, Black RE. Undernutrition as an underlying cause of child death's associated with diarrhoea, pneumonia, malaria, and measles, *Am J Clin Nutr,* 2004, 80:193–198.

[18] Kalokerinos A. Interview for International Vaccine Newsletter, June 1995.

[19] Sommer A. Vitamin A prophylaxis, *Arch Dis Child,* 1997, 77:191-194.

[20] World Bank. World development report 1993: Investing in health, Washington DC: World Bank/New York: Oxford University Press, 1993.

[21] National strategies for overcoming micronutrient malnutrition. 45th World Health Assembly (agenda item 21), 1992. World Health Organisation, Geneva.

[22] Horrobin DF. Science is God, 1969, ISBN 85200 000 pp. 96 – 98.

[23] USAID, USAID Forward, https://www.usaid.gov/usaid-forward. Accessed March 2019.

[24] Andrus JK, Crouch AA, Fitzsimmons J, et al. Immunization and the Millennium Development Goals: Progress and challenges in Latin America and the Caribbean, *Health Affairs*, 2008, 27(2): Disparities: Expanding the Focus.

[25] United Nations Children's Fund, Progress for Every Child in the SDG Era, Available at: https://data.unicef.org/wp-content/uploads/2018/03/Progress_for_Every_Child_V4.pdf. Accessed May 2019.

[26] Hundreds of Nigerian parents refuse polio vaccines, *The Star*, 2nd August 2011, https://www.thestar.com/news/world/2011/08/02/hundreds_of_nigerian_parents_refuse_polio_vaccines.html. Accessed March 2019.

[27] Global Press News Service, Anti-vaccine parents in Uganda face jail time under new law, *The Seattle Globalist*, 23rd August 2016.

[28] Yolisizira Y. 10 arrested over polio immunization, *The Monitor*, 3rd June 2016

[29] Uganda 2016 International Religious Freedom Report, https://www.state.gov/documents/organization/268952.pdf. Accessed March 2019.

[30] Ibid. See reference #28.

[31] Saifi S, Botelho G. Over 500 Pakistani parents arrested for children's failure to get polio vaccine, *CNN*, 4th March 2015.

[32] Chiriac M. Romania parents face fines for refusing child vaccinations, *Balkan Insight*, 3rd August 2017.

[33] Larson HJ, de Figueiredo A, Xiahong Z, The state of vaccine confidence 2016: Global insights through a 67-country survey, *EBioMedicine*, 2016, 12:295 – 301.

[34] Toor A. France looks to curb its growing anti-vaccination movement with a new law, *The Verge*, 13th July 2017.

[35] Germany vaccination: Fines plan as measles cases rise, *BBC News*, 26th May 2017, https://www.bbc.com/news/world-europe-40056680. Accessed March 2019.

[36] Tan J. Anti-vaxx parents looking at fines, The NewPaper, 28th May 2016, https://www.tnp.sg/news/singapore/anti-vaxx-parents-looking-fines. Accessed March 2019.

[37] Police and parents clash in Jiangsu after 145 children get sick from expired vaccines, Asia News, 11th January 2019, http://www.asianews.it/news-en/Police-and-parents-clash-in-Jiangsu-after-145-children-get-sick-from-expired-vaccines-45954.html. Accessed March 2019.

[38] Farmer B. Polio worker gunned down in Pakistan trying to persuade family to vaccinate children, *The Telegraph*, 9th April 2019.

[39] Farooq Khan O. People set hospital afire in Peshawar, *Times of India*, 23rd April 2019.

[40] Janjua H. Afghan clerics in talks with ISIS to break polio vaccine myths, *The Guardian*, 27th March, 2018.

[41] ABC News. Vaccine Boycott Grows in Northern Nigeria, 24th February, 2004.

[42] Kenya Conference of Catholic Bishops: Press Statement by the Kenya Conference of Catholic Bishops, http://www.kccb.or.ke/home/news-2/press-statement-by-the-kenya-conference-of-catholic-bishops/. Accessed March, 2019.

[43] Oller JW, Shaw CA, Tomljenovic L, et al. HCG Found in WHO tetanus vaccine in Kenya raises concern in the developing world, *Open Access Library Journal,* 2017, 4:e3937.

[44] McVeigh T. Nigeria battles to beat polio and Boko Haram, *The Guardian*, 7th May 2017.

[45] Helleringer S et al. Supplementary polio immunization activities and prior use of routine immunization services in non-polio-endemic sub-Saharan Africa, *Bulletin of the World Health Organization*, 2012, https://www.who.int/bulletin/volumes/90/7/11-092494/en/. Accessed February, 2019.

[46] Measles and Rubella Initiative, SIA Schedule, https://measlesrubellainitiative.org/resources/sia-schedule/, Accessed February, 2019.

[47] Edwards M. R & D in Emerging Markets: A new approach for a new era, McKinsey & Company, 2010, https://www.mckinsey.com/industries/pharmaceuticals-and-medical-products/our-insights/r-and-38d-in-emerging-markets-a-new-approach-for-a-new-era, Accessed February, 2019.

[48] Joelving F. Many drugs for US kids tested in poor countries, *Reuters*, 23rd August 2010,

[49] Kulkani P. Malaria Vaccine trials in Africa: Dark saga of outsourced clinical trials continues, *Newsclick,* March 2018.

[50] Muchangi J. Kenyan children to get first malaria vaccine in the world next month, *The Star*,14th February, 2019.

[51] Ibid. See reference #49.

[52] UNICEF, Global Task Force on Cholera Control marks a year of progress toward ending cholera worldwide, https://www.unicef.org/press-releases/global-task-force-cholera-control-marks-year-progress-toward-ending-cholera. Accessed February, 2019.

[53] MedicalExpress, 38 children hospitalised after meningitis shot in Chad, https://medicalxpress.com/news/2013-01-

children-hospitalised-meningitis-shot-chad.html#jCp. Accessed February, 2019.

[54] England C. Minimum of 40 children paralyzed after new meningitis vaccine, VacTruth, https://vactruth.com/2013/01/06/paralyzed-after-meningitis-vaccine/. Accessed February 2019.

[55] Ward Hackett D. Ebola vaccinations expanding in Central Africa, https://www.precisionvaccinations.com/v920-ebola-vaccine-now-deployed-drc-uganda-and-south-sudan. Accessed February, 2019.

[56] Liu A. China approves domestic Ebola vaccine developed from recent outbreak, FiercePharma, https://www.fiercepharma.com/vaccines/china-approves-self-developed-ebola-vaccine-from-2014-outbreak-virus-type. Accessed February, 2019.

[57] Gordon M. Trial kicks off in Malawi: First child vaccinated with typhoid conjugated vaccine in Africa, http://www.coalitionagainsttyphoid.org/trial-kicks-off-in-malawi-first-child-vaccinated-with-typhoid-conjugate-vaccine-in-africa/. Accessed February, 2019.

CHAPTER 10: VACCINE OPPOSITION

[1] Durbach, N. They might as well brand us: Working class resistance to compulsory vaccination in Victorian England, *The Society for the Social History of Medicine*, 2000, 13:45-62.

[2] Sermon against the dangerous and sinful practice of inoculation. Preach'd at St. Andrew's Holborn, on Sunday, July the 8th, 1722. / By Edmund Massey, M.A. Lecturer of St. Alban Woodstreet, Available at: http://name.umdl.umich.edu/N02782.0001.001, Accessed May 2019.

[3] Storm AE, Religious Conviction and The Boston Inoculation Controversy of 1721, Available at: http://scholar-works.wm.edu/cgi/viewcon-tent.cgi?referer=https://scholar.google.com/&httpsre-dir=1&article=1409&context=honorstheses. Accessed May 2019.

[4] Porter D, Porter R. The politics of prevention: anti-vaccinationism and public health in nineteenth-century England, *Med Hist*, 1988;32(3):231-252.

[5] Gibbs J. Compulsory Vaccination Briefly Considered in its Scientific, Religious and political Aspects, London, 1856, pp 50.

[6] Ibid. See Reference #1.

[7] Ibid. See reference #4.

[8] Williamson S. Anti-vaccination leagues: One hundred years ago, *Arch Dis Child*, 1984, 59: 1195-1196.

[9] Crookshank EM, The history and pathology of vaccination, 2 vols, 1889, HK Lewis, London.

[10] Wolfe, R.M., Sharpe, L.K. Anti-vaccinationists past and present, *BMJ*, 2002d;325:430-432.

[11] Ibid. See reference #8.

[12] Leicester Mercury, 10th March, 1884.

[13] Leicester Mercury, 10th June, 1884.

[14] Leicester Mercury, 30th January, 1884.

[15] Leicester Mercury, 3rd July, 1884.

[16] Ibid. See reference #8.

[17] Wohl A. Endangered Lives: Public Health in Victorian Britain, 1984, Methuen, London, pp. 134-135.

[18] Ibid. See reference #1.

[19] Ibid. See reference #10.

[20] Albert M, Ostheimer KG, Breman JG. The last smallpox epidemic in Boston and the vaccination controversy, *N Engl J Med*, 2001, 344: 375-379.

[21] Gostin L. Jacobson vs. Massachusetts at 100 years: Police powers and civil liberties in tension, *AJPH*, 2005, 95:576-581.

[22] Baker J. The pertussis vaccine controversy in Great Britain, 1974-1986, *Vaccine*, 2003, 21:4003-4011.

[23] Millward G. A Disability Act? The Vaccine Damage Payments Act 1979 and the British government's response to the pertussis vaccine scare, *Soc Hist Med*, 2016, 30(2):429–447.

[24] Pollock TM, Miller E, Lobb J. Severity of whooping cough in England before and after the decline in pertussis immunisation, *Arch Dis Child,* 1984, 59:162-165.

[25] Stewart GT. Whooping Cough and Pertussis Vaccine: a comparison of risks versus benefits in Britain during the period 1968-83, *Dev Biol Stand*, 1985, 61:395-405.

[26] Wakefield AJ, Murch SH, Anthony A, et al. Ileal-lymphoid-nodular hyperplasia, non-specific colitis, and pervasive development disorder in children, *Lancet*, 1998, 351(9103): 637-641.

[27] Professor John Walker Smith vs General Medical Council [2012] EWHC 503, http://www.eastwoodslaw.co.uk/wp-content/uploads/2013/03/Walker-Smith.pdf. Accessed May, 2019.

[28] Horvath K, Medeiros L, Rabszlyn A, et al. High prevalence of gastrointestinal symptoms in children with autistic spectrum disorder (ASD), J Pediatr Gastroenterol *Nutr,* 2000, 31:S174.

[29] Horvath K, Perman JA. Autistic disorder and gastrointestinal disease, *Curr Op Ped*, 2002, 14:583-587

[30] Ashwood P, Anthony A, Torrente F, Wakefield AJ. Spontaneous mucosal lymphocyte cytokine profiles in children with regressive autism and gastrointestinal symptoms: Mucosal immune activation and reduced counter regulatory interleukin-10, *J Clin Immunol*, 2004, 24:664-673.

[31] Torrente F, Anthony A, Heuschkel RB, et al. Focal-enhanced gastritis in regressive autism with features distinct from

Crohn's and helicobacter pylori gastritis, *Am J Gastroenterol*, 2004, 4:598-605.

[32] Singh VK. Neuro-immunopathogenesis in autism. In: Berczi I, Gorczynski R, eds. Neuroimmune Biology: New Foundation of Biology. New York, Elsevier Science BV, 2001, pp. 447–458.

[33] Singh VK, Lin SY, Yang VC. Serological association of measles virus and human herpesvirus-6 with brain autoantibodies in autism, *Clin Immunol Immunopathol*, 1998, 89:105–108.

[34] Singh VK, Lin SX, Newell E, Nelson C. Abnormal measles-mumps-rubella antibodies and CNS autoimmunity in children with autism, *J Biomed Sci*, 2002, 9:359-364.

[35] Ibid. See reference #21.

[36] Kim SS, Frimpong JA, et al. Effects of maternal and provider characteristics on up-to-date immunization status of children aged 19-35 months, *Am J Public Health*, 2007, 97(2):259-266.

[37] Gullion JS, Henry L, Gullion G. Deciding to opt out of childhood vaccination mandates, *Pub Health Nurs*, 2008, 25(5):401-408.

[38] Aubusson K, Butt C. Sydney postcode has Australia's worst vaccination rate for five year old children, *Sydney Morning Herald*, 8th June, 2017.

[39] Butt C, Spooner R. Melbourne vaccination data: immunisation rates not improving in wealthy inner-city suburbs, *The Age*, 7th June, 2017.

[40] Killoran M. Inner-city Brisbane suburbs have some of the worst vaccination rates in Queensland, *The Courier Mail*, 6th May, 2017

[41] Chai C. Who are the anti-vaxxers in Canada? New poll profiles resistant group, *Global News*, 9th March, 2015.

[42] Martin M, Badalyan V. Vaccination practices among physicians and their children, *Open J Ped*, 2012, 2:228-235

[43] McCauley MM, Kennedy A, Basket M, Sheedy K. Exploring the choice to refuse or delay vaccines: a national survey of parents of 6- through 23-month olds, *Acad Pediatr*, 2012, 12(5): 375-383.

[44] Robison SG, Groom H, Young C. Frequency of alternative immunization schedule use in a metropolitan area, *Pediatrics*, 2012, 130(1):31-38.

[45] Tidman Z. Vaccination law amendment fuels protests, *The Italian Insider*, 17th July 2017.

[46] Vaccine Confidence Project, State of Vaccine Confidence in the EU 2018, https://www.vaccineconfidence.org/wp-content/uploads/2018/10/EU_state_of_vaccine_confidence_2018.pdf. Accessed February, 2019.

[47] VaccinesToday, MMR Rates Fall in Poland – Despite Mandatory Vaccination Rules, 18th January 2018, https://www.vaccinestoday.eu/stories/mmr-rates-fall-poland-despite-mandatory-vaccination-rules/. Accessed April 2019.

[48] Chasmar J. State Farm drops Rob Schneider over anti-vaccine views, *The Washington Times*, 24th September 2014.

[49] Bever L. 'Bring back our #ChildHoodDiseases,' White House official's wife says as she criticizes vaccines, *The Washington Post*, 15th February, 2019.

[50] Siddiqui S. Wife of White House communications chief goes on anti-vaccine tirade, *The Guardian*, 14th February, 2019.

[51] Ward M. 'Questions that need to be asked': Pete Evans endorses anti-vaxxer, *Sydney Morning Herald*, 14th March, 2019.

[52] Yahoo Sport, 'Dangerous clown' Anthony Mundine slammed over controversial anti-vax claims, 10th April, 2019.

[53] Healy CM, Pickering LK. How to communicate with vaccine-hesitant parents, *Pediatrics*, 2011, 127(1):S127-S133.

[54] Edwards KM, Hackell JM. Countering vaccine hesitancy, *Pediatrics*, 2016, 138(3):e20162146.

[55] Rochman B. Should Paediatricians 'Fire' Patients Whose Parents Don't Vaccinate? *Time Magazine*, 4th August, 2011.

[56] BlueShield, 2016 Performance Recognition Program, Available at: http://www.whale.to/c/2016-BCN-BCBSM-Incentive-Program-Booklet.pdf. Accessed April, 2019.

[57] WHO, Ten threats to global health in 2019, https://www.who.int/emergencies/ten-threats-to-global-health-in-2019, Accessed March, 2019.

[58] Editorial Board. How to Inoculate Against Anti-vaxxers, *The New York Times*, 19th January 2019.

[59] Adam Schiff. Schiff sends letter to Google, Facebook regarding anti-vaccine misinformation, https://schiff.house.gov/news/press-releases/schiff-sends-letter-to-google-facebook-regarding-anti-vaccine-misinformation. Accessed May, 2019.

[60] Alexander J. Jack Dorsey's endorsement of anti-vax podcaster highlights Twitter's misinformation problem, *The Verge*, 13th March 2019.

CHAPTER 11: THE FUTURE OF VACCINES

[1] Pharmaceutical Research and Manufacturers of America (PhRMA), Medicines in development: Vaccines, http://phrma.org/press-release/medicines-in-development-vaccines, Accessed May, 2019.

[2] Hull M, Sadowsky C, Arai H, et al. Long-term extensions of randomized vaccine trials of ACC-001 and QS-21 in mild to moderate alzheimer's disease, *Curr Alzheimer Res*, 2017, 14(7):696-70.

[3] Azegami T, Yuki Y, Sawada S, et al. Nano-gel based nasal ghrelin vaccine prevents obesity, *Mucosal Immunol*, 2017, 10(5):1351-1360.

[4] Kublin JG, Mikolajczak SA, Sack BK, et al. Complete attenuation of genetically engineered plasmodium falciparum sporozoites in human subjects, *Sci Transl Med*, 2017, 9(371).

[5] Kosalaraksa P, Watanaveeradej V, Pancharoen C, et al. Long-term immunogenicity of a single dose of Japanese Encephalitis chimeric virus vaccine in toddlers and booster response 5 years after primary immunization, *Ped Infect Dis J*, 2016, 36(4):e108-e113.

[6] Erasmus JH, Auguste AJ, Kaelbar JT, et al. A chikungunya fever vaccine utilizing an insect-specific virus platform, *Nat Med*, 2017, 23(2):192-199.

[7] Poore EA, Slifka DA, Raue HP, et al. Pre-clinical development of a hydrogen peroxide-inactivated West Nile virus vaccine, *Vaccine*, 2017, 35(2):283-292.

[8] Frenck RW Jr, Creech B, Sheldon EA, et al. Safety, tolerability and immunogenicity of a 4-antigen Staphylococcus aureus vaccine (SA4Ag): Results from a first in-human randomized, placebo-controlled phase 1/2 study, *Vaccine*, 2017, 35(2):375-384.

[9] Seledtsova GV, Shishkov GV, Kaschenko EA, Seledtsov VI. Xenogeneic cell-based vaccine therapy for colorectal cancer: safety, association of clinical effects with vaccine-induced immune responses, *Biomed Pharmac*, 2016, 83:1247-1252.

[10] Rello J, Krenn CG, Locker G, et al. A randomized, placebo-controlled phase II study of a pseudomonas vaccine in ventilated ICU patients, *Crit Care*, 2017, 21(1): 22.

[11] Wei M, Meng F, Wang S, et al. 2-year efficacy, immunogenicity, and safety of Vigoo enterovirus 71 vaccine in healthy

Chinese children: a randomized, open-label study, *J Infect Dis*, 2017, 215(1):56-63.

[12] Posgai AL, Wasserfall CH, Kwon KC, et al. Plant-based vaccines for oral delivery of type-1 diabetes-related auto-antigens: evaluating oral tolerance mechanisms and disease prevention in NOD mice, *Sci Rep*, 2017, 7:42372.

[13] Keenan BP, Saenger Y, Kafrouni MI, et al. A listeria vaccine and depletion of T-regulatory cells activate immunity against early stage pancreatic intraepithelial neoplasms and prolong survival of mice, *Gastroenterology*, 2014, 146(7):1784-1794.

[14] Wang CY, Hua R, Liu L, et al. Immunotherapy against metastatic bladder cancer by combined administration of granulocyte macrophage-colony stimulating factor and interleukin-2 surface modified MB49 bladder cancer stem cells vaccine, Cancer Med, 2017, 6(3):689-697.

[15] Fragoso C, Hernandez M, Cervantes-Torres J, et al. Transgenic papaya: a useful platform for oral vaccines, *Planta*, 2017, 245(5):1037-1048.

[16] Cohut M. A new vaccine could wipe out acne, *Medical News Today*, 31st August 2018.

[17] Elliot D. Preventing Mental Illness with a Stress Vaccine, *The Atlantic*, 26th Nov, 2016.

[18] Moore J. Tired of the common cold? A new vaccine could prevent it, *WSB-TV*, 3rd November 2017.

[19] National Institutes of Health, News Releases: NIH begins first in-human trial of a universal influenza vaccine candidate, 3rd April, 2019.

[20] Tang DC, DeVit M, Johnston SA. Genetic immunization is a simple method for eliciting an immune response. *Nature*, 1992, 356(6365):152-154.

[21] Ulmer JB, Donnelly JJ, Parker SE, et al. Heterologous protection against influenza by injection of DNA encoding a viral protein, *Science*, 1993, 259(5102):1745-9.

[22] Kutzler MA, Weiner DB. DNA vaccines: ready for prime time? *Nat Rev Gen*, 2008, 9(10):776-788.

[23] Mor G, Singla M, Steinberg AD, et al. Do DNA vaccines induce autoimmune disease, *Hum Gene Ther*, 2008, 8(3):293-300.

[24] Zhou Q, Wang F, Zhang Y, et al. Down-regulation of Prdx6 contributes to DNA-vaccine induced vitiligo in mice, *Mol Bio Syst*, 2011, 7(3):809-16.

[25] Feltquate DM, Heaney S, Webster RG, Robinson HL. Different T helper cell types and antibody isotypes generated by saline and gene gun DNA immunization, *J Immunol*, 1997, 158(5):2278–2284.

[26] Justewicz DM, Webster RG. Long-Term Maintenance of B Cell Immunity to Influenza Virus Hemagglutinin in Mice Following DNA-Based Immunization, *Virology*, 1996, 224(1):10–17.

[27] Liu HF, Li W, Lu MB, Yu LJ. Pharmacokinetics and risk evaluation of DNA vaccine against Schistosoma japonicum, *Parasitol Res*, 2013, 112(1):59-67.

[28] US Department of Health and Human Services, Types of vaccines, https://www.vaccines.gov/basics/types/index.html, Accessed May, 2019.

[29] McAleer WJ, Buynak EB, Maigetter RZ, et al. Human hepatitis B vaccine from recombinant yeast, *Nature*, 1984, 307(5947):178-180.

[30] Vesikari T, Matson DO, Dennehy P, et al. Safety and efficacy of a pentavalent human-bovine (WC3) reassortant rotavirus vaccine, *N Engl J Med*, 2006, 354(1):23-33.

[31] National Institute for Biological Standards and Control. New polio vaccines, http://www.nibsc.org/science_and_research/virology/polio/new_polio_vaccines.aspx, Accessed May, 2019.

[32] Gu R, Shampang A, Nashar T, et al. Oral immunization with a live coxsackievirus/HIV recombinant induces gag p-24-specific T cell responses, *PLoS One*, 2010, 5(9):e12499.

[33] Bishop DHL. The release into the environment of genetically-engineered viruses, vaccines and viral pesticides, *Trends Eco Evol*, 1988, 3(4):12-15.

[34] Chan VS. Use of genetically modified viruses and genetically engineered virus-vector vaccines: environmental effects, *J Toxicol Enviro Health*, 2006, 69(21):1971-1977.

[35] CDC. Vaccine excipient and media summary, https://www.cdc.gov/vaccines/pubs/pinkbook/downloads/appendices/B/excipient-table-2.pdf. Accessed May, 2019.

[36] Bosse D, Praus M, Kiessling P, et al. Phase 1 comparability of recombinant human albumin and human serum albumin, *J Clin Pharmacol*, 2005, 45(1):57-67.

[37] Bulletin of the World Health Organization: China enters the global vaccine market. http://www.who.int/bulletin/volumes/92/9/14-020914/en/. Accessed January, 2017.

[38] BBC News, China "fake milk" scandal deepens, http://news.bbc.co.uk/2/hi/asia-pacific/3648583.stm. Accessed September, 2017.

[39] New York Times, From China to Panama, a trail of poisoned medicine, http://www.nytimes.com/2007/05/06/world/americas/06poison.html. Accessed September, 2017.

[40] USA Today: Pet food maker to pay for vet bills, https://usatoday30.usatoday.com/news/nation/2007-03-23-poison-pet-food_N.htm. Accessed September, 2017.

[41] Greenemeier L, Heparin Scare: Deaths from tainted blood thinner spur race for safe replacement, *Scientific American*, 4th November, 2008.

[42] Branigan T. Chinese figures show five-fold rise in babies sick from contaminated milk, *The Guardian*, 2nd December, 2008.

[43] VOA News, China's melamine milk crisis creates crisis of confidence, https://www.voanews.com/a/a-13-2008-09-26-voa45/403825.html. Accessed September, 2017.

[44] Financial Times, Beijing scrambles to contain vaccine scandal, https://www.ft.com/content/3954a690-f0ae-11e5-aff5-19b4e253664a. Accessed September, 2017.

[45] TIME: China's food safety problems go deeper than pet treats, http://time.com/107922/china-pet-food-contamina-tion-recall-video/. Accessed September, 2017.

[46] New York Times, China's vaccine scandal threatens public faith in immunizations, https://www.ny-times.com/2016/04/19/world/asia/china-vaccine-scan-dal.html. Accessed September, 2017.

[47] Caixin: Authorities investigate claims of cadmium-laced wheat from central China, http://www.caixinglobal.com/2017-06-22/101104603.html. Accessed 2017.

[48] Caixin, Tianjin probes counterfeit ring that produced toxic soy sauce, http://www.caixinglobal.com/2017-01-19/101046873.html. Accessed September, 2017.

[49] Spencer R, Foster P. Chinese ordered coverup of tainted milk scandal, *The Telegraph*, 24th September, 2008.

[50] TIME, China has begun cracking down on parents protest-ing substandard vaccines, http://time.com/4302878/china-

vaccines-scandal-immunizations-protest-detained/. Accessed September, 2017.

[51] Financial Times, WHO urges China to build trust in vaccines after safety scandal, https://www.ft.com/content/281a19e6-f590-11e5-803c-d27c7117d132. Accessed September, 2017.

[52] Xueqiu, Are China's vaccines ready for the world, https://xueqiu.com/1624730572/20733076. Accessed September, 2017.

[53] Fox News, WHO approves China flu vaccine, lauds growing industry, http://www.foxnews.com/health/2015/06/12/who-approves-china-flu-vaccine-lauds-growing-industry.html. Accessed May, 2019.

[54] Marsteller D. As drug making goes global, oversight found lacking, *USA Today*, 21st October, 2012.

Got feedback or comments? I'd like to hear them! Feel free to get in contact, via www.theothersideofvaccines.com

Regards,

Kate William

www.ingramcontent.com/pod-product-compliance
Lightning Source LLC
Chambersburg PA
CBHW072128170526
45158CB00004BA/1294